T0293324

Complete Revision Guide for MRCOG Part 3

Justin C Konje FWACS, FMCOG (Nig), FRCOG, MD, MBA, LLB, PgCert Med Ed
Emeritus Professor of Obstetrics and Gynaecology
University of Leicester, UK
Professor of Obstetrics and Gynaecology
Weill Cornell Medicine-Qatar, Qatar
Senior Attending Physician
Sidra Medicine, Qatar

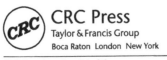

CRC Press
Taylor & Francis Group
Boca Raton London New York

CRC Press is an imprint of the
Taylor & Francis Group, an **informa** business

First edition published 2021
by CRC Press
6000 Broken Sound Parkway NW, Suite 300, Boca Raton, FL 33487-2742

and by CRC Press
2 Park Square, Milton Park, Abingdon, Oxon, OX14 4RN

© 2021 Taylor & Francis Group, LLC

CRC Press is an imprint of Taylor & Francis Group, LLC

ISBN: 978-0-367-61168-2 (pbk)
ISBN: 978-0-367-61169-9 (hbk)
ISBN: 978-1-003-10445-2 (ebk)

Typeset in Times LT Std
by Deanta Global Publishing Services, Chennai, India

Contents

This book is dedicated to my wonderful, loving father – Papa Tabe Augustine Konje, who passed on to another world in December 2014. He sacrificed the pleasures of his life to see my siblings and I educated. His dream lives on.

1
Preface to *Complete Revision Guide for MRCOG Part 3*

In my preface to the *Complete Revision Guide for MRCOG Part 2*, I stated that 'The Membership of the Royal College of Obstetricians and Gynaecologists (MRCOG) examination remains one of the most internationally recognised postgraduate examinations in the specialty'. Such an international appeal means that not only those who are trained in the UK sit this examination.

Part 1 examination focuses on basic sciences and how these are applied clinically, while Part 2 focuses predominantly on knowledge and its clinical application. Part 3, on the other hand, aims to address important aspects of Miller's education skills triangle – 'knows how, shows how, and in some cases does'. It is therefore obvious that communication is central to this examination. Clinicians have traditionally been poor communicators, often talking down to patients. This is no longer acceptable as patients increasingly demand (and rightly so) to be involved in decision making about their care. For this to happen, there must be equity in understanding, and the clinician is required to ensure that this is achieved through communication, in as much detail as possible and to a level that will guarantee understanding. Without this, the concept of equity will be unachievable. In the Part 3 examination, therefore, communication is assessed in several domains. Of course, the clinician must first be knowledgeable to be able to communicate with the patients to allow them to make informed choices about their care. Finally, while communication is important, patient safety remains the *raison d'être* of healthcare. It should therefore be a given point that this domain is assessed in all the tasks in this examination.

Uncoupling Part 2 into Parts 2 and 3 has allowed for a better assessment of applied clinical knowledge and communication skills. Part 3 examination consists of 14 tasks, each assessing one of the 14 core modules in the curriculum. Each task assesses specific skills, which may include all or some of 'Information Gathering, Communication with Patients and Families, Communication with Colleagues, Patient Safety and Applied Clinical Knowledge'. Not all the tasks will lend themselves to assessing all these domains – for example, in the discussions with the examiner, it may not be possible to assess communication with patients and families.

There is a general recognition that while candidates' performance at the examination should be judged by experienced clinicians (the examiners), ultimately the simulated patient (who is in place of the real patient) should have a say on how good the candidate's approach to dealing with patients is. Attempts to address this in the past included asking the simulated patients (role players) to award an overall mark for each of the stations. This has further evolved so that in the Part 3 examination, there are trained lay examiners who assess candidates, especially in the domains of communication with patients and families. This is important, as ultimately, it is the patients who are on the receiving end of our communication. While this is only incorporated in a few tasks at the moment, I foresee a time when most of the examiners will be lay members of the public.

In the Part 2 MRCOG book, I generated four sample examinations; the same principle has been adopted in writing this book. There are four main sample diets, and in each of them, attempts have been made to cover all the 14 modules in the core curriculum. I must admit that I have left out some of the modules in one or two of the samples. This is probably because I take the view that it is better to include questions on the difficult modules than cover all the modules in each of the samples. At the end of the four diets, there is an additional chapter with random tasks, which should help with your preparation.

I have kept to the concepts of all my books for the examination, once again giving general advice on how to prepare for the examination and also giving 'tips' on how to fail it. I must state here that the contents of the book, including the statements and interpretation of evidence, are personal, and I accept responsibility for inaccuracies and mistakes. It is important that you verify whatever information is in this book and also accept that there will be errors, some of which will be glaring omissions and others as a result of misinterpretation on my part.

I hope that not only will trainees find this book useful but trainers and examiners will also find the content useful in guiding trainees and also help them generate good questions for examinations.

When I embarked on writing the third edition of my complete revision guide, I envisaged this would be a quick project, but as I began to write, it was obvious that the tasks were far greater than I had anticipated. Furthermore, it was imperative to separate the two parts since these are now distinct examinations. I am glad that this has finally been completed. I am hoping that any subsequent revisions will be less arduous than this.

I would like to thank my family for resolutely supporting me throughout this project. They have endured hours and hours on end of me sitting in front of the computer at home, tapping on keys. I am sure that finally closing this chapter will be welcome to them. Thank you Mrs Joan Kila Konje, not only for being an adorable and the best wife but for also being very understanding, encouraging and not losing your cool too often. Thanks to my wonderful kids – Dr Swiri Konje, Monique Konje and Justin Jr Konje – for bearing with your dad and not complaining too much about ignoring you and not being in touch that often.

I could not have wished for better children. I am truly blessed.

I would like to personally thank Dr Wafaa Belail, who has not only been very encouraging but has provided very useful input into the contents of the book, read and suggested changes to the structure, edited the manuscript and contributed a chapter from a recent trainee's perspective. She has been a great support, and I value her friendship and support.

I would like to thank the publisher for being so patient with me. The manuscript was meant to have been submitted shortly after Part 2 was completed, but it has taken me almost one year to complete!

Finally, I am most grateful to God, my creator and our Almighty Father in Heaven, for giving me the belief and patience. This would not have been possible without His blessings.

2
How to Use This Book

This book is only a guide to preparing for Part 3 examination. It cannot replace face-to-face practice, especially in supervised clinical settings. As you prepare for the exams, I suggest you pay particular attention to the following:

1. Guidance on how to prepare for the exams
2. Tips on communication
3. How to explain various surgical procedures to patients
4. How to explain investigations to patients
5. First-hand experience of how I prepared for Part 3 exams by Dr Wafaa Ali Belail Hammad

Once you have done these, you should go through each of the tasks diligently and identify the key expectations from candidates. These are only guidances and should be used as such. You should then take these into a clinical scenario or one with a simulated patient and put it into practice. If you are able to cover most of the points in each of the domains, you are most definitely on your way to passing the exams.

Come back to these as often as possible, and by the time you have completed each of the domains and the additional tasks, you should be prepared for the examination.

I hope that some of the layman's explanations I have provided for various medical terminologies, including diagnosis, investigations and treatment, will come in handy in your day-to-day clinical activities.

I wish you the very best of luck in your preparations and hope that you find the book useful.

3
An Overview of the Part 3 MRCOG Examination

Introduction

This part of the examination assesses knowledge and how this is applied in clinical practice (i.e. clinical skills). The assessment is based on the 14 knowledge-based modules of the RCOG obstetrics and gynaecology curriculum. These modules are shown in Table 3.1, and more details can be found on the RCOG website (www.rcog.org.uk).

The examination itself is undertaken in circuits of 14 tasks (stations) – each task lasting 12 minutes, of which 2 minutes is for an initial reading of the information for the particular task. In effect, the candidate has 10 minutes to perform each task. The total duration of the examination is

Table 3.1 Modules of Part 3 examination and their link to the corresponding core curriculum module

Part 3 Module Name	Corresponding Core Curriculum Module
1. Teaching	2 (teaching part only)
2. Core surgical skills	5
3. Post-operative care	6
4. Antepartum care	8
5. Maternal medicine	9
6. Management of labour	10
7. Management of delivery	11
8. Postpartum problems (the puerperium)	12
9. Gynaecological problems	13
10. Subfertility	14
11. Sexual and reproductive health	15
12. Early pregnancy care	16
13. Gynaecological oncology	17
14. Urogynaecology and pelvic floor problems	18

therefore 168 minutes, of which 140 minutes is for performing the tasks themselves. Each of the 14 tasks is assessed on the following five domains:

1. Information gathering
2. Communication with patients and families
3. Communication with colleagues
4. Patient safety
5. Applied clinical knowledge

In most of the tasks, there is not a very clear demarcation between the various domains, as, for example, in assessing patient safety, your knowledge must be sound and the same will apply to communication with either the patient and her relatives or colleagues. However, an attempt is made to ensure that at least three or four of these domains are assessed for each of the tasks.

4
Logistics of the Exams

Most candidates sit for the examination in London at the RCOG; however, there may be overseas centres. The exams may be run on more than one day, depending on the number of the candidates who apply to sit for the examination. There are often several circuits per day, running in the morning and afternoon. The tasks are the same for a particular day but differ from one day to another. While the tasks are different, assessment is independent to ensure that no set of candidates is disadvantaged.

There are two types of tasks – the simulated patient or colleague task (role player task) and a structured discussion (often with the examiner). The simulated patient task is commonly akin to the clinical interface between the doctor and the patient (the role of the patient being played by an experienced role player or actor and that of the doctor being played by the candidate). It is important for the candidate to always remember that this is an assessment of their clinical skills, and, where there is uncertainty, it's best to default to what one will do in a clinical setting. The examiner at these stations (tasks) is supposed to be passive, and indeed their presence should be ignored by the candidate. Candidates should therefore not ask the examiner any questions or additional information unless it is indicated in the instructions. The simulated patient (in place of a patient) in some scenarios will exhibit various emotions such as anger, frustration, distress and doubt and even lack of confidence in the examinee. These should be regarded as normal clinical behaviours, and while these should not be ignored, they should not significantly influence or alter the course of the exams. It is highly likely that you would have encountered such a scenario in your clinical experience. Remember that at the simulated patient station, no attempts are made to match the role player to the characteristics of the role they are playing – for example, a 24 year with a BMI of 22 kg/M^2 may be playing the role of an obese postmenopausal woman. Some candidates may find this off-putting, but my advice is that, with practice, candidates should try to imagine the simulated patient in their role rather than relate who is in front of them to the role. Most tasks involving colleagues are to do with teaching and communication. It is important to know that two tasks (stations) may be linked, i.e. one following on from the other (assessing different aspects of the module but with the same simulated scenario). For example, the scenario for the assessment of one task may then lead to the assessment of the next task.

Each task is assessed in real time (i.e. as the task is being performed) by either experienced examiners or lay persons. In order to ensure consistency in assessment, all the examiners from the different circuits for the same task meet before the start of the examination to be briefed (usually by a member of the examination committee) and to review the task and the marking scheme. Similarly, the simulated patients (role players/actors) meet to ensure that there is consistency in the way they interact with the candidates (i.e. the tasks are performed in the same way). In some of the patient-simulated tasks, a lay examiner will assess communication with the patient and relatives. These lay examiners are not clinicians but have undergone training to ensure standardisation and consistency of this process. They tend to assess alongside the clinician examiner, but there is a discussion of marks awarded for each of the tasks.

Unlike the previous oral examination, a component of the then Part 2 examination, the assessment of the Part 3 examination is based more on attaining the minimum standards expected of an average year five trainee rather than on a scale of 20 marks. Each of the domains is assessed as pass, borderline or fail, with awarded marks of 0 for fail, 1 for borderline and 2 for pass (or meeting the minimum standards), respectively. The pass mark is then computed based on the standards set for the particular composition of the examination.

5

Guidance on How to Prepare for the Part 3 MRCOG Examination

Candidates often ask what seems an obvious question – 'how do I prepare for the examination'? The answer should also be obvious to both the candidates and the examiners, but often I am surprised at how ignorant some candidates appear to be. The best preparation for the Part 3 examination is making the best of being a clinician – in your role as a trainee. If you take almost every clinical patient encounter you have from the time Part 2 examination results are announced to the time you sit for the Part 3 examination as a 'potential task', it's very likely that you would have in a busy job encountered most of the tasks you will be tested on. The worst preparation, in my view, would be taking weeks/months off clinical duties to study; while this might have helped with your preparation for Part 2, it is less likely to be as helpful with this part. The following are my simple guidance points to ensure you are well prepared for the examination.

1. Make sure that your clinical duties cover most aspects of the specialty rather than just one, especially the highly specialised areas of the 14 modules (i.e. teaching, core surgical skills, antepartum care, maternal medicine, management of labour, management of delivery, postpartum problems, gynaecological problems, subfertility, sexual and reproductive health, early pregnancy care, gynaecological oncology and urogynaecology and pelvic floor problems, elective gynaecology, labour ward, antenatal and postnatal clinics and wards).
2. For each patient you see, ask yourself, how would I be assessed in the five domains – patient safety, communication with the patients and families, communication with colleagues, information gathering and applied knowledge – this should be a routine. It will be useful to ask more experienced/senior colleagues to give you regular drills on some of the patients you see.
3. Familiarise yourself with the contents of the following documents:
    a. GMC Good Medical Practice
    b. MBBRACE – the most recent publication
    c. Informed consent – RCOG and GMC (including Fraser and Montgomery principles)
    d. Clinical governance
4. Attend one of the courses run nationally/internationally. I believe the RCOG course offers the best value for money.
5. Have a sparring partner – someone you are not afraid to criticise or be honest with and practice as many tasks as possible.
6. Familiarise yourself with what is required to be a good teacher.
7. Speak to colleagues who have just been successful in Part 3 examination.

8. At the examination itself:
   a. Read through the information for each task thoroughly, making sure that you understand the instructions and the domains to be assessed in. Focus on the parts of the task on which you will be assessed.
   b. Make sure you know what the question is not asking – this is very difficult. Most candidates will make assumptions and answer the questions they believe the task is about, rather than what is being asked. For example, counselling someone about prenatal diagnosis is not the same as counselling them about invasive testing.
   c. Use the note pad you have with you to make a plan – it is useful to have subheadings for your history and the key investigations you would like to undertake. Finally, have an overview of how you will manage the problem, always having alternative options should your preferred option be declined.
   d. Start by introducing yourself – your name, your position and why you are there. You should always confirm the patients details. This is an important patient safety point. It is useful to ensure that you know how to address the simulated patient/role player. Asking how they would like to be addressed is not just common sense but makes them relax. However, this is not imperative, as it does not earn you any marks.
   e. Listen to the simulated patients' questions, following verbal as well as body language cues.
   f. Open-ended questions will allow the simulated patient/role player to provide more information than do closed-ended questions. However, you must be careful as this could eat into your time, especially with the simulated patient who cannot stop talking.
   g. Explain yourself in a language that the patient understands (layman's language). It is often useful to support your explanations with illustrations. If you are unsure of the equivalent layman's phrase/word to use, try several words and ask whether the simulated patient has understood.
   h. Be sympathetic to the patient and show empathy, an understanding of emotional reaction – especially to bad news – but do not show emotions yourself, such as crying when the simulated patient shows extreme emotions!
   i. If you are completely lost, do what you do in the clinic – follow basic principles of clinical care. Everyone will have come across a patient in the clinic with a complaint they had no clue about, but they did not send the patient home. You should have been able to spend time and made the patient comfortable in the knowledge that you were in the process of helping them. Apply the same principles to the examination, and you would not be wrong, so long as you do not make glaring errors that could result in severe harm to the patient. Also remember that there may be occasions when you refer on to an expert in the area, a more senior colleague, or offer to find out more information. This is not a weakness but a demonstration of honesty and good clinical practice. There is nothing wrong with saying, for example, 'I am sorry I am unable to answer your question or provide more answers now but will find out and get back to you'.
   j. Always be prepared to repeat yourself.
   k. NEVER end a station with a simulated patient without asking whether there are any questions, and always affirm plans and that the patient understands.
9. For those who have never worked in the UK, I would strongly recommend that, if possible, find an opportunity to visit and observe the UK practice for a minimum of one week. Remember that this is a UK-standards practice exam. This will help you with communication with patients, relatives and colleagues (especially GPs (General Practitioners) and midwives) and to also understand the hierarchy of care and training in the UK.

6
Overview of the Five Domains of Assessment

In this short overview, the focus will be on the key issues candidates should focus on in their preparation. The five domains assess core clinical skills as detailed in the RCOG curriculum (referred to previously and available on the RCOG website).

Information gathering: This will take place in various forms, including obtaining a relevant history for purposes of informing diagnosis; gathering information; e.g. from previous records (in the same hospital or other institutions); requesting for and interpreting results of investigations, operations or cardiotocographs; making a management plan; or counselling. With regard to taking a history, there is usually not enough time to take an unfocussed history, and so it is useful to have a systematic approach to this task. Tasks in this domain may include taking a history from a patient, discussing with the examiner or patient, investigations that would provide information to make a diagnosis or help manage a patient, interpretation of results of investigations, gathering information in order to undertake a root cause analysis or reviewing a clinical incident and making a plan to gather information in order to undertake a root cause analysis.

- Have an approach to obtain relevant/focussed history from patients over a period of 8–10 minutes. I recommend having headings so as not to forget anything
- Practice with a colleague, bearing in mind the limitations of time which are part of the examination (i.e. limiting each task to 10 minutes)
- Review and practice various types of information gathering scenarios as detailed above with colleagues (sparring partners)
- Work with senior and junior colleagues using Case Base Discussions (CBD)s as an opportunity to gather information

Communication with patients and families: Central to this is the ability to take the patient to a level where they are able to understand what is happening to them and use information provided to make an informed choice. Most patients we see are frightened of what we may tell them and what we may offer them in terms of treatment. Making the patient feel less frightened ought to be integral to our clinical responsibilities. A well-informed patient is easier to manage. Do not forget that this particular domain may be assessed by a lay examiner. The keys to successful communication include introducing yourself and your role in the care of the woman; referring to the patient by her name (ask what she wishes to be called); listening and answering questions (i.e. being attentive); making use of both visual and auditory clues; sympathising and empathising if appropriate; understanding anxieties; not imposing (e.g. patients who disagree with advice/recommended treatment option); exercising patience and never losing your temper with those who are angry, aggressive and abusive (this is unlikely to happen in exams, but it is a reality in clinical practice); and avoiding medical jargon and abbreviations (i.e. using language that the lay examiner and therefore the patient/simulator understands). The lay person in the UK has been legally defined as the person on the 'Clapham Bus' – a London City bus. In most Trusts, clinicians are encouraged to use language that would be understandable to an 11- to 12-year-old. The following is a suggested approach to simulate tasks.

- Introduce yourself and your role (e.g. I am Dr XXX, the Specialist Trainee year 5, etc.) and confirm the simulated patient's name and, if possible, ask how she/he would like to be addressed. Explain why you are there (e.g. I will be asking you a few questions and then explaining the symptoms you have and the investigations/tests we will like to undertake). How this role is explained will depend on the tasks
- Work out the best way to communicate in non-medical terms
- Be prepared to justify everything you say, which includes being able to make an argument for and against including convincing a patient to change her mind but at the same time be prepared to acknowledge differences and accommodate concerns of the patient
- Avoid giving too much information at the same time (this could potentially confuse the patient) – break it up and pause to ensure there is an understanding
- Pause to take questions and always ask if there is an understanding
- Conclude by asking if there are any unanswered questions (often the simulated patient has a list of questions and may forget to ask)
- Summarise the session to ensure that all the points have been covered and ensure that these have been understood. Do not hesitate to repeat yourself

Communication with colleagues: Communication with colleagues is just as important as that with patients and relatives. The main difference is that this is with professionals and therefore the language should be professional. Key to this is brevity (being very precise and knowing just what is and is not relevant). Communication could be with colleagues at the trainee level; senior colleagues in the same specialty; colleagues in other specialties, e.g. in the form of referrals, handovers or seeking additional expert opinion; Midwives, or GPs in the form of letters, discharge summaries or referrals. Here it is important that the candidate is able to write a good letter and understands what the contents of such a letter should be, as from time to time they may be asked to review and comment on letters written by colleagues.

The most common form of communication is between colleagues from one shift to another or with a senior colleague about a patient being managed contemporaneously. A common communication tool is the 'SBAR', which provides the best basis for handing over patients. This acronym refers to **S**ituation, **B**ackground, **A**ssessment and **R**ecommendation. A not-uncommon means of assessing communication with colleagues is teaching – this may involve explaining a task to a learner, often a junior colleague or another professional, e.g. a midwife/nurse. Here the principles of teaching must apply – ensuring that objectives are set and that there is feedback from the teaching process to ensure an understanding of what has been taught or explained:

- Understand what good communication with colleagues should be like – content, wording and specific, and not leaving room for interpretations which may be wrong and therefore affect the care of patients
- Know when and with whom to communicate, especially in the context of multidisciplinary team working

- Use the SBAR as often as possible – only including relevant and useful information that will inform colleagues of what has happened and may happen going forward
- Work with a colleague as you prepare for this task, including sharing of summaries, teaching or debating about care options

Patient safety: This is central to our duty of care and has several strands to it. These include understanding your responsibilities and limitations, knowing when to seek for assistance, respecting patient confidentiality (in the context of data protection, sharing or not sharing information with family members, and when to do so especially in the context of the Mental Capacity Act, and dealing with patients who have not attained the age of maturity – 16 years in England) and being able to undertake tasks expected (safe prescription, appropriate investigation of patients and interpretation of results and instituting the right treatment, managing complications ensuing, etc.). Other examples that should be covered under this domain include respecting the patient's dignity – the role of chaperone for intimate examinations, understanding and respecting religious beliefs, e.g. Jehovah's Witness and blood transfusion, cultural diversity and implications for OBGYN, e.g. female genital mutilation (FGM) and the law with respect to FGM – safeguarding children, clinical governance with an emphasis on audit (knowing the principles of audit, the audit cycle, being able to use audit reports such as Mothers and Babies, Reducing Risk through Audit and Confidential Enquiries (MBRRACE) etc.) and incidence reporting and how to manage incidences (what are near-misses, never events, etc.) and triaging patients (on the labour wards, clinics and waiting lists – often described as prioritisation – being able to justify decisions irrespective of whether these are right or wrong as per General Medical Council (GMC) recommendation). Be familiar with the following:

*RCOG and GMC guidelines and documents on consent – when and how to obtain it, when is it valid and the principles of obtaining consent. Have a look at a consent form in your unit. These tend to be the same nationally and are available on the internet for those not working in the UK. Visit www.nhs.uk/conditions/consent-to-treatment/ and read 'Consent to treatment' and also review NHS Consent Form 4 (for adults who lack the capacity to investigate and treat).

*RCOG and national guidelines/documents on clinical governance, especially audit – how to undertake audits (components of the audit cycle); how to produce protocols, guidelines and incident (adverse event) reporting; how to respond to these including MDTs (multidisciplinary teams) and never events (https://improvement.nhs.uk/documents/2266/Never_Events_list_2018_FINAL_v5.pdf); and how to deal with these.

- Local/national documents/guidelines on safeguarding children and those with learning disabilities and the Mental Capacity Act
- Safe practices such as prescribing (right drug, right dose, right route and right time – 4Rs) and being able to identify errors on drug and monitoring charts
- The WHO safety checklist and where it applies

Applied clinical knowledge: This domain is the essential core of training and should form the basis of the various domains. The candidate is expected to demonstrate not only the acquired minimum knowledge but its application in clinical practice. For example, you might have read the evidence (NICE or RCOG guidelines), but how do you apply these to a clinical scenario? How do you interpret and act on a result based on not only knowledge but the clinical scenario for which the test was undertaken? Here independent clinical thinking is encouraged, including being critical of evidence and understanding that application could vary from one patient to another. You are not expected to say that the recommendation or treatment being offered is derived from NICE/RCOG Guideline etc. and therefore must be accepted to demonstrate that you are using this as the basis of your overall management. The best way to prepare for this domain is to have a thorough reflection on the cases managed, asking the following questions:

a. Were the investigations requested appropriate? What is the evidence to support my requests?
b. Were the management plans the most up-to-date, and did they provide value for money?
c. Could I justify the management options discussed with the patients with colleagues?
d. Were there any obvious omissions in information gathering, investigations or managements?
e. Were the most suitable colleagues involved in the woman's care?

7
How to Fail the Part 3 MRCOG Examination

In as much as I would like to believe that no one sets out to fail this examination deliberately, it is not difficult to understand and appreciate how some candidates by default indeed embark on the road to failure. For these candidates, the following clues would make the whole process of failing easier! For the others, fully understanding these clues should ensure that you avoid them.

1. Once you pass Part 2, assume that you are good enough to pass Part 3 and make no relevant preparations

2. Do not make any attempt to attend one of the Part 3 courses (after all, these are expensive and you are a very good trainee)

3. Take time off from work (a few weeks to months before the exams and only concentrate on your books) until you are able to sit for the Part 3 examination

4. Work independently and do not use the consultants and seniors you work with, as they do not know the changes that have happened in the exams over the last few years. Furthermore, some of them will demotivate you with their negative comments

5. Pay no attention to clinical governance and aspects of care that promote patient safety, such as audit and duty of care, including recommendations from recent investigations of hospitals, major incidence and the guidance from the GMC

6. At the simulated station or during the exams
    a. Do not read the instructions thoroughly – after all this is a clinical examination
    b. Do not introduce yourself to the role player
    c. Use language that is professional as this makes you gain more respect from the role player
    d. Talk down to your patient and be patronising – you are more knowledgeable and the patient ought to listen to you
    e. Tell the patient what they like to hear rather than what is an honest and frank discussion about the issues
    f. Do not listen to the patient but impose what you believe is the right approach to managing the problem
    g. Do not be logical in your approach of communication with patients, relatives or colleagues
    h. Ask as many irrelevant questions as possible, as this will put the patient at ease
    i. At the exams, you should never admit ignorance or say you do not know and will have to find out
    j. By the end of each task, the simulated patient must be left in no doubt that you have solved her/his problems and with absolute certainty.

8
Examples of Possible Tasks under the Various Domains

Information Gathering

1. History
2. Interpretation of results
3. Ordering investigations/tests
4. From other sources – RCOG, NICE, FSRH, SIGN etc.
5. Recovering/reviewing information from records in the same or other hospitals
6. Encouraging questions and offering timely and rational answers

Communication with Patients and Families

1. History taking
2. Discussing diagnosis
3. Communicating results
4. Breaking bad news
5. Knowing when, where, what and how to and not to communicate
6. Dealing with a teenager/patients that lack the capacity
7. Dealing with an angry patient/relative
8. Demonstrating how to check understanding and encouraging questions and providing appropriate answers

Communication with Colleagues

1. Teaching others (e.g. junior colleagues, nurses, midwives and medical students)
2. Letters to GP (General Practitioner)
3. Handover – SBAR (Situation, Background, Assessment and Recommendation)
4. MDTs (knowing what the composition of the multidisciplinary teams should be)
5. Sharing information (with patients, GPs, Midwives, other healthcare providers, etc.)

Patient Safety

1. Issues on Data Protection Act, Mental Capacity Act, Child Protection
2. When the candidate can call for help
3. Issues of confidentiality
4. Cultural and religious factors involving care
5. Audit and clinical governance
6. WHO safety checklist
7. Safe prescription and prescribing errors
8. Confirming that results belong to the patient (confirming that the details on the results are the patients')
9. Unlicensed medication
10. Ensuring that patients' health is not jeopardised (contraindications to management etc.)
11. Complications arising from treatment or failure to treat
12. Consenting for surgery – who, what and when to consent
13. Prioritisation of care – inpatient/outpatient/labour ward/waiting list
14. Prioritisation of referral letters
15. Prioritisation of results

Applied Knowledge

1. Evidence bases of practice
2. Limitation of evidence
3. How to generate evidence
4. How are guidelines and protocols developed
5. Familiarity with current literature and guidelines

9
What Are the Examiners Looking for in Each of the Tasks?

Module 1: Teaching

The most likely domains to be assessed are in italics. Here the examiner is looking for good communication between the candidate and the trainee (*information gathering, communication with patients and families, communication with colleagues, applied clinical knowledge and patient safety*). It is important to recognise the level of the trainee being taught and that the candidate understands the principles of teaching. A very good candidate will know when to compliment and encourage the trainee to improve on skills. In order to teach, the candidate must be knowledgeable and be conscious of patient safety. All these have to be taken into consideration during the 10-minute session. Examples of topics that could be covered here include:

1. Teaching on practical skills based on OSATS
   a. Making surgical knots
   b. Episiotomy repair
   c. Instrumental deliveries
   d. Vaginal breech deliveries
   e. Conducting vaginal twin deliveries
   f. Manual removal of placentas
   g. Laparoscopy
   h. Hysteroscopy
2. Others
   a. Conducting a tutorial
   b. How to consent a patient for surgery
   c. How to conduct an audit
   d. Electrosurgery/diathermy
   e. Fetal blood sampling
   f. Evacuation of retained products of conception
   g. Teaching how to read a protocol and how to produce guidelines
   h. Conduction of a 'fire drill' (e.g. on eclampsia, cord prolapse and massive PPH)
   i. Giving feedback (for example, on training, consent forms, letters to GP and MDT oncology letters)
   j. Conducting an appraisal
   k. Inserting a urinary catheter or pessary
   l. Dealing with bullying, undermining and underperforming colleagues

Module 2: Core Surgical Skills

In this module, the candidate is expected to demonstrate an understanding of the principles of safe surgery and how these are applied to specific operative procedures to the level of a Specialist Trainee 5 (ST5). These principles cover pre-operative assessment including pre- and post-operative ward rounds, intraoperative procedures and complications arising thereof and their management. Consenting for surgical procedures, WHO safety checklist and knowledge of the various surgical instruments used in the most common obstetrics and gynaecological procedures are assessed in this module. Candidates should be able to understand and discuss the principles of managing complications of surgery, such as a perforated uterus, bladder, bowel, ureteric and other visceral injuries. For some of these complications, it is not expected that the candidate will be able to manage them but an understanding of how these are managed immediately (who to call and what they may do for example) and in the long term, including counselling, incident reporting and risk management, would be tested. Examples of potential areas for assessment include:

1. Surgical procedures
   a. Caesarean section (CS) (especially when there are associated pathologies such as adhesions, fibroids and placenta praevia)
   b. Hysterectomy – vaginal and abdominal
   c. Diagnostic laparoscopy and laparoscopic surgical procedures for common gynaecological problems such as ectopic pregnancies and adnexal pathology
   d. Evacuation of retained products of conception and complications including uterine perforation
   e. Ovarian cystectomy – laparoscopic and open
   f. Complications of surgery such as bowel, bladder and ureteric injuries
2. For complications of surgery
   a. Recognition or suspicion – who to inform and when (team in theatre, consultant and the speciality involved)
   b. If procedure is under regional anaesthesia – informing the patient prior to embarking on exploration/investigation to confirm and manage the injury
   c. Dealing with the surgical complication e.g. haemorrhage, collateral damage etc.
   d. Managing the complication immediately and outlining plan for care after
   e. Incident reporting – Datix, etc.
   f. Debriefing of patient
   g. Communication with the GP

Module 3: Post-Operative Care

As a member of the team managing women after surgery, it is an expectation that candidates will be able to understand the principles of post-operative care including counselling (usually about what happened at surgery, what to expect immediately after surgery, on leaving the hospital and at follow-up), debriefing, medication, thromboprophylaxis, fluid balance, catheter management and indeed management of complications arising from surgery, and the rationale for the specified length of hospital stay (the benefits versus risks of short and long hospital stay, day care surgery and care in the community). The candidate should understand the principles of enhanced recovery following surgery and be able to demonstrate this to the examiner. The assessment of communication here is likely to be with the patient, family and colleagues. Examples of areas that could be assessed include:

1. Discussing post-operative care of women who have undergone various surgical procedures, such as hysterectomy with or without bladder injury, exploratory laparotomy, unplanned procedures and complications
2. Updating a patient information leaflet about a surgical procedure such as laparoscopy, hysterectomy, tubal ligation, etc.
3. Care of women who have undergone complicated obstetric procedures such as caesarean hysterectomy, ruptured uterus, classical CS, massive PPH managed by Brace suture, etc.

Module 4: Antenatal Care

This module is one with a wide range of topics that can be assessed. Important here is an understanding of the principles of routine antenatal care (as outlined in NICE guidelines): why and when is care classified as low-risk (midwifery care) or high-risk (consultant care), how plans are made and varied as determined by risk factors (which are these) and the concept of multidisciplinary care (communicating with midwives, GPs and various professionals, e.g. colleagues from other specialties, etc.). A very common form of assessment here is with simulated patients where history taking (obtaining information and communicating with the patient and colleagues) is undertaken. Examples of areas for assessment here include:

1. Medical disorders, e.g. diabetes mellitus, thyroid and other endocrine, cardiac, gastrointestinal, pulmonary, renal, autoimmune, connective tissue and neurological disorders in pregnancy
2. Pregnancies complicated by growth abnormalities (small for gestational age, growth restriction, macrosomia and polyhydramnios)
3. Complicated pregnancies – hypertension, pre-eclampsia, multiple pregnancies (monochorionic and dichorionic), placental abnormalities, breech presentation, obstetric cholestasis and antepartum haemorrhage
4. Ultrasound scan fetal abnormalities
5. Prenatal diagnosis (screening tests, amniocentesis, chorionic villus sampling (CVS) and non-invasive prenatal testing/non-invasive prenatal diagnosis (NIPT/NIPD))
6. Preterm prelabour rupture of fetal membranes (PPROM)

In preparing for this module, there should be a focus on taking a relevant history, initiation of appropriate investigations and being able to justify these; providing information to the woman and her partner and family; making a plan for management including timing of delivery and being able to justify your plans. It is important to recognise that there are controversies in care and that the opinion of the patient is important in decision making.

Module 5: Maternal Medicine

This module is similar to Module 4 in that it is able to assess the candidates on any of the five domains (patient safety, information gathering, communication with the patients and families, communication with colleagues and applied clinical knowledge). Here, however, the student is expected to demonstrate an understanding of the aetiology and pathophysiology of most of the maternal medical complications of pregnancy, such as the common endocrine, haematological, renal system (including transplant), cardiovascular (e.g. cardiac disease, hypertension), respiratory (e.g. asthma), gastrointestinal (e.g. inflammatory bowel disease – Crohn's and ulcerative colitis), neurological (e.g. epilepsy and headaches) and musculoskeletal (e.g. spina bifida and pubic symphysis dysfunction) disorders. Assessments in this module will include tasks aimed at the candidates' ability to provide or understand the rationale for preconception care, antenatal and often multidisciplinary care, including intrapartum and postpartum care. It is important to remember that for most of these medical problems there is usually a two-way approach to their management – the effects of pregnancy on the condition and that of the condition on the pregnancy. Examples of tasks in this module include:

1. Endocrine problems in pregnancy – diabetes, thyroid and Cushing's syndrome
2. Respiratory problems – asthma
3. Gastrointestinal – ulcerative colitis and Crohn's disease
4. Musculoskeletal – arthritis that affects the pelvis and spina bifida
5. Connective disorders – systemic lupus erythematosus (SLE), Marfan's syndrome and antiphospholipid syndrome
6. Cardiovascular – hypertension (essential or otherwise), cardiomyopathy, various congenital cardiac malformations and Eisenmenger's syndrome
7. Haematological – sickle cell, thalassaemia, anaemia, bleeding disorders (especially inherited), ITP and TTP
8. Transplant – renal/cardiac transplant
9. Renal – chronic renal failure on dialysis
10. Neurological – epilepsy, headaches and intracranial hypertension
11. Infections in pregnancy – cytomegalovirus, HIV, chickenpox, herpes, hepatitis, syphilis etc.

Module 6: Management of Labour

This is probably one of the most critical modules in the specialty, as most trainees will be expected to have played a central role in the management of various intrapartum cases – complicated and uncomplicated. This module therefore allows for the assessment of the five domains, particularly patient safety and communication. Obviously a very sound knowledge of the process of labour and how it affects various physiological and pathological changes associated with pregnancy is crucial to the management of labour. Here applied knowledge is essential. Communication is central to effective care of women on the labour ward, and this happens at various levels – with patients and their partners and with staff (senior, junior, midwifery, other specialties like anaesthesia, haematology, chemical pathology, microbiology, virology, blood bank and neonatology) at various stages and during handovers. Here the SBAR acronym is very useful. Recognising normal and abnormal labour and how to manage these are central and so too is prioritisation of tasks on the labour ward – something which an average ST5 should have dealt with on more than one occasion. Examples of tasks under this module include:

1. Induction of labour
2. Unstable lie
3. Vaginal birth after caesarean section (VBAC)
4. Poor progress in labour
5. Precipitate labour
6. Prioritisation board

7. Management of complications of labour
8. Previous difficult labours (e.g. PPH, 3/4th perineal tears, shoulder dystocia and ruptured uterus)
9. Preterm labour

Module 7: Management of Delivery

This is a continuation of Module 6 and again lends itself nicely to each of the five domains of assessment. Here your decision making and its timing are critical and will be assessed. The trainee must be well versed with the management of normal and abnormal delivery, including complications resulting from these. Important to this module is risk management and patient safety, especially with regard to counselling after poor outcomes including breaking bad news. Examples of the tasks include:

1. Labour dystocia
2. Forceps delivery
3. Ventouse delivery
4. Elective CS
5. Emergency CS
6. CS in the second stage
7. PPH
8. Uterine rupture
9. Preterm labour
10. Intrauterine fetal death – delivery and management
11. Retained placenta
12. Uterine inversion

Module 8: Postpartum Problems (The Puerperium)

Having delivered the baby, it is not unusual for problems to arise after. These could be maternal or neonatal. For the trainee, the focus of assessment under this module is mainly maternal, although occasionally there may be a task on a neonatal problem. Irrespective of the problem, you should not forget to communicate with the midwife and the patients' GP (through discharge summaries and letters). Ultimately these are members of the healthcare team that would be involved in the care of the woman. Typical problems include:

1. Maternal collapse
2. Retained placenta
3. PPH – primary and secondary
4. Lactation problems – poor lactation and lactation suppression in those opting not to breast feed. Mastitis in women breastfeeding
5. Appropriate contraception
6. Perineal trauma management – now and in future pregnancies
7. Infections and management

8. Wound infections
9. Psychiatric problems
10. Bladder problems
11. Neonatal jaundice and feeding problems

Module 9: Gynaecological Problems

This module covers a variety of gynaecological problems – elective and emergency. Assessments here would easily cover the five domains detailed earlier. Gynaecological exposure for trainees is limited, but it is the expectation that an average ST5 would be able to manage most emergencies independently but not some of the uncommon gynaecological problems. For these unusual cases, applied knowledge would be assessed. Examples of potential tasks, including those with simulated patients for this module, include:

1. Menstrual disorders (primary and secondary amenorrhoea, dysmenorrhoea, irregular periods and oligomenorrhoea)
2. Developmental abnormalities of the genital tract including congenital malformations
3. Paediatric and adolescent gynaecology including puberty and pubertal disorders
4. General gynaecological endocrine disorders
5. Emergency gynaecology
   a. Adnexal accidents
   b. Miscarriages
   c. Ectopic pregnancies
6. Menopause and hormone replacement therapy (HRT)
7. Pelvic pain and endometriosis
8. Vaginal discharge
9. Benign tumours (fibroids and ovarian cysts)

Module 10: Subfertility

This module covers all aspects of infertility – seeking information from couples attending with infertility, investigations and making a diagnosis and counselling and providing appropriate treatment. In this module, patient confidentiality is very important and equally important are the ethical aspects of assisted reproduction. An average ST5 should be able to take a good history, initiate investigations and understand when and how various aspects of assisted reproduction technology, including ovulation induction, IVF, ICSI, etc., are offered. Equally important is an understanding of the investigation and management of couples presenting with recurrent implantation failure and pregnancy losses.

Examples of tasks that can be assessed under this module include:

1. Female infertility
2. Male infertility
3. Counselling about various aspects of assisted reproductive techniques (ART)
4. Ethical aspects of ART
5. Recurrent pregnancy failures

Important to consider here are:

1. Confidentiality issues around investigation results from couples
2. Gamete donation – confidentiality and ethical aspects
3. Offering ART for social reasons, importance of age, etc.
4. Gamete storage and the ethics of this in single women/men or couples delaying childbirth
5. Ethics of treating same-sex couples

Module 11: Sexual and Reproductive Health

This module covers contraception, including understanding the United Kingdom Medical Eligibility Criteria (UKMEC), sexual health (including sexually transmitted infections, same-sex relationships and their associated problems) and termination of pregnancy (TOP) (including the laws governing this as well as the procedures for TOP). Safeguarding vulnerable women and children forms part of this module, and an understanding of these is important for assessment. Examples of areas that can be assessed include:

1. Choice of contraception and when to discontinue in the over 40s
2. Options for contraception in women with various co-morbidities or contraindications to some of the options
3. Surgical contraception
4. Long-acting reversible contraction (LARC)
5. Complications of various contraceptive options
6. Emergency contraception – immediate, medium and long-term counselling
7. Sexually transmitted infections (STIs)
8. Problems of same-sex relationships

Module 12: Early Pregnancy Care

This module focuses on early pregnancy complications and their management. An average ST5 should not only be very knowledgeable about each of these complications but should be able to demonstrate how to manage these, including how to perform surgical procedures and also discussing the options of care with the patients. The topics covered in this module include nausea and vomiting in pregnancy and hyperemesis gravidarum, miscarriages (the different types), ectopic pregnancies and trophoblastic disorders. Possible tasks from this module include:

1. Management of a molar pregnancy (scan with a complete mole)
2. Hyperemesis gravidarum
3. Ectopic pregnancy – diagnosis and management options
4. Cervical and caesarean scar ectopic pregnancies
5. Various types of miscarriages – threatened, inevitable, complete, incomplete and septic
6. Review of histology reports and appropriate management (e.g. complete/incomplete mole, ectopic pregnancy but no chorionic villi in tube or evidence of decidualisation in endometrial curettage)

Module 13: Gynaecological Oncology

At the ST5 level, most trainees will not be expected to manage gynaecological oncology problems, independently; however, they will be expected to understand the principles of premalignant screening (for vulval, vaginal, cervical and endometrial cancers), the staging of these cancers, how these are investigated and the various treatment options, especially in the context of a multidisciplinary team (MDT), as well as cancer targets in the UK, including timelines from referral to treatment. The principles of chemotherapy and palliative care, including psychological support, would form part of this module. Examples of tasks in this module include:

1. Explanation of the results of investigations to patients and management (e.g. breaking the news that the patient has cervical, endometrial, ovarian, vulval cancer, etc.)
2. Management of an abnormal cervical cytology
3. Investigations and management of ovarian, cervical, endometrial and vulval cancers
4. Management of choriocarcinoma
5. Chemotherapy and radiotherapy – principles, indications and complications
6. Principles of palliative care, including pain control and dying

Module 14: Urogynaecology and Pelvic Floor Problems

As the population is ageing, there is the expectation that upon completion of training, an average specialist should be able to manage most urogynaecological problems initially and only refer where first options have failed. An average ST5 should therefore understand the anatomy and physiology of the pelvic floor and the urinary tract (especially the bladder), the pathologies that arise when there is abnormality in either anatomy or function, how these are investigated and the treatment options including medical and surgical. Complications arising therefore should be understood as well as how these can be managed. Trainees are expected to interpret urogynaecological investigations and appreciate when to seek information to inform decisions on managing women with bladder outflow problems or overdistension. Some of these problems may arise as complications of deliveries or surgery, in which case there may be an overlap with some of the other modules. Examples of tasks in this module include:

1. Urinary incontinence
2. Pelvic organ prolapse
3. Urinary retention
4. Investigations of urinary incontinence – urodynamic investigations – discussion with the patient and management options

Below are general tips for each of the modules structured under the various domains.

Module 1: Teaching

- Information gathering – background of the student – skill and knowledge levels and definition of deficiencies
- Communication with patients and families – introduction of self and task, explanation of role and that of tutee, obtaining consent for teaching or supervision of task

- Communication with colleagues – using language and other tools to teach, setting objectives and demonstrating appropriate steps in teaching to accomplish task objectives and giving feedback
- Patient safety – ensuring patient safety is maintained throughout teaching and knowing when to stop
- Applied clinical knowledge – demonstrating use of knowledge to define teaching objectives and using evidence to support the approach to teaching and giving feedback

Module 2: Core Surgical Skills

- Information gathering – pre-operative assessment – history, physical examination and investigations; appropriateness of investigations for surgery; appropriate review of notes
- Communication with patients and families – able to counsel patients appropriately using non-directional techniques and enabling patients to make the right surgical choice
- Communication with colleagues – appropriate documentation of procedures, demonstrates ability to teach surgical skills, knows what to do and when to call for help and communicate where on the surgical ladder of a procedure has a complication occurred with colleagues; knows how to prioritise patients on a waiting list
- Patient safety – principles of consenting for surgery and capacity, WHO safety checklist, perioperative thromboprophylaxis and antibiotic prophylaxis and post-operative care including complications; knows when and who to call for help; demonstrates understanding of the use of blood products in surgery
- Applied clinical knowledge – application of clinical knowledge including evidence to support decisions on various surgical (gynaecological and obstetrical) procedures including risks, complications and alternatives to surgical treatment

Module 3: Post-Operative Care

- Information gathering – being able to institute appropriate investigations and taking the necessary actions from these
- Communication with patients and families – appropriate communication of operative findings and procedures performed to patients and families, including the course of post-operative care and follow-up; involving patients and relatives in all aspects of their care
- Communication with colleagues – appropriately handing over of patients and involving others in the care of patients, especially when complications arise (using SBAR)
- Patient safety – demonstrating understanding of risk management, especially in dealing with complications and involvement in aspects of post-operative care that influence patient safety, such as prescribing, fluid management, thromboprophylaxis, care of catheters and antibiotics including drug allergy
- Applied clinical knowledge – management of routine post-operative patients and complications and demonstrating the use of evidence to support decisions about care

Module 4: Antenatal Care

- Information gathering – able to obtain a detailed and focussed history from the patient and initiate appropriate investigations; knows what to do when appropriate records are not available (missing information on care given in previous pregnancies or medical records unavailable in the unit); demonstrates ability to review records of previous pregnancies to influence choice/care

- Communication with patients and families – able to discuss with patients and relatives their care, including issues around difficult topics such as FGM, domestic violence and substance misuse; communicates care pathways, including investigations (when and why) with enough justification with patients and relatives
- Communication with colleagues – able to demonstrate that antenatal care is multidisciplinary (involving midwife, hospital and GP and other specialties where appropriate) by sharing care plans/pathways
- Patient safety – able to demonstrate aspects of care that could affect the safety of the baby and mother – e.g. investigations (how are these affected by pregnancy), dual effect of drugs and risk management when indicated, and what are the principles of prioritisation to ensure that patient safety is not compromised
- Applied clinical knowledge – able to demonstrate the use of clinical knowledge in the planning and care of uncomplicated and complicated pregnancies (e.g. fetal growth restriction, fetal macrosomia, polyhydramnios, multiple pregnancies, fibroids and other tumours in pregnancy, etc.)

Module 5: Maternal Medicine

- Information gathering – able to obtain a good history, initiate appropriate investigations (and interpret and act accordingly) and to obtain information about past obstetric and medical histories from other sources
- Communication with patients and families – able to communicate effectively with patients and their relatives about their disorders and how these affect pregnancies and vice versa
- Communication with colleagues – able to work with colleagues a plan of care within an MDT (other specialties, midwives, GPs, social workers, etc.)
- Patient safety – in addition to the comments on antenatal care, able to recognise the value of pre-pregnancy care and counselling, especially in the context of optimising health before and during pregnancy
- Applied clinical knowledge – to use evidence to plan and manage pre-pregnancy and antenatal care

Module 6: Management of Labour

- Information gathering – able to review records for relevant information that may influence intrapartum care, including the partogram and CTG – fetal and tocographic monitoring; know when to initiate investigations and interpret them
- Communication with patients and families – able to ensure that the patient and the family are well informed about the course of labour and any interventions (including benefits and risks) instituted
- Communication with colleagues – able to know when to involve colleagues (seniors and juniors and from other specialties) in the care of labour; able to prioritise cases on the labour ward including delegation of tasks; able to teach others procedures like instrumental delivery, repair of episiotomies/perineal tears, breech delivery, caesarean section, etc.; able to manage emergencies such as shoulder dystocia, cord prolapse, maternal collapse and eclampsia; able to conduct twin vaginal delivery and manage a retrained placenta

- Patient safety – able to demonstrate an understanding of all aspects of patient safety in labour – where to labour (e.g. standalone low-risk, alongside or consultant units), appropriate analgesia, fluid balance, fetal health (CTG) management, prescribing and how it may affect the neonate and risk management
- Applied clinical knowledge – able to demonstrate the use of evidence (guidelines, protocols, etc.) to make decisions about care of patients

Module 7: Management of Delivery

- Information gathering – able to use patient records to obtain information that would inform on delivery options; order appropriate investigations to assist with delivery options and interpret them appropriately
- Communication with patients and families – able to explain delivery options and obtain consent, recognising the views of the woman and her family
- Communication with colleagues – able to work with colleagues to effect a safe delivery; able to understand and demonstrate involvement of multidisciplinary teams in delivery (especially operative delivery and how these are classified) and management of ensuing complications (e.g. haemorrhage, uterine rupture, inversion, collapse and fetal distress) including teaching and triaging of patients
- Patient safety – able to demonstrate aspects of safe delivery both for the mother and the baby – critically appraising delivery options and making the right choices and ensuring that the environment is safe for the mother and the baby; prioritisation of patients requiring delivery and ensuring that safety remains paramount in decision making
- Applied clinical knowledge – able to demonstrate application of knowledge in the management of delivery – technical skills and dealing with multiple pregnancies, preterm delivery, breech presentation and shoulder dystocia

Module 8: Postpartum Problems (The Puerperium)

- Information gathering – able to use information from antepartum and intrapartum periods to plan postpartum care, including the management of complications; knowing which and when to initiate investigations and timely and appropriate response to abnormal results
- Communication with patients and families – able to communicate about postpartum care (including a pathway of care), taking into consideration factors that may affect this
- Communication with colleagues – able to work with colleagues (midwives, GPs, neonatologists, anaesthetists, etc.) on clear pathways of care
- Patient safety – able to demonstrate awareness of safety around prescription, care of vulnerable women and neonates and clinical governance around postpartum care
- Applied clinical knowledge – able to use knowledge of postnatal care from clinical guidelines and protocols and appropriately manage normal and complicated postnatal care

Module 9: Gynaecological Problems

- Information gathering – able to take a comprehensive and relevant history, obtain information from present and past records that would influence care and initiate relevant investigations and interpret them to support management options
- Communication with patients and families – able to communicate with patient and family about their care, including diagnosis, investigations and management options, recognising the principles of autonomy

- Communication with colleagues – able to work with colleagues in the care of women through handovers, consultations and MDT working
- Patient safety – able to demonstrate risk management in gynaecology, recognising limitations and when to call for senior support and how to use the WHO safe surgery checklist
- Applied clinical knowledge – able to use evidence critically to support decisions about care (including investigations, plan of care and treatment options) and counselling about these

Module 10: Subfertility

- Information gathering – able to sensitively take a detailed history from couples and initiate timely and appropriate investigations; interpreting these and using them to plan care and being able to seek additional information from other sources to help with care
- Communication with patients and families – able to communicate with patients and their family/families in a sensitive manner around the issues of fertility, investigations, treatment and complications, including the legal framework for treatment in the UK
- Communication with colleagues – able to involve MDT where appropriate and knowing when to refer for specialist care, including a clinical psychologist
- Patient safety – able to understand the safety issues involved in the treatment of subfertility – prescribing for super-ovulation and multiple pregnancies; embryo storage and freezing of gametes; the legal framework for assisted reproductive techniques (ART), including the provisions of the Human Fertilisation and Embryology Act (HFEA) for treatment
- Applied clinical knowledge – able to use evidence critically to inform management of couples, including constraints of care, for example, in those with one partner with a child, age, same sex couples, etc. Understands the contribution of male and female factors to subfertility and how these are managed

Module 11: Sexual and Reproductive Health

- Information gathering – able to take a detailed sexual history sensitively; initiate timely and appropriate investigations and use these to formulate a well thought out management pathway, including contact tracing and contraception
- Communication with patients and families – this is a very sensitive area and the trainee must be able to show an ability to communicate, bearing in mind sensitivities (such as the subject itself, beliefs, societal perception and labels, sexual diversity and age of maturity), diagnosis, treatment and contact tracing, including implications for fertility
- Communication with colleagues – able to communicate with colleagues especially from the GUM and family planning services about differential diagnoses and treatment
- Applied clinical knowledge – able to demonstrate the use of critical evidence to manage patients including the correct application of laws on termination of pregnancy (the Abortion Act) and the Sexual Offences Act
- Patient safety – able to demonstrate issues of clinical governance around this subject

Module 12: Early Pregnancy Care

- Information gathering – able to take a good history to allow for diagnosis; initiation of investigations and the interpretation of results thereof to help plan appropriate and timely management; demonstrate the ability to use other sources to obtain information to help management

- Communication with patients and families – able to communicate with patients and their families sympathetically about diagnosis, management plans and follow-up
- Communication with colleagues – able to involve colleagues appropriately in care of women with early pregnancy complications, recognising the limitations of the trainees' abilities
- Patient safety – able to demonstrate an understanding of clinical governance around this topic including audit and triaging of patients; able to prescribe safety in ongoing early pregnancies and understand the impact of treatment (medication or otherwise) on ongoing pregnancy
- Applied clinical knowledge – able to use evidence to support overall care of patients, including miscarriages, ectopic pregnancies, molar pregnancies and recurrent pregnancy loss; able to make reasoned arguments for and against various approaches to management, for example, expectant, medical, versus surgical management of miscarriages and ectopic pregnancies

Module 13: Gynaecological Oncology

- Information gathering – able to take a comprehensive history, initiate investigations and interpret them appropriately
- Communication with patients and families – able to give information to patients and families about suspected diagnosis, investigations and treatment options, including referral to specialist care; able to deal sensitively with breaking bad news and providing psychological support
- Communication with colleagues – able to understand and demonstrate involvement of an MDT in the care of women with malignancies; recognise that most of the care is highly specialised and demonstrate an understanding of the pathway for cancer care in the UK
- Patient safety – able to demonstrate an understanding of clinical governance as applies to oncology, cancer treatment and referral pathways for the UK, including recommendations for timelines of care, and able to show an understanding of the aspects of care that could improve or compromise safety, e.g. prescription of chemotherapeutic agents/drugs
- Applied clinical knowledge – able to use critically appraised evidence (including from guidelines, various oncology society guidance, etc.) to inform all aspects of care (investigations, diagnosis, treatment, prognosis including 5-year survival), counselling and follow-up

Module 14: Urogynaecology and Pelvic Floor Problems

- Information gathering – able to take a detailed urogynaecological history, initiate investigations, including a fluid diary, and use these appropriately to initiate treatment and follow-up; know when to refer to tertiary level care and the limitations in providing care to these women
- Communication with patients and families – able to provide patients and families information about urogynaecological problems and the psychological effects of these on lifestyle and their management; recognise that there are sensitivities around this subject with women
- Communication with colleagues – able to involve colleagues in care, including communication of information about care
- Patient safety – able to demonstrate an understanding of clinical governance in urogynaecology and safety with regard to treatment options, including medications, and especially that of devices such as meshes which are associated with class actions
- Applied clinical knowledge – able to use evidence critically to justify options for the care of women with urogynaecological problems

10
How to Prepare for the MRCOG Part 3: A Personal Perspective
Wafaa Ali Belail Hammad*

In this chapter, I outline how I prepared for the exams; I hope that you will find it useful in your preparations. What worked for me may not work for you, but please modify my approach to meet your own needs and ensure that you are ready on the day of the exams. Good luck!

Key Resources – What's Involved

When it comes to preparing study material, it is important to bear in mind how this will help you in dealing with the exam scenarios. I have therefore provided some resources and guidance on some key technical areas that you will need to be aware of as you embark on your study journey.

1. *Patient information leaflets*. Talking to the patient in a manner that is understandable is the key to effective communication. Leaflets will help you become more accustomed to the layman's language you will use while counselling. There are plenty of cases/topics, and they all have leaflets on them. There are also many leaflets on the RCOG website and the NHS. For NHS leaflets, you will need to search for the name of the topic ending with NHS; for example, 'Down syndrome NHS'.

2. *RCOG Green Top guidelines, NICE guidelines and TOG articles*. These are important for the applied clinical knowledge and patient safety domains. Your knowledge has to be up to date, and these provide the basis for this. They can be very helpful in you providing the right and most up-to-date information to the patient, in addition to the leaflets.

3. *Stratog*. This RCOG resource has case studies which should be utilized in your preparations. They also have 14 full exam scenario videos for the Part 3 MRCOG – one case per module.

4. *Online groups (Telegram and Facebook)*. It is important to join a learning community that will help keep your finger on the pulse of the subject matters that are relevant to the exam. Joining those groups can open up discussions and cases that you may not have thought of. It is also a great place to get support from colleagues who are in the same boat with you. These groups are full of people who have sat through the exam – some who have passed and some who have not – and their collective experiences can be useful for your study journey

---

* Specialist Trainee (Clinical Attachment) in Obstetrics & Gynaecology. Derby, UK

and will give you insights you may have never thought of. The key is to maximize your exposure.

Process of Study/Methodology

Finding a Study Partner from the Beginning Is Crucial. Why?

It may be hard to find a partner who 'clicks', and you may go through a few until you find the partner who is on the same wave length – having an understanding and willingness to help, does not slow you down, and willing to incorporate your study styles into theirs and vice versa.

I, personally, had two study partners from different countries. With work commitments and time zone differences, I managed to study with each of them around two to three times a week. We built a very strong bond and shared information with each other. On my own time, I practiced alone either in front of the mirror or recording my stations and frequently listening to them; this helped me appreciate my weaknesses.

Duration for Preparation

I believe that this should take on an average of 4–5 months. This is not just a random number. It is 4–5 months because I found that it typically took approximately 1 week to comfortably complete a module. This being the case, it should take three and a half months to complete the modules, leaving you 6 weeks to revise and repeat your case studies.

Study Plan

Go through the MRCOG Part 3 syllabus from the RCOG website, focusing on the modules. This will give you an idea of exactly what you will have to go through and ultimately need to retain in memory. Set a timetable for each of the 14 modules; ideally you should set aside 1 week for each module, remembering that some smaller modules may take only 3 days to complete. I recommend that you print the syllabus out and highlight the areas you have covered as you go along. The process of 'checklisting' what you have studied is useful as both a mental and an organizational exercise. The example below shows how you should prepare for each of the modules.

Module: Early Pregnancy. The early pregnancy care module is one of the smallest but is at the same time challenging as it has elements of breaking bad news. Topics under this module include miscarriage, ectopic pregnancy, molar pregnancy, pregnancy of unknown location and hyperemesis gravidarum.

Start with ectopic pregnancy – go through the guideline with the aim of extracting the necessary information needed to counsel and plan for the recommended treatment in accordance to the patient's needs. Ideally, you would want to know the symptoms, examination findings, investigations and criteria for each treatment option to be offered and discussed. It should not take more than 1 hour to write down these points. The headings can include the following:

1. Symptoms
2. Examination
3. Investigations

4. Expectant management: criteria, risks
5. Medical management: criteria, contraindications, risks
6. Surgical management: criteria, risks
7. Recurrence and future advice

Having done that, go to the patient RCOG information leaflet on ectopic pregnancy and read it thoroughly. It has all the patient-friendly language you need in terms of explaining what ectopic pregnancy is and what are the management options available. Incorporate these two sources together to build up the case.

Formulate your case from the leaflet in points such as:

1. Introduce myself
2. Confirm the aim of the consultation (from scenario/GP letter)
3. Break the bad news in steps – displaying empathy
4. Explain ectopic pregnancy and draw pictures to help understanding
5. Further history/investigations needed
6. Each management options with risks and benefits: expectant, medical (methotrexate) and surgery
7. Effect on fertility and future pregnancy (recurrence) and need for scan early next pregnancy
8. Contraception
9. Involve consultant
10. Offer leaflet

Points 4, 5, 6, 7, 8 and 9 will be from the guideline and leaflet. The other points are communication skills that you will learn from watching audiovisual case examples. This will be further elaborated upon under communication skills below.

You are then ready to practice it with your study partner for 10 minutes, who will thereafter give you feedback. I would recommend that you record the practice with your partner and then listen to it alone on your spare time. This will allow you to pinpoint your weaknesses. For example, after listening to my practice I noticed I said the word 'OK' repetitively around 17 times in one case and realised I was doing it subconsciously. By listening to a recorded case, I was able to easily identify the repetition and take the necessary steps to address it.

It's difficult to get the perfect case study for the first time, but with continuous practice, talking and giving feedback, you will sharpen your communication skills and consolidate your knowledge.

Tips while Studying

Have a separate notebook for the layman terminologies you find difficult to remember and slowly you will build a bank of terminologies that you can call on for the required case. Use a board with sticky notes containing communication phrases that you come across. You can use them while you are performing a case.

I will encourage group studies and discussion as well. Studying in groups gives insights into how cases are being approached by your peers. This is a double-edged sword as you will be able to go through a variety of cases studies with peers either as examinees or as examiners but will not always be able to identify a good performance example. This is why it is important to cross reference with your resources.

How to Improve Your Communication Skills

Out of all the other domains, I chose to elaborate specifically on this one, because as an overseas candidate, it was what I struggled with the most at the beginning. Later, I found out you could actually easily get a good grip on it, and it is not that difficult after all; but yes, it does require plenty of practice. You can memorize knowledge but you can never memorize communication. It has to be a habit in you, and it will become so with practice, working on your pronunciations, paying attention to your body language and most importantly, adapting yourself to listening and responding to patients.

Communication with a patient ranges from building a rapport and managing their expectations to handling sensitive situations and learning to assert yourself without appearing aggressive. You have to be clear and direct. Dealing directly with real patients in hospital environments is the best way to sharpen your communication skills.

People who reside in the UK should take advantages of opportunities in front of you. If you are not working in the UK, you should get an attachment (if possible), as this will put you in a hospital environment where you will listen to communication between patients and experienced staff members. I will suggest you shadow nurses because they spend more time speaking to the patient. This is not a must to pass the exam but it is helpful.

For those outside the UK, be aware that in certain parts of the world, communication between patient and doctor may fall below the standards required for the examination. Not surprisingly, this is one area of the exams in which most overseas candidates struggle. After understanding the principles of good communication and counselling, apply these to patients in your clinic or hospital. It is very useful to get feedback as this will help identify areas where you need to make improvements. Such feedback can come from patients as well as colleagues who are happy to observe you.

Whether you are in the UK or not, practicing with your study partner is extremely important, as it provides one of the best preparations for the exam. This is because, over time, with repetition on real patients, you will subconsciously develop more effective communication skills that will be transferred to the exam. Whether your first language is English or not should not matter when it comes to counselling, as long as the information is correct, the correct procedures are followed, and when needed, empathy is shown; however, in the exams, this has to be in English.

Challenging Communication Skills

Not every patient simulated task is the same; therefore, it is vital to address the communication needs of each task and adapt your behaviour accordingly to support effective communication.

I will work through examples of three communication scenarios below; these may sound difficult at first but all that it requires from you is repetitive practice on the tone of voice along with facial expressions and body language. So I advise that you write down all the communication sentences you would use in such cases, record yourself, listen to it and keep repeating the process. For practice, bring a friend/family member and tell them you are going to give them bad news, for example, 'IUFD'. Ask them for an honest feedback on how they felt when you were breaking the news and giving them management options.

Helpful sources to learn how to tackle such cases will be available as videos on YouTube – search for 'dealing with an angry patient' or 'breaking bad news to a patient'.

Such cases in the exam depend largely not just on the medical implications of the situation but rather the way the information is delivered and expectations are managed. If your information is conveyed in a cold and insensitive way to the patient, this can result in you failing the task even if the medical diagnosis and information given are correct.

1. *Breaking bad news.* All patients who suffer tragic losses of their babies or whose babies have serious/lethal anomalies or who receive news about their health such as a diagnosis of cancer need to have the best possible care and support. News given to them must be done in stages by using phrases such as 'I'm afraid I don't have good news' or 'I'm sorry to say the results are not what we expected'.

   The care received must make their experience more manageable rather than exacerbating the pain and distress at this devastating moment. Good communication is essential. You must be mindful of your tone, express genuine concern and empathy, be sensitive, non-judgmental, use warm open body language and maintain eye contact when providing them with information on management plans.

   Use simple language and encourage the patient to ask questions, as some patients may feel shocked and find it difficult to understand information or think clearly. If there is a lot to discuss, ask if they would like another appointment to discuss additional details.

2. *Dealing with an angry patient/parent/husband.* Learning how to deal with angry patients and/or relatives is a valuable skill we can develop. Given the nature of the healthcare environment, you may encounter these situations in the exam. Patients can become angry for many reasons – they may have been left to wait for a long time before being seen in clinic, an error has been made by the medical/surgical team, they have received bad news or their expectations are not met.

   You must show empathy, reassurance or an apology, depending on what the patient is feeling and what events have occurred.

   While sitting, adopt a professional yet relaxed posture, and so un-cross your arms and legs with both feet on the floor. Keep a calm tone of voice, stay composed, speak slowly and clearly and do not raise your voice if the patient is shouting. Demonstrate active listening skills – eye contact, nodding and verbal responses, e.g. 'mmm'.

   Allow the patient to completely vent their anger if needed. Give them plenty of space to speak and avoid Interruptions. Apologize for any errors/delays but be aware that sometimes despite our best efforts and excellent communication skills, patients may still remain very angry over what has occurred.

3. *Dealing with a difficult patient.* It's a common scenario to come across a patient who is asking for a specific treatment plan that is not recommended; for example, a request for sterilization, vaginal delivery for a breech baby, requesting to deliver at home or requesting hormonal replacement therapy, with a history of breast cancer on treatment. Similarly, a patient can refuse a recommended management plan or procedure which is considered a standard of best practice, such as refusing all non-expectant management options for a symptomatic ectopic pregnancy.

   In situations like this, you should not forget that time is limited and this could potentially add more pressure on you. Potentially all these could lead to a situation in which you put the patient into a position of having to approve a treatment plan. If the information that you give is well put together and complete, this can give the patient the confidence in making the right and safe choice for themselves.

   Despite this, they can still insist on a choice that you disagree with. So, it is important to recognize your limitations as an ST5 and refer to a consultant. This also communicates the gravity of the situation to the patient, in that the consultation must be referred to a higher authority. This is not a reflection of your failure in communication; in fact, it is quite the opposite.

The Exams Are Nearly Here – What Should You Be Doing?

1. *Last week before the exam*. When it comes to the last week of the exam, I will suggest reducing the amount of study on a day-to-day basis in order to put your mind in a calmer state. You should simulate the exam conditions with your study partner as much as possible. You have to remember that your exam will run for 3 hours. You need to train your mind to be able to stay focused for 3 hours and change from one topic to another as you move through your stations.

   In order to do that, I would recommend you set a time table with your study partner just to revise and repeat the cases you already know in order to consolidate the information you have learned and become more confident around the topic. Practice 14 cases on a daily basis to train your mind and body to go through that process. This on its own will simply improve your ability to recall the information when required.

2. *The night before the exam – to revise or not?* Some people find that not engaging in intense revision the night before the exam helps them coalesce what they have learned, whilst others prefer to go over much more information to ensure it is as fresh as possible in their minds. Whether you prefer to do one or the other, we can all agree the night before the exam is an important night as we have to deal with the stress of the upcoming exam, as well as retain all the required knowledge.

   I have always preferred to study/review on the last night, but this session is different from other study days, and how I study and review in this crucial night is slightly different. I found that listening to recordings and videos works better than deep dives into heavy text. Audiovisual learning is easier to take in without making you feel stressed or overwhelmed, in addition to using more than one sense to process information.

   I do not go into study groups in the last days before the exam. Everyone is different the day before the exam, and some people can have a negative impact on your process, as some candidates may panic you by bringing up a subject area that you are not confident in or studied well. As you can imagine, this may inadvertently affect your performance by taking away focus from the areas that you have studied and can affect your recall of them during the exam. For this reason, it is ideal to stay away from study groups a week before the exam.

   Despite this, you can accidently find yourself in this situation; the most important thing is not to panic and start making decisions that are not objective. When you have two options, either try to look up and learn the subject area in a short space of time or stick to your original study plan.

   So, given the lack of time, what is the best way to approach this, should you find yourself in this situation? For me personally, and for the most part, I stuck to the study plan, but I am human and I cannot help but feel concerned and I would certainly want to look up the subject area just in case. I am not going to recommend that you do this but if you do, be objective and time sensitive.

   Preparations that are too demanding and overstretch you the night before an exam can cause distress and slow you down on the morning of the exam; you need to allow yourself time to wake up and get ready with ease and peace of mind. Have your outfit ready and allow yourself to get enough sleep, which is probably more than you usually get. Go to bed after a good meal and well hydrated. These may seem like basic things on their own but they are highly important to do and all contribute towards creating the right environment for you on the day of the exam.

3. ***The day of the exam***. Wear appropriate clothes; remember the exam is 3 hours long and you need to make sure your formal dress is comfortable as well as appropriate. Eating breakfast is essential before a long test. Hunger is just another distraction that you do not need. You want your mind to be ready but you do not want to psych yourself out before the test. Cramming – both the night before and the morning of the exam can have a negative effect on the information that you have already stored.

Allow ample of time to travel to the exam centre; arrive early. Allow time for traffic and unexpected delays so that you can arrive at the testing location with time to spare. This allows you to get comfortable with your surroundings and calm down before you embark on the exam.

4. ***During the exam***. This day is going to bring together all you have done in that last few months in your preparations over a short 3 hour period of examination. In these 3 hours, you will demonstrate what you have practiced and studied over the last few months, so it is important to be relaxed.

During the exam you will be given a note book and pencil at each station. You have two minutes to read the scenario and write down the points you wish to cover with the patients/examiner. Utilize these 2 minutes carefully as you have 10 minutes in each case to effectively and efficiently counsel the patients/answer the examiner on the key areas of the exam.

A key point to recognize while you are taking the exam is the possibility that you may come across a task on a topic/case that you find difficult and may end up questioning your performance. STOP – it is highly important that you do not do this whilst in the exam. You must develop the ability to keep calm, move on to the next station and leave the previous ones behind.

In Summary

- Understand your modules, the domains under each of them and the principles behind effective communication, especially those related to the module.
- While taking a history, it is better to start with an open-ended question and try to involve the patient more in the discussion.
- When offering to examine the patient, take permission; offer a chaperone, as there is always a nurse or midwife with you in the clinic or the ward.
- When explaining a diagnosis, relate it to the patient's symptoms as it improves understanding.
- When discussing management options, give the patient a brief overview of what you are going to discuss.
- Always communicate (loop back) with a health professional in the community setting (GP, midwife, nurse, etc.).

11
Common Tips on Communication

Approaching Tasks with Fetal Anomalies

In these scenarios, it is typical that you are the ST5 in the team and the consultant is away or has asked you to see someone who has just had an ultrasound scan by sonographers. This is because if the scan had been performed by a fetal medicine consultant, management would have be taken over rather than sending her to the general clinic. The following are my personal approaches to these tasks:

1. Introduce yourself as usual, as well as the role you are there to play. For example, 'I am Dr Kross, Mrs Quantien's ST5 in the clinic and I am here to discuss your ultrasound scan and how we are going to manage you'.
2. Confirm her name and date of birth – to make sure that you have addressed an important aspect of *patient safety* – one of the domains being assessed (it is not uncommon to forget to do this).
3. You could apologise for the unavailability of the consultant (if she/he is away) and then move straight to explain the findings. It is not very sensitive to start asking questions about LMP, social history, drug history, past medical history, etc., when the patient is expecting you to explain the results of her ultrasound. Furthermore, in clinics, you would have had the time to review notes and have all that information. Most patients will immediately interrupt you and ask that you please proceed and explain the ultrasound findings. You could say to the patient that as you do not have her notes, 'I will first explain the ultrasound findings and then ask you some questions that will give me some background information to help plan your management'. This is particularly useful if the instructions include a focused history.
4. Bad news may be (a) very bad news (abnormality incompatible with life or one compatible with life but with major consequences on the quality of life) or (b) one with a minor or no impact on the quality of life. Furthermore, these could either be correctable or not. This will determine the tone and the type of empathy you offer and how you broach the subject of breaking the news. If it is (a), it would be useful to ask if she has someone she would like to call or reach out to before you break the news, but this may not be necessary for (b). In almost all cases, the patient will either ask you to proceed or say she will call someone to come but would still like you to go ahead and break the news.
5. Break the news and give time for the patient to react. If the information is complicated, break it down and deliver it in parts so that the understanding is improved. Encourage questions and confirm understanding at each stage (you do this by checking that what you have said is understood and there are no questions). It is not unusual for the patient to be so distraught by the news that any more information will just be 'hitting a brick wall'. In this case, you must be able to help bring her back to the problem. There are two approaches to breaking bad news – (a)

implosive or (b) indirect. I prefer the implosive approach – you go straight to the bad news. It is also what most patients prefer. The other approach involves coming to the news slowly and indirectly. This can create a lot of anger and resentment from the patient. I will strongly recommend that you use the note pads available with you at the exams to help explain things to the patient. Some examples of phrases/sentences you may use to break the news: (1) I am sorry what I am about to tell you is not good news. (2) I am sorry I have some bad news to tell you about your baby. (3) I have been asked to come and explain the ultrasound findings and I am afraid to say that what I will be telling you is not good news. (4) Unfortunately, I have bad news about your baby. (5) The ultrasound scan you have just had unfortunately has picked up major problems or a major problem with the baby. I am afraid this is not good news. These are some of the ways I approach this and remember others may do it differently. Whatever the approach you chose, make sure you are comfortable with it.

6. Having broken the news, the next and most important question is 'What are the implications of the findings?' This will depend on the abnormality. I have examples of the various malformations discussed below. The implications are four-fold: (a) the abnormality is not compatible with life, and therefore termination is an option; (b) it is compatible with life (with or without a major impact on quality) and not correctable and termination may be an option; (c) it is compatible with life (with or without a major impact on quality and correctable; or (d) it has minimal or no consequence on the fetus, and it's either correctable or not. Finally, irrespective of the options above, is it one that requires further investigations like karyotyping? Most types of abnormalities you will encounter in the exams will require karyotyping, except for things like gastroschisis.

7. Who is required in the MDT to counsel and manage antenatally? First, the fetal medicine consultant should be involved (here their role is two-fold – to confirm the fetal abnormality and exclude other subtle abnormalities and therefore confirm implications and also initiate/perform additional investigations which you would have mentioned (like amniocentesis/CVS)). If it is an abnormality that will require surgical correction, involve the appropriate speciality antenatally (paediatric surgeon, neurosurgeon, plastic surgeon, orthopaedic surgeon, etc.). Consider involving the clinical geneticists, especially where the prognosis is guarded or unknown or the malformation may be part of a syndrome. Support from a clinical psychologist or counsellor should always be considered, especially for the lethal abnormalities that are associated with severe consequences for the baby. Finally, do not forget the triangulate back to the GP and the community midwife. There are several support groups for various malformations, and you will not be wrong if you offer to link the patient up with a support group and also provide her with information leaflets on the abnormality.

8. Discussions on investigations should focus on the fetus and then the mother if appropriate. In discussing these, timing, the procedure itself (if applicable), complications, availability of results and how the results will be delivered must be discussed, including the accuracy and what will be done after results are available.

9. When results are available, there are usually two options depending on the result. If normal or the patient wishes to continue with the pregnancy irrespective of the result, then discuss antenatal care and delivery. If the option is the termination of pregnancy, counsel appropriately and then discuss this in detail. Do not forget that some patients may decline investigations and opt for termination.

10. Finally provide the patient with a contact number, in case she has questions and arrange a follow-up appointment with her partner or family member. This may be on the same day or as soon as it is feasible to discuss and agree on management plans. If a management plan has been agreed on, discuss timescales and ensure a buy-in from the consultant (i.e. inform the consultant – *communication with colleagues*).

Describing a Fetal Abnormality

It is not unusual for a clinician to be called upon to explain an ultrasound scan finding to a couple/woman. Often these are simple abnormalities that do not have a significant impact on the outcome of the pregnancy – i.e. these are not abnormalities that may lead to a termination of pregnancy or may have a significant long-term effect on the baby. Occasionally, these abnormalities are either lethal or have a major bearing on the decision the couple/woman has to make about continuing or terminating the pregnancy. Ensuring that there is a clear understanding of not only the abnormality but the implications is crucial. Under such circumstances, it is useful to remember that referral to an expert is always expected, although this should not stop you from explaining to the woman/the couple. In preparing to counsel women/couples with fetal abnormalities, you should think about the possible questions you may be asked. In the examples below, some of such questions are discussed.

1. Anencephaly

What is the problem with my baby, or what is wrong with my baby? Your baby has a major abnormality in the head. This abnormality is known as anencephaly and is characterised by the absence of most of the baby's head. Essentially, the upper part of the baby's skull and brain has not developed (that is, a major part of the brain, skull and scalp). The baby will, therefore, be born without the front part of the brain (forebrain) and the thinking and coordinating part of the brain (cerebrum). This abnormality is not compatible with life. In fact, babies with anencephaly are stillborn (i.e. born dead) in about 75% of cases. Those born alive only survive for a few hours, days or weeks before they die. The remaining parts of the brain are often not covered by bone or skin.

Why does my baby have anencephaly (what causes anencephaly)? In most cases, the cause is unknown. There are, however, some cases in which the baby has anencephaly because of a change in their genes or chromosomes or the mother has been exposed to certain factors in the environment such as what she eats or drinks or takes (especially some medications) in the early weeks of pregnancy. We may not be able to give you an answer until all the tests have been carried out, and even then, we may never know.

What tests are you talking about? As some of the cases of anencephaly may be associated with abnormal chromosomes, we would like to offer you a test to check the baby's chromosomes. This test is called an amniocentesis (explained much later in this chapter). If you do not want to have this test now, we can still collect some tissue from the baby after it has been born to check its chromosomes. Unfortunately, the tissue may sometimes fail to allow the chromosomes to be determined.

Is there any treatment for it? There is no known cure or standard treatment for anencephaly. Almost all babies born with anencephaly will die shortly after birth.

Does it run in families? Most cases of anencephaly are sporadic, which means they occur in people with no history of the disorder in their family. A small percentage of cases have been reported to run in families; however, the condition does not have a clear pattern of inheritance.

Is it likely to occur again? Following the delivery of a baby with anencephaly, it is often estimated that there is a 1 in 25 chance of this happening again in another pregnancy. This recurrence rate is essentially that for a neural tube defect (NTD), so the baby may have a spina bifida instead of anencephaly.

Can this be prevented? There is no way to prevent this 100%; however, eating food that is rich in folic acid (getting enough folic acid before and during early pregnancy can help prevent neural tube defects, such as anencephaly). The standard recommendation is to take folic acid at least one month before you start to try for pregnancy and continuing with this for the first three months of pregnancy. This has been shown to reduce the risk of the baby developing a neural tube defect, of which anencephaly is a part. As you have had a baby with anencephaly, the recommended dose of folic acid is 5 mg daily (this is slightly more than 10 times the recommended dose for someone who has not had a baby with such an abnormality).

What are the options for managing this pregnancy? You can elect to continue with the pregnancy or go for termination of pregnancy. If you decide to continue with the pregnancy, you will be followed up regularly, as there is a risk of you having excessive water around the baby (we call this polyhydramnios). Furthermore, you may go past your due dates, in which case we may have to start your labour with a risk of caesarean section, as the baby may not be lying the right way. If you wish to have a termination of pregnancy, this will be performed in a sensitive way as we will do for other terminations.

2. Holoprosencephaly

What is the problem with my baby, or what is wrong with my baby? Your baby has a major abnormality involving the development of the brain. This abnormality is called holoprosencephaly. Normally, the **brain** divides into two halves (hemispheres) during early development. **Holoprosencephaly** occurs when the **brain** fails to divide properly into the right and left hemispheres. Where the abnormality is so severe, the babies tend to die before birth, but in the less severe cases, the babies are born with normal or near-normal brain development and facial deformities that may affect the eyes, nose and upper lip. There are three types of this abnormality, depending on how severe the abnormality is. These types are (a) alobar, where the brain has not divided at all, and it is the one that typically is associated with facial features; (b) semi-lobar, where the division of the brain into hemispheres (or lobes) is incomplete; and (c) lobar, in which there is a separation of the hemispheres. In some cases of lobar holoprosencephaly, the baby's brain is nearly normal.

What causes holoprosencephaly? Is it hereditary? Although this condition is well known to be associated with chromosome abnormalities, it is not always possible to find a cause. This condition can be inherited, but this is not always the case. Inherited causes include certain types of chromosome abnormalities (especially extra chromosome 13 in a condition known as Patau syndrome) and changes in single genes called mutations that cause a combination of problems in the same person known as syndromic disorders. Some cases are sporadic (that is they occur out of the blue). It would be useful for you to undertake some tests to help us answer the questions you are asking. I should say here that it is not always possible to find a reason or associated problems. In that case, it will be considered sporadic (that is happening out of the blue).

If it is inherited, how does this happen (in other words, how is it inherited)? The risk for a family member to have holoprosencephaly depends on the specific cause of this condition in the family, if known. For example, non-syndromic holoprosencephaly is usually inherited in an autosomal dominant manner. This means that having a variation (mutation) in only one copy of the responsible gene in each cell is enough to cause the condition.

How likely is it to occur again in a future pregnancy? You are much more likely to have a normal, healthy baby in your next pregnancy than to have another baby affected with holoprosencephaly. There is, however, a small risk of this happening again, and this will depend on the reason why your baby had the condition. A genetic specialist will provide more information about the recurrence risk in future pregnancies.

Is there a treatment for holoprosencephaly? Each child has a unique degree of malformations. Treatment must be individualised, although common problems occur. In general, treatment is largely symptomatic and supportive. Involvement in support groups is helpful as it may give you help on what to expect and how to cope. There is no cure for this abnormality, and therefore the treatment is focused on dealing with the symptoms and giving support. Where there are associated abnormalities, especially those of the face, these can be corrected. These abnormalities include cyclopia (single eye), median cleft lip (harelip) and palate and missing front teeth. Those affected may also suffer from seizures and have a small head and multiple hormone deficiencies, feeding difficulties and developmental delays. These can be managed by appropriate experts with much support.

What is the life expectancy of someone with holoprosencephaly? This depends on the type of abnormality. Those with the most severe forms are often born dead or die shortly after birth. For those with less severe forms, for example, more than 50% of those with semi-lobar or lobar holoprosencephaly without significant malformations of other organs will be alive till the age of 12 months. The life expectancy for individuals with semi-lobar holoprosencephaly depends on the underlying cause of the condition and the presence of associated anomalies.

Can its occurrence be prevented? There is no way to prevent its recurrence. If it is inherited, then there is the possibility of screening the embryos before putting them in the womb using a technique called pre-implantation genetic diagnosis. For this to happen, the exact gene or chromosome responsible for this must be known.

3.   Ventriculomegaly

What is the problem with my baby, or what is wrong with my baby? Your baby has an abnormality called ventriculomegaly, which simply means there is more than usual fluid in the baby's brain. Normally the brain and the spinal cord are surrounded (bathed) by a fluid called cerebrospinal fluid (CSF). This fluid, which is clear, is also found throughout the ventricles (or brain cavities and tunnels). The fluid cushions the brain and spinal cord from jolts and rapid movements, thereby protecting the brain and the spinal cord. This fluid is produced in certain structures in the brain and flows through the brain and the cord freely. Ventriculomegaly occurs when the fluid-filled structures (lateral ventricles) in the brain are too large. This is diagnosed when the sizes of the ventricles measured on the ultrasound scan are more than 10 mm. Sometimes the ultrasound will only show one of the ventricles, even though there are two (one on the right and one on the left side). Ventriculomegaly seems to occur more often in male fetuses than in female fetuses. The mild to moderate types (where the size of the ventricle is 10-15mm) occur in approximately 1% of pregnancies.

What causes ventriculomegaly? There are many causes of ventriculomegaly, but, in a large number of cases, the cause is unknown. Amongst the known causes are structural brain abnormalities, especially those that cause an obstruction to the circulation of the fluid or conditions that lead to overproduction of the fluid. The most common causes include structural brain and spine abnormalities and infection and chromosomal abnormalities, which are present in about 10% of fetuses with isolated ventriculomegaly.

How will you know the cause of this condition in my baby? You will be offered a test to check the baby's chromosomes. This test is called an amniocentesis (explained below with risks). You will also be offered a blood test to check for certain infections that may cause ventriculomegaly. It is important to remember that in most cases the investigations fail to find a cause.

What is the outcome for the baby? The outcome depends on several factors including (a) the actual size of the ventricles, (b) whether or not there are any other abnormal findings on the ultrasound (in the brain or elsewhere that may affect the outlook for the baby) and (c) whether the baby's chromosomes are normal or not. In general, the outcome is worse when the ventricles are larger, the chromosomes are abnormal or there are other problems seen on the ultrasound. The best outcome is typically observed when the ventriculomegaly is mild (measures between 10 and 15 mm in size) and isolated. In this case, there are no other problems seen on ultrasound and the baby's chromosomes are normal. The exact outcome for your child's health is difficult to know. The most common effect in the child is a developmental delay. This seems to be related to the size of the ventricles. Doing a fetal MRI may help experts predict the degree of disability and may provide families with more information on what to expect for their child's health and development. This information will help parents make decisions during pregnancy and prepare in advance for challenges their child and the family may face.

What are my options now? In the first instance, there is a need to have the baby scanned by an expert in fetal medicine. They will look for any other abnormalities that may have been missed. Once this is done, it would be advisable for you to have a test to check the baby's chromosomes, as this may influence what you may want to do. If you do not want to have the test or if the test is normal, you will be asked to see a neurosurgeon (someone who will most likely deal with your baby's problem after birth) for discussions on what will happen after birth.

Is there any treatment during this pregnancy? There is no treatment before the baby is born. After-birth treatment involves managing the child's symptoms. It is important that during pregnancy a more detailed ultrasound scan is done by a fetal medicine expert and an amniocentesis (to check the baby's chromosomes discussed and performed if acceptable). During a follow-up, an MRI of the baby's brain will help to determine if there are any additional problems and how severe this enlargement is. If the chromosomes are abnormal or the ventriculomegaly is judged to be severe enough to affect the quality of the baby's life, termination of pregnancy can be considered.

What is likely to happen if I decide to continue with the pregnancy? In some cases, the baby will develop hydrocephalus (a condition in which the baby's head grows bigger). This is usually in cases where the fluid is not draining well. Hydrocephalus is the build-up of cerebrospinal fluid, which causes pressure on the brain. In such a situation, after delivery, the fluid is shunted into the baby's tummy (called the peritoneum) in a procedure called a ventriculoperitoneal shunt (VP shunt). This surgery is not done immediately after birth, but the baby will be monitored and, in most cases, we will know by 6 months.

What are the chances of this happening again in the next pregnancy? This will depend on the cause of the ventriculomegaly. Where it is sporadic (i.e. it occurs out of the blue), the recurrence risk is low. If there is a genetic abnormality, then the recurrence risk will depend on the recurrence risk of the genetic/chromosome abnormality. If there is a genetic/chromosomal cause, you will be referred to the clinical geneticist for further information on recurrence.

4. Congenital diaphragmatic hernia (CDH)

What is the problem with my baby, or what is wrong with my baby? Your baby has an abnormality called congenital diaphragmatic hernia. This is an abnormality that occurs when there is a gap (defect) in the muscles that make up the sheet that separates the chest from the abdomen (known as the diaphragm). As a consequence, some of the structures that are normally in the abdomen, such as the stomach, the intestines and sometimes the liver, push through this gap into the chest. Because of these additional structures in the chest, the baby's heart is pushed to one side and the lungs may not develop as well. Most of the hernias are on the left, but they may also occur on the right.

What causes a diaphragmatic hernia? The cause is unknown in more than 80% of cases (isolated CDH). In less than 20% of cases, the cause is a problem with the baby's chromosomes or a genetic disorder. Here the baby may have additional medical problems or organ abnormalities. In an isolated CDH, the primary concern is how much this affects the development of the lungs (the degree of smallness of the lungs or pulmonary hypoplasia) caused by the defect. In order to determine if CDH is isolated and to provide the correct information about the disease, genetic testing is required. In the other cases that are caused by a problem with the baby's chromosomes or a genetic disorder, in addition to the problems with the lungs, those specific to the genetic/chromosome abnormality will have implications for the outlook for the baby.

What tests will be performed to help find the reason for this abnormality? The only test that can be performed is called an amniocentesis. It allows for the chromosomes of the baby to be determined. In most cases, the chromosomes will come back as normal. This is important as it means everything can be done to help the baby when it is born.

How will the baby be managed? There are certain centres in the world where treatment in the womb is possible. This procedure is known as Fetoscopic Tracheal Occlusion (FETO). The basis of this treatment is that the baby's lungs produce fluid that leaves the body through the baby's mouth. If this outflow of fluid is blocked, it has nowhere else to go and as such swells up in the affected lung. When this occurs over a period of 4–5 weeks, the lung expands and its function appears to improve. This type of blockage can be achieved by temporarily blocking the fetal windpipe (trachea) with a balloon for a period of time. This is done through keyhole surgery (typically around 30 weeks) when a tube with a balloon is put down the windpipe of the baby and the balloon is blown up. The balloon is then deflated and removed with the tube at about 34 weeks. It is believed that FETO works by increasing the lung maturation and reversing some of the damaging effects of CDH on lung function. As this is not available in all centres in the UK, you may be referred to the centre in London (Kings College) which does this. If this procedure is not available, your baby will be monitored and delivered as planned, but at the time of delivery, every attempt will be made to stop the baby from breathing on its own as this will allow air to be swallowed into the stomach and stop the lungs from expanding. Surgery can then be planned to close the defect.

Will it recur in the next pregnancy? If the congenital diaphragmatic hernia is isolated, then the recurrence risk is low. If it occurs as a feature of a genetic syndrome or chromosomal abnormality, then the recurrence risk will depend on the chromosomal abnormality or the syndrome, and in this case, you will be referred to the clinical geneticist for appropriate counselling and information about recurrence.

How will I be delivered? This abnormality is not an indication for caesarean section. You will be offered a caesarean section if it is indicated for obstetric reasons. However, it is important that you deliver in a unit where there are experts in managing the baby at the time of delivery. It may be better to plan the delivery so that the baby is born during working hours rather than at night. Some units prefer this and therefore offer the women an elective caesarean section.

5.   **Gastroschisis**

What is the problem with my baby, or what is wrong with my baby? Your baby has an opening (or defect) on its belly (abdominal wall) through which its intestines have come out and all lying in the water that surrounds the baby (amniotic fluid). This abnormality typically occurs to the side of the spot where the umbilical cord enters the baby (belly button of the baby), and the defect is not covered so the intestines are exposed to the amniotic fluid. How much of the intestines that come out depends on the size of the defect. It is more commonly seen in younger mothers, particularly those who are less than 20 years old. The outcome for the babies with this abnormality is very good, and the overall survival for live-born infants with gastroschisis is over 90%, if it is the only problem the baby has.

Why did my baby have this condition? The exact cause of gastroschisis is not known. What is known is that it is more common in younger mothers and also those who smoke. There is also an association with the use of recreational drugs.

Are they any tests that I should have now? Unless your baby has other abnormalities in general, no additional tests are undertaken on mothers like you. This is mainly because isolated cases are sporadic (that is, there is no obvious reason for them).

What will happen to me from now onwards? First, the baby will be scanned again by an expert (fetal medicine consultant), and if this is the only problem, then the baby will be monitored regularly with ultrasound scans usually every 2–4 weeks to check the growth of the baby, as some of the babies with this condition may not grow as well as those without this malformation. You will also be referred to see the paediatric (children's) surgeon, who will discuss the management of the baby after delivery.

How will I be delivered? This condition is not an indication for having a caesarean section. If the baby is growing well and you do not have any complication(s), there is no reason why you cannot deliver on your own. A significant number of women whose babies have this condition will go into labour before their due date, and some may deliver early (before 37 weeks). It is ideal for you to have the baby in a unit where there are surgeons to manage the baby's condition; otherwise, the baby will be transferred to such a unit after delivery.

Will it happen again in my next pregnancy? Almost all isolated cases are incidental, meaning the risk of recurrence is low. If there are associated abnormalities, then the recurrence risk will depend on these abnormalities.

Is this an inherited condition? Gastroschisis is not inherited, especially if it is not associated with any other problem. If, however, there are associated abnormalities, it would be necessary to check the baby's chromosomes. If these are abnormal, then the recurrence risk will depend on the chromosomal abnormality.

What will happen to my baby at delivery? The baby's lower body will be placed in a special, clear plastic bag to make sure that fluid loss through evaporation is kept to a minimum. This also helps keep the exposed intestines moist. The intestines will be supported by sterile gauze to keep them from becoming kinked. The exposed bowel will be covered with sterile gauze specially coated in petroleum jelly, similar to Vaseline. In order to stop the baby from swallowing air, which will cause the bowel to distend, a tube may be placed through the baby's nostrils and down the oesophagus to the stomach and connected to suction. Surgery on your baby will then be carried out to replace the intestines and close the defect. Occasionally this will not happen at one go, especially in those cases where significant amounts of intestines are outside.

6. **Exomphalos/Omphalocele**

What is the problem with my baby, or what is wrong with my baby? Your baby has an abnormality called exomphalos or omphalocele. This is due to a weakness on the baby's abdominal wall at the point where the umbilical cord gets into the baby. Because of this weakness, the structures inside the abdomen, especially the intestines and the liver, may protrude outside through this point into a loose sac with the cord attached (inserting) to the top of this sac.

What causes exomphalos? The cause of this condition is unknown. It is rare and occurs in about 2–4 in every 10,000 births. Up to 80% (8 in 10) of babies with exomphalos will have other serious problems such as abnormalities in the heart and kidneys and chromosomal problems. We will recommend some tests to help but always remember that these may not show any reason for the cause.

What tests will be offered? First, you will need to have a more detailed scan performed, especially by experts such as fetal medicine consultants, so as to identify some of these abnormalities. Because of an increased risk of chromosomal abnormalities (up to 30% of these babies will have a chromosome abnormality), you will be offered a test known as an amniocentesis (taking a small amount of fluid around the baby) to help determine if the baby's chromosomes are normal or not.

What will happen at the time of delivery? There is no reason for you not to deliver normally; although if the sac containing the structures is fairly large, it may break at the time of delivery, and in this case, a caesarean section may be preferred. Your baby will be transferred to the newborn baby (neonatal) unit soon after delivery. After your baby is born, the sac will be wrapped in a protective film to reduce heat and fluid loss. A drip will be inserted into a small vein so that intravenous fluids can be given. A tube will be passed through your baby's nose into the stomach to drain away green fluid (bile) that collects in the stomach. This lessens the risk of your baby vomiting and reduces discomfort. Your baby will be examined in order to identify any problems with other body systems and may need further tests. If there are associated lung problems, assistance may be required with breathing.

Is this an inherited condition? Exomphalos may be inherited, especially if it is not associated with chromosome problems. If the chromosomes are normal but there are associated abnormalities, the baby may have a syndrome (a combination of problems). If abnormalities (chromosome or syndrome) are present, then the recurrence risk will depend on these. You will be asked to see a clinical geneticist who will provide more information on recurrence in the next pregnancy.

7. **Congenital pulmonary (cystic) airway malformation (CPAM) formerly congenital cystic adenomatoid malformation (CCAM) of the lung**

What is the problem with my baby, or what is wrong with my baby? Your baby has an abnormality known as congenital pulmonary airway malformation (CPAM). Everyone has five parts to their lungs. These are known as lobes, with two on the left and three on the right. Occasionally a problem occurs during development, resulting in one of the lobes containing fluid space(s) (cysts) rather than lung tissue. These cysts are usually confined to one lobe but may occasionally affect more than one lobe. The cysts can be detected on ultrasound before birth and have various appearances ranging from a small number of large cysts to a large number of small cysts. When this happens, the baby is said to have CPAM, which is what your baby has.

Why causes this condition? We do not know why this happens, but we know that it is very rare. It occurs in about 1 in 10,000 babies. You can be assured that there is no evidence to suggest that it is caused by anything you have done or have not done during the pregnancy.

What tests will be offered? Because we do not know the cause of this abnormality, there are no specific tests to find the reason why it happens. You will, however, be sent to an expert in fetal medicine who will do a thorough ultrasound scan and thereafter offer you follow-up regular scans.

Will it affect my baby before delivery? In some babies, the cysts can enlarge quite rapidly during pregnancy resulting in major problems for the baby before birth. Occasionally babies with this condition do not survive the pregnancy. More often, however, the cysts do not grow rapidly and may not grow at all. In fact, in some cases, the cysts may actually disappear completely before birth, and the baby will be born with no problems whatsoever. For this reason, it is important that you have regular ultrasound scans throughout the pregnancy.

Will it affect how and when I deliver? This condition is not an indication for a caesarean section. If there are no other complications in your pregnancy, you should be allowed to labour and deliver in the same way as any other woman whose baby does not have this condition.

What will happen to the baby after the delivery? *This will depend on whether your baby has breathing difficulties or not.*

- *Your baby has no breathing difficulty:* Most babies with this condition will have no breathing difficulties after delivery. For these babies, a chest X-ray will be performed on the first day or two to determine whether any treatment is necessary.
- *Your baby does have breathing difficulty after delivery:* In some babies, the cysts press on the rest of the lung, causing difficulty in breathing for the baby. In this case, he/she will be admitted to the newborn baby (Neonatal) unit for observation and management, which may include helping the baby with breathing and sometimes surgery.

8. Talipes equinovarus

What is the problem with my baby, or what is wrong with my baby? Your baby has an abnormality in its foot/feet known as Talipes or clubfoot. This is an abnormality in which your baby is born with his/her foot/feet pointing downwards and inwards. It is twice as common in males as in females (2:1). It may affect one or both feet (50% are bilateral; that is, it affects both feet). This may be isolated (that is, it's the only problem the baby has), or it may be associated with other problems, which may be genetic/chromosomal or abnormalities of some other parts of the body.

What causes clubfoot? In most cases, the cause is unknown (idiopathic). There is, however, a familial tendency noted (some members of the family have a gene that causes it, and this has been passed onto the baby). It may also occur in combination with other abnormalities, and in these cases, the baby will have a specific syndrome. Some of the associated disorders or syndromes include poorly developed hip joint(s) (developmental hip dysplasia), spina bifida, joint problems (arthrogryposis) or muscle weakness (myotonic dystrophy).

What tests will be offered? In a small number of cases, the baby may have a chromosome abnormality. You will, therefore, be offered a test to check the baby's chromosomes. This test is known as an amniocentesis (details below).

Will it happen in the next pregnancy? Your chance of having another baby with clubfoot is about 1 in 25 (about 4%). If you do not have a family member with a clubfoot, and none of your other children have clubfoot, then the chance of having a child with clubfoot (random occurrence), is 1 in 1,000. However, as you already have a child with clubfoot, their future children have a 3% (3 in 100) chance of having the same abnormality. If you had clubfoot yourself, then you have a 20–30% chance of having a child with clubfoot.

What happens from now onwards? You will be referred to a fetal medicine consultant, who will scan the baby again to make sure that there are no other abnormalities that have been missed. You will be advised to have a test to check the baby's chromosomes and then asked to see an orthopaedic surgeon, who will explain what will happen to the baby when it's born. Some of the babies may need surgery, while others will not. If the baby's chromosomes are abnormal, you will have further discussion on options, including the termination of pregnancy.

How will my baby be delivered? Clubfoot is not an indication for a caesarean section. Your pregnancy will be managed as before, and you should deliver normally, unless there is an obstetric reason.

9. Cleft palate and lip

What is the problem with my baby, or what is wrong with my baby? Your baby has an abnormality known as cleft lip. This is a birth defect in which the baby's upper lip is not formed completely and has a gap in it. This may be on one side of the face or may involve both sides. A cleft lip may occur on its own or may be associated with a cleft palate, which is the presence of a gap in the roof of the mouth. It can also be left, right or bilateral. Approximately 1 in 700 children are affected.

What causes facial clefts? The exact cause is not known; however, it is associated with certain risk factors which include taking certain medicines during pregnancy, smoking during pregnancy, certain infections during pregnancy, changes in genes (genetic mutations) during pregnancy, mutated genes (genes that changes in parents) that are passed from parents to the child and not getting enough folic acid before pregnancy.

What will happen from now onwards? You will be referred to a fetal medicine consultant for a further ultrasound scan to make sure that any other subtle abnormality has not been missed. You will then be offered an opportunity to have your baby's chromosomes checked by a test called amniocentesis. If these are normal or you do not wish to have the test, you will be referred to a plastic surgeon who will explain what will happen after the baby is born. At some stage, you will be shown pictures of babies that had this problem before and after surgical correction.

You will also need to see a neonatologist to explain how the baby will be looked after when it is born, especially with respect to feeding.

Will it affect how I deliver? All being well, you should aim for a normal vaginal delivery unless there are other obstetric complications and indications. A facial cleft is not an indication of a caesarean section.

What are the chances of it happening again? The recurrence risk child depends on the severity of the cleft and the presence or absence of family history. The recurrence risk for a cleft lip on one side (unilateral) is about 2–3%, and if it is lip and palate, this risk rises to about 4%. If the cleft and palate are on both sides, the risk of recurrence is 5–6%. If one parent is affected, the risk is about 4%; however, if both parents are affected or two siblings are affected, the recurrence risk is 10%.

Can I do anything to reduce this recurrence risk? In your next pregnancy, you will be advised to take folic acid 5 mg (starting 1 month before you start trying for a baby and continuing until 12 weeks or for the first 3 months). Folic acid is a vitamin that can help protect your baby from birth defects of the brain and spine called neural tube defects. It may also reduce the risk of oral clefts by about 25%.

10. Spina bifida

What is the problem with my baby, or what is wrong with my baby? Your baby has an abnormality of the spine called spina bifida. This occurs when the baby's spine and spinal cord do not develop properly in the womb, causing a gap in the spine. Spina bifida is a type of neural tube defect. The neural tube is the structure that eventually develops into the baby's brain and spinal cord.

There are four different types of spina bifida. These are myelomeningocele, meningocele, spina bifida occulta and closed spina bifida. (a) Myelomeningocele is the most severe type, and here the baby's spinal canal remains open along several vertebrae in the back (portions of the backbone or spine), allowing the spinal cord and the membrane that surrounds it to push out and form a sac in the baby's back. (b) Meningocele is the second type in which the membranes around the spinal cord (meninges) push out through a defect in the spine, but the spinal cord usually develops normally so that surgery can often be used to remove the membranes without damaging the nerves. (c) Spina bifida occulta – this is the most common and mildest type of spina bifida. Here one or more vertebrae are not formed properly, but the gap in the spine is very small. It does not usually cause any problems, and most people are unaware that they have it. (d) *Closed spina bifida* – this consists of a diverse group of defects, in which the spinal cord is marked by malformations of fat, bone or meninges. In most of those with closed spina bifida, there are few or no symptoms; however, in a few, the malformation causes incomplete paralysis with urinary and bowel dysfunction.

What causes spina bifida? The exact cause of spina bifida is unknown, but a number of factors can increase the risk of a baby developing the condition. These include (a) low folic acid intake during pregnancy, (b) having a family history of spina bifida and (c) medication – taking certain medications during pregnancy has been linked to an increased risk of having a baby with spina bifida.

Will it happen again? The incidence of spina bifida, which is part of abnormalities collectively known as neural tube defects (NTDs), varies with race, geographic location and various other predisposing factors. In the United States, for example, the incidence is approximately 1–2 cases per 1,000 live births, whereas the incidence in the UK is about four (4–8/1,000 live births) times greater. Following the introduction of fortification of grain products in 1996, the incidence of NTDs has decreased by about 25%. The risk of recurrence is 10-fold higher after having a child with NTD without intervention. If the defect in the first affected pregnancy was anencephaly, a risk for the recurrence of anencephaly is higher than for the recurrence of spina bifida.

How will my pregnancy be managed from now on? Your pregnancy will be managed normally, with regular ultrasound scans to monitor the baby, especially the water around the baby and the baby's head. Sometimes the baby's head may become large (a condition called hydrocephalus), and there may be excessive water around the baby (polyhydramnios). Some women, following counselling, may opt for termination of pregnancy. It is important that before this decision is made, you meet with experts who will provide information about the impact of spina bifida on the long-term health of the baby. These experts include a fetal medicine consultant, who will rescan the baby (to make sure that there are no subtle abnormalities that have been missed), a neonatologist (newborn baby doctor), a neurologist (brain surgeon), a geneticist and a developmental paediatrician.

How will this affect how I deliver? If there are no complications and the baby is lying the right way, there is no reason why you cannot deliver normally. However, if there are additional complications, you may have to have a caesarean section. Spina bifida, on its own, is not an indication for a caesarean section.

Can this be prevented next time? Women thought to be at a higher risk of having a child with spina bifida need to be prescribed a higher (5 mg) dose of folic acid by their GP.

Women at a higher risk include those with a family history of neural tube defects, a partner with a family history of neural tube defects, have had a previous pregnancy affected by a neural tube defect, have diabetes and/or are taking medication such as that for epilepsy, which increases the risk of the baby having an NTD. As you fall into one of these high-risk categories, you should take folic acid 5 mg for 1 month before you start trying for a baby, and and continue with it for the first 3 months when you are pregnant.

11. Complex cardiac abnormality

What is the problem with my baby, or what is wrong with my baby? There are many complex cardiac abnormalities, and no specific one will be described here. However, a general approach will be provided.

Your baby has an abnormality in its heart. Before I proceed to explain this to you, I would like to describe what a normal heart looks like. The heart is divided into two sides (left and right), separated by a wall with no gap or hole in it, and on each side, there are two compartments – an upper and lower compartments. The upper compartments are known as atria and receive blood. This is then passed to the lower compartments (known as ventricles), which then pump it out. The blood from the right ventricle goes to the lungs, where oxygen is added and carbon dioxide is removed. This blood comes back through the left atrium into the left ventricle, which then pumps it to the rest of the body, where the oxygen is used.

Valves control the flow of blood into and out of the ventricles. There are two on each side of the heart. These valves make sure that blood moves forward and not backward, especially between contractions. The valve between the right atrium and right ventricle is called the tricuspid valve, while that between the right ventricle and the pulmonary artery (the blood vessel taking blood to the lungs) is called the pulmonary valve. On the left side, the valve between the left atrium and the left ventricle is called the mitral valve, and that at the entrance to the aorta (the blood vessel taking blood to the body) is called the aortic valve.

Every cardiac abnormality should be confirmed by an echo, preferably by a paediatric cardiologist or a fetal medicine consultant, followed by karyotyping to exclude a chromosomal abnormality.

Abnormalities that are not compatible with life, such as a hypoplastic right heart, should be managed jointly with clinical geneticists, paediatrician, paediatric cardiologist and counsellors.

What tests will be offered? The cause is unknown in most cases. In a small number of cases, these are associated with a chromosome problem. It is for this reason that you will be advised about having an amniocentesis (a test to check the baby's chromosomes).

Will it happen again? The population risk for congenital heart disease is about 1%. The risk of recurrence is greater in your next pregnancy as you have an affected child, and this risk will even be higher if you have more than one child with a congenital heart abnormality. For parents with one affected child, the recurrence risk is between 2% and 5%. For parents with two affected children, the recurrence risk is 10–15%.

How will my pregnancy be managed from now on? Your pregnancy will continue as normal, but the baby will be monitored with regular ultrasound scans, looking out for complications that may arise as a result of the cardiac abnormality. These include the growth of the baby.

How will this affect how I deliver? Labour and delivery will not be affected if your baby is diagnosed with congenital heart disease. Most babies will tolerate labour and delivery without any problems. There is no need to do a caesarean section for a baby with congenital heart disease.

12. Hydrops

What is the problem with my baby, or what is wrong with my baby? Your baby has an abnormality called hydrops fetalis. This is a condition in which there is an abnormal accumulation of fluid in two or more fetal compartments (parts of the body) such as ascites (fluid in the abdomen or tummy), pleural effusion (fluid around the lungs), pericardial effusion (fluid around the heart) and skin oedema (fluid under the skin). In some patients, it may also be associated with polyhydramnios (excessive fluid around the baby) and placental oedema (a swollen placenta)

What causes hydrops fetalis? There are two main types of hydrops – immune and non-immune. The immune causes are commonly because of incompatibility between elements in the mother and baby's blood. In this case, the mother reacts to the baby's blood by producing antibodies which pass back to the baby through the placenta and destroy the baby's blood, causing anaemia and heart failure. The most common type of this is known as Rhesus isoimmunisation, where the mother is Rhesus negative and the baby is Rhesus positive. Among the non-immune causes are infections (commonly viral infections), chromosomal abnormalities, structural abnormalities (like severe heart problems) and syndromes (the combination of problems together). In a significant number of cases, the cause is unknown.

Will it happen again? Whether hydrops fetalis happens again or not depends on the cause. If the cause is immune, then there is a high chance that it will happen again, depending on the baby's blood group. If it is non-immune, then the recurrence risk will depend on the cause. If this is genetic, then this will be determined by the recurrence risk of the genetic condition, and for this you will be referred to the geneticist for details about recurrence.

How will my pregnancy be managed from now on? A series of investigations will have to be performed to see whether the cause of the hydrops can be identified. These will include a more detailed scan by a fetal medicine expert, taking blood from you to check for infections and also looking for antibodies that may be crossing back into the baby and destroying its blood cells (in most cases, this would have been suspected as it is standard practice to check your blood group when you book for antenatal care). Additionally, a test will be performed to determine the baby's chromosomes. This test is called an amniocentesis (taking a small amount of fluid around the baby).

Following the investigations, you will have a discussion with the consultant about the options available, and this will be influenced to a large extent by the results and the cause identified. If the hydrops is very severe and the outcome for the baby is very poor, then termination will be one option. If the cause is infection, it may be possible to transfuse the baby to correct the anaemia. Where the cause is a chromosomal abnormality or a severe structural abnormality, termination of pregnancy will be an option to consider.

How will this affect how I deliver? This will depend on the chances of the baby surviving after it is born. If the lungs are very small and the baby, therefore, has a very small chance of surviving when it is born, you will be encouraged to have a vaginal delivery. In this case, it may be inadvisable to monitor the baby during labour as an abnormal heart rate will necessitate an emergency caesarean section, which would be inappropriate. Hydrops fetalis is not an indication for a caesarean section, and, therefore, you may be allowed to go into labour if you wish. However, most experts will opt to deliver the baby early and not allow you to go past 37–38 weeks.

Can this be prevented in the next pregnancy? As most causes are incidental or unknown, it would be difficult to prevent them. However, if it is immune, it is known that if the next pregnancy is affected, this will happen earlier, and hence the baby will be monitored closely much earlier. Furthermore, you will undergo a blood test to check the baby's blood group to see whether it is incompatible with yours. This will be done early around 10 weeks by a simple blood test (non-invasive prenatal diagnosis or NIPD). In very rare cases, when it is recurrent, pre-implantation genetic diagnosis can be done and an embryo that is not be affected is replaced (IVF followed by testing of the embryo/baby in the laboratory and identifying unaffected ones and putting them back into the womb).

13. Duodenal atresia

What is the problem with my baby, or what is wrong with my baby? Your baby has an abnormality known as duodenal atresia. This is an abnormality in which there is blockage at the beginning of the first part of the small intestines (called the duodenum). This is the part of the small intestines that connects to the stomach. Because of this blockage, your baby is unable to swallow water, and, as a result, the amount of water around the baby is increased (what we call polyhydramnios). This condition is rare and occurs in around 1 in 10,000 births.

What causes duodenal atresia? There is no known cause, but it can be associated with other abnormalities. Approximately, one-third of babies with duodenal atresia will have a chromosomal abnormality known as Down syndrome (mongolism).

What will happen to me and the baby? You will be asked to have another ultrasound scan by a fetal medicine consultant to make sure that there are no other abnormalities associated with this condition. You will then be offered a test to check the baby's chromosomes. At this stage, the test will be an amniocentesis. What happens next will depend on the result of the chromosome test. If this is normal, you will be asked to see a paediatric surgeon, as well as the neonatologist, to discuss the management of the baby after birth. If it is abnormal, you will have the option to terminate or continue with the pregnancy.

What happens at the delivery? It should be possible for you to deliver your baby in the normal way unless there are other reasons for requiring a caesarean section. We would recommend, however, that you deliver in a unit where there is an expert to manage the baby after delivery. Because of the block, you will not be able to feed your baby after delivery, as it will vomit, and this may cause severe problems in the lungs, including infections. Consequently, the baby will have a drip through which fluids containing nutrients will be given until the baby has had corrective surgery and is able to feed.

Will this occur in my next pregnancy? This is unlikely to recur (i.e. the risk of you having another baby with duodenal atresia is not significantly higher than that of a woman who has not had a baby with duodenal atresia), if it is isolated. If there is an associated abnormality (structural or chromo-somal), this may influence the recurrence risk, and liaising with a geneticist will enable counselling about the exact recurrence risk of the genetic/chromosomal abnormality.

14. Abnormal NT

The fluid behind your baby's neck is more than average for this stage of pregnancy. This means that the risk of your baby having chromosome abnormalities is higher than normal. Not every baby with an increased fluid behind the neck has abnormal chromosomes. A significant number have normal chromosomes. Where the chromosomes are normal, the baby will be at an increased risk of structural abnormalities, especially those of the heart.

You will be offered a test to determine your baby's chromosomes. At this stage, the test that will give you a definitive answer is called a chorionic villus sampling (CVS). If the chromosomes are normal, you will be referred for a detailed scan by a fetal medicine consultant, who will also have a thorough examination of the baby's heart.

If the chromosomes are abnormal, you would have the option to undergo termination of pregnancy.

What does this test entail, and are there any risks? The test involves a needle being inserted into your uterus and taking a small sample of what will become the placenta. A local anaesthetic will be given to numb the area before the needle is inserted. The test has some complications, the most common of which are infections, bleeding and miscarriage. A procedure-related miscarriage risk is about 1%. In 1% of cases, the result will be inconclusive and a more definitive test will have to be performed. This inconclusive test is known as mosaicism.

Is there an alternative to this test? At this stage, a non-invasive prenatal test (NIPT) could be performed. This is not a diagnostic test, but it gives a very high detection rate for common chromo-some abnormalities that are seen at birth. It is a simple blood test. It will not, however, exclude all chromosome abnormalities, and a further invasive test may have to be performed.

Another alternative to a chorionic villus sampling is amniocentesis, a test also in which a needle is passed through your tummy into the sac housing the baby and a small sample (less than 2 oz.) of fluid that surrounds the baby is taken and sent to the lab. This test is performed at a more advanced stage of pregnancy – the earliest time it can be performed is 15 weeks. The test also has risks; the most important of which are infections, bleeding and miscarriage. The procedure-related miscarriage rate is 1%. Although very rare, the test may fail to generate a result.

Chromosomes and Chromosomal Abnormalities

Chromosomes are the things that carry genes. Each of us has 46 of these, and they are in pairs – that is there are 23 pairs (the 23rd pair is made of chromosomes that determine the gender (sex) of the baby and are called sex chromosomes). Each parent gives 23 chromosomes to their child – hence the 23 pairs. These are present in the sperm (from the father) and egg (from the mother). A male child's chromosomes are written as 46XY, while those of a female child are written as 46XX. This simply means that they have 46 chromosomes with two normal sex chromosomes.

Abnormalities in chromosomes are common and typically occur at the time eggs, and sperms are formed. A typical way in which these occur is through a process called translocation. Translocation Down syndrome, for example, is the only type of Down syndrome that can be passed down from a parent who does not have the features of Down syndrome. If a parent has a balanced translocation, there is up to 15% chance of having another child with Down syndrome. A balanced or chromosomal translocation is a condition in which part of a chromosome has broken off and reattached in another location. This is usually the case for reciprocal (or balanced) translocation, a type of chromosomal translocation that increases the risk of recurrent miscarriages. The other type of translocation is Robertsonian translocation.

The resulting baby will have an abnormal chromosome. Most of the chromosomal abnormalities end in very early miscarriages, but some are compatible with the continuation of pregnancy or life. A significant number of these will have associated unique structural abnormalities that an ultrasound scan will identify or produce abnormal hormones that routine tests in pregnancy will pick up and a definitive test will lead to a diagnosis. Some of these are described below.

a. **Down syndrome (Trisomy 21):** This is a condition in which there is an extra chromosome 21. The chromosomes are written as 47XX + 21 (if it's a girl) or 47XY + 21 (if it's a boy). Another name for this is mongolism. Baby's with this condition may have various abnormalities that ultrasound scan may identify. However, in a large proportion of these babies, it may not be possible to identify abnormalities during pregnancy. Those with this condition have learning difficulties, which could be very severe in some cases.

b. **Edward syndrome (Trisomy 18):** This is a condition in which there is an extra chromosome 18. The baby's chromosomes will be written as 47XY + 18 or 47XX + 18, depending on whether it's a boy or a girl. These babies have a number of abnormalities, especially of the heart, that an ultrasound scan may pick up. Most babies with Edward syndrome will die before or shortly after birth. Some with the less severe form, for example, those with a mixture of normal and abnormal chromosomes (called a mosaic or partial trisomy 18), do survive beyond a year and, very rarely, into early adulthood. They are, however, likely to have severe physical and learning disabilities.

c. **Patau syndrome (Trisomy 13):** This is a condition in which there is an extra chromosome 13. The baby's chromosomes will be written as 47XY + 13 (if male) or 47XX + 13 (if female). Babies with this condition are likely to have various structural abnormalities that ultrasound may pick up during pregnancy. These include problems especially in the face (such as cleft lip also known as harelip and cleft palate, small eyes and small distance between the eyes) and the head (small head size or poor development of the brain). The life expectancy of Patau syndrome for those born alive ranges on average from 7 to 10 days, and 90% will die in the first year of life. Survival is often attributed to mosaicism (where there is a combination of normal and abnormal chromosomes) and the severity of associated malformations.

d. **Turner syndrome:** In this condition, instead of the baby having a pair of sex chromosomes, one of these is missing and the baby therefore only has one. The one that is usually present is the X or female chromosome. This means that all babies with Turner syndrome are female (girls). The chromosomes are written as 45XO. They may have various abnormalities in the womb, and these may include a swelling around the next (called a cystic hygroma) and heart problems (especially narrowing of the aorta – the big blood vessel that takes blood from the heart to the rest of the body). About 30% of children with Turner syndrome have extra folds of skin on the neck (webbed neck), a low hairline at the back of the neck, puffiness or swelling (lymphoedema) of the hands and feet, skeletal abnormalities or kidney problems. Turner syndrome is not a cause of mental retardation. They are more likely to be employed than other adult women. Life expectancy is slightly shorter than average but may be improved by paying attention to associated chronic illnesses, such as obesity and hypertension. The most common feature of Turner syndrome is short stature, which becomes evident by the age of 5. Females with Turner syndrome are infertile as they do not produce eggs but are able to carry pregnancies with donor eggs if their wombs are stimulated to grow with hormones.

e. **Klinefelter syndrome (KS):** This is a condition in which there is an extra X chromosome in a male fetus. The chromosomes are written as 47,XXY or XXY. The babies tend not have any abnormalities that are identified during pregnancy. In fact, most often the diagnosis is made when investigating infertility. The primary features are infertility and poorly functioning testicles. Often, symptoms may be subtle, and many people do not realise they are affected. They typically have the following features: (a) taller than average stature; (b) longer legs, shorter torso and broader hips compared with other boys; (c) absent, delayed or incomplete puberty; (d) after puberty, less muscle and less facial and body hair compared with other teens; (e) small, firm testicles and small penis; and (f) enlarged breast tissue (gynaecomastia). The life expectancy is usually normal, and many people with KS have a normal life. These conditions, which are often called 'variants of Klinefelter' syndrome, usually have more serious problems (intellectual disability, skeletal problems and poor coordination) than classic Klinefelter syndrome (47,XXY). The vast majority of men with Klinefelter syndrome are infertile and can't father a child the usual way (between 95% and 99% of XXY men are infertile because they do not produce enough sperm to fertilise an egg naturally), but sperms are found in more than 50% of men with KS.

How to Counsel about Termination of Pregnancy: An Example

Counselling about Termination of Pregnancy

You have a primigravida who has been diagnosed with an abnormality at 21 weeks of gestation and, following counselling, wishes to have termination of pregnancy.

In offering a patient termination of pregnancy, it is often difficult, if not heart breaking, for the parents to be told that you are offering them termination of pregnancy. While this may be acceptable to most couples, others may find this difficult, and therefore, it would be being sensitive if our counselling is phrased to be less traumatic. Below is an example of how I will approach this with my patients. I am not saying this is the only correct approach, but I find that couples are more accepting of this than just saying the pregnancy will be terminated.

'One of the options you have is to end the pregnancy. Unfortunately, at this stage of the pregnancy, you will have to deliver the baby. We recommend that the baby is given an injection so that he/she is not born alive. It also helps to reduce the pain and suffering by the baby. It is recommended that we do this for all babies that are more than 20 weeks.

Following this you will be given a tablet to take in the hospital. You will then be allowed to go home and come back after 2 days (48 hours) to have some tablets put in your vagina. You may have these put in more than once.

You will then start having pains (contractions), and these will result in you delivering the baby. It is important that the afterbirth (placenta) is also delivered. Very occasionally, this may not come out on its own, in which case, we will have to remove it either surgically or by using the hand.

When you start having pains, there will be various options available to you for pain relief. This will include "gas and air" or Entonox, injections of strong pain killers, or you may instead wish to have an epidural.

Complications include bleeding that may be severe enough to require blood transfusion and surgery to remove especially parts of the placenta and infections'.

Explaining Some Gynaecological Diagnoses

1. **Early pregnancy**

Ectopic pregnancy. You have what we call an ectopic pregnancy. In this situation, the pregnancy unfortunately is not inside your womb but is in the fallopian tube. Because the wall of the tube is much thinner than that of the womb, as the pregnancy grows, the tube will burst, leading to bleeding. The symptoms you have are partly because of the stretching of the tube by the pregnancy and the bleeding into your tummy. Blood in your tummy causes irritation and pain. Sometimes if the blood is large enough it will move up when you are lying down to irritate the diaphragm (the wall between your chest and the tummy), leading to pain at the tip of your shoulder. If the bleeding is severe enough, you may also feel dizzy.

There are three options of treating you, and these include (a) expectant management, (b) medical management and (c) surgical management.

The first option (expectant management) is normally reserved for those in whom this diagnosis is made incidentally; they have no symptoms and the levels of hormones that are produced in pregnancy are falling. Part of this treatment is to have repeated blood tests to make sure that this hormone called human chorionic gonadotrophin (hCG) is falling and that you do not develop symptoms. There is a small chance that this may not succeed, in which case medical treatment or surgery will be the next option.

The second option (medical treatment) involves you having an injection called methotrexate. This injection will stop the pregnancy tissues from growing and, indeed, should cause it to gradually reduce and then disappear. This treatment is given to women with this type of pregnancy, who meet very specific criteria (this includes the size of the pregnancy sac, no active bleeding and the levels of hormones do not exceed an upper limit). Apart from these, you must be prepared to come to the hospital regularly for a blood test in the knowledge that the injection may be repeated. There is also a small risk that this may not work, and you may then require surgery. The chances of success with this type of treatment are about 70–80%. There are several advantages including the fact you will not require surgery (if it's successful), and you do not need to stay in the hospital.

The third option – surgery – is reserved for those who do not wish to have medical treatment (for one reason or the other) or do not meet the criteria for medical treatment (including severe symptoms, bleeding or contraindications for the medicine). Surgery is in most cases keyhole, in which one of three things could happen – (i) the tube may be removed (this depends on how damaged the tube is by the pregnancy and also what the tube on the other side looks like); (ii) opening the tube and removing the pregnancy and stopping the bleeding from the pregnancy bed; and (iii) squeezing the pregnancy out of the tube (called milking). Again, the choice of one of these will be determined at the time of surgery. If any of the options other than the removal of the tube is performed, you will have to have a blood test to make sure that all pregnancy tissues have been removed and your hCG level has fallen back to normal.

Miscarriages. Bleeding in early pregnancy is very common. It complicates about 15–20% of all pregnancies that are 6 weeks or more. There are different types of miscarriages, and these include (a) threatened miscarriage, (b) missed miscarriage, (c) inevitable miscarriage, (d) incomplete miscarriage, (e) complete miscarriage and (f) septic miscarriage.

a. **Threatened miscarriage:** In this type of early pregnancy complication there is bleeding, which is typically painless. The neck of the womb (cervix) is closed when you are examined internally, and an ultrasound scan will show a live fetus. Very occasionally there may be a small blood clot around the pregnancy sac (called a haematoma). The presence of this blood clot does not mean that you will lose the pregnancy. Most women with a threatened miscarriage go on to have a baby. It is important that you are followed up regularly to identify any complications that may occur. You have a slightly increased risk of delivery before your due date.

b. **Inevitable miscarriage:** This is a type of miscarriage where you present with bleeding often associated with pain, and when you are examined the neck of the womb (cervix) is opened. This means that even if the baby is still alive you will go on to miscarry. If you have this diagnosis, you will be given the option of waiting for the process to be completed naturally or to have either medical treatment or surgery.

c. **Incomplete miscarriage:** This is when you have passed some of the pregnancy tissues but not all. Some of them are still in your womb. Your management will depend on whether you are bleeding, whether you have pain and your wishes. In most cases waiting will allow nature to complete the process, but if there is bleeding then this process may be expedited by surgery (called an evacuation – see below for a description of surgical evacuation). If you are not bleeding or the bleeding is very slight, you may also elect (choose) to have medical treatment (See below for details).

d. **Missed miscarriage:** This is when you have had an ultrasound scan that shows a pregnancy sac without a fetus (baby), and the sac is greater than the minimum size. Most of these happen because the fetus has not developed properly. There are three options to deal with these – (a) expectant management, (b) medical treatment and (c) surgery.
    • With expectant management, you will wait for nature to take its course. This usually takes about 3 weeks. You will have to be patient with this option and also in the knowledge that if it does not work, you will have to either go for medical management or surgery.

- In medical management, you are given tablets followed by pessaries (put in the vagina) – typically 2 days after the tablets. You must be prepared to come for the pessaries and also accept that you may need surgery. The success rate with this type of management is about 80–90%. A small proportion of women will have an incomplete miscarriage and require surgery.
- The surgical treatment is called surgical evacuation. There are two approaches to this – one is called manual vacuum evacuation, and the other is called suction evacuation. In the first option a cannula called Karman is attached to a plastic tube that is put into your womb. The pregnancy is then sucked out into the cannula. This can be done without putting you to sleep (but with sedation and injecting a local anaesthetic around the neck of the womb). The main advantage is that you are not put to sleep, and therefore recovery is faster. In the surgical suction evacuation, you are put to sleep and the neck of the womb (cervix) is stretched – what we refer to as dilation – and a plastic tube is passed into the womb, and suction pressure is applied to remove the pregnancy. The main complications of these surgical procedures are perforation of the womb (making a hole in the wall of the womb), bleeding, infections and injury to the cervix.

e. **Septic miscarriage:** This type of miscarriage is rare, but here some of the pregnancy tissues remain in the womb, and there is also an infection of these products. The woman presents with bleeding which may be dirty brown and smelly and a temperature with lower tummy pain. Treatment is antibiotics and removal of the remaining pregnancy tissues by evacuation. You will need to have the antibiotics injected into your vein for a few hours before the surgery is performed.

f. **Complete miscarriage:** This is a type of miscarriage where all the pregnancy tissues have come out and there is no need to do anything else.

2. **Swyer syndrome.** This is a condition in which the individual has 46XY chromosomes but develops as a female. They typically have normal female external genitalia, identify as female and are raised as girls. They are thus externally female but have streak (non-functioning thin line tissue) gonads and, if left untreated, will thus not experience puberty. Swyer syndrome is caused by mutations in a gene known as the DHH gene. It is inherited in an autosomal recessive condition, which means both parents pass this mutation to their child (i.e. copies of the gene in each cell have mutations). The parents of an individual with this autosomal recessive condition, therefore, carry one copy of the altered gene (which is why they are not affected).

It affects sexual development. Sexual development is usually determined by an individual's chromosomes (with the genes on the Y chromosome being crucial in driving male sex differentiation); however, in Swyer syndrome, sexual development does not match the affected individual's chromosomal makeup. People usually have 46 chromosomes in each cell. Two of the 46 chromosomes, known as X and Y, are called sex chromosomes because they help determine whether a person will develop male or female sex characteristics. Females typically have two X chromosomes (46, XX karyotype), males usually have one X chromosome and one Y chromosome (46, XY karyotype). In Swyer syndrome, individuals have one X chromosome and one Y chromosome in each cell, the pattern typically found in boys and men but have female reproductive structures. *This is because the important genes that drive male sex differentiation are absent.* People with Swyer syndrome have typical female external genitalia. The uterus and fallopian tubes are normally formed, but the gonads (ovaries or testes) are not functional; affected individuals have undeveloped clumps of tissue called streak gonads.

Because of the lack of development of the gonads, Swyer syndrome is also called 46,XY complete gonadal dysgenesis. The residual gonadal tissue often becomes cancerous, so it is usually removed surgically early in life. People with Swyer syndrome are typically raised as girls and have a female gender identity. Because they do not have functional ovaries, affected individuals usually begin hormone replacement therapy during adolescence to induce menstruation and develop female secondary sex characteristics such as breast enlargement and uterine growth. Hormone replacement therapy also helps reduce the risk of reduced bone density (osteopenia and osteoporosis). Women with this disorder do not produce eggs (ova) but may be able to become pregnant with a donated egg or embryo.

3. **Androgen insensitivity syndrome (AIS).** This is when a person who is genetically male (i.e. has one X and one Y chromosome) and is resistant to male hormones (or androgens).
   In offering this explanation, it is advisable not to refer to the patient as a man as this could have a very significant psychological effect on her.

   A typical human has 46 chromosomes of which 2 are sex chromosomes. Men are typically 46XY, while women are typically 46XX. A very small proportion of women will have 46XY chromosomes, while a very small proportion of men will have 46 XX chromosomes. The small proportion of women with 46 XY chromosomes has a condition called androgen insensitivity syndrome (AIS). In these women, the gonads (what should have been ovaries) are not normal and, in most cases, may not be found where most women's ovaries are. As a result, they do not produce the normal hormones that ovaries produce. The womb is therefore not developed, and as such they are not able to have periods and cannot have children. Because the gonads are abnormal, there is a great risk that they may develop into cancer. These will therefore have to be removed and following that you will need hormone replacement until you reach the age of change (menopause).

4. **Molar pregnancy.** A molar pregnancy is an abnormal pregnancy in which the fetus does not form properly in the womb, and the baby does not develop. Instead, lumps of abnormal cells grow in the womb. This growth is called a 'hydatidiform mole', of which there are two types (a) a complete mole, where there's a mass of abnormal cells in the womb and with no fetus. The pregnancy, in this case, is made of abnormal tissue (which grows from what would have become the placenta [afterbirth]) that contains very tiny swollen cysts which together resembles grapes (when they are removed from the womb they often appear like a bunch of grapes), and (b) a partial mole, where an abnormal fetus starts to form, but it does not survive or develop into a baby. The tissues in this abnormal pregnancy produce the hormone called human chorionic gonadotrophin (hCG) that pregnant women produce in very high quantities and as such may cause severe sickness (excessive vomiting).
   This condition is important because there is a small chance that it may progress to cancer, and hence it is important that you are monitored for a period of time before you become pregnant again. This is very important as the hormones that a normal pregnancy produces are similar to those produced by persistent disease or cancer, which may confuse your follow-up and cause confusion between what is an ongoing pregnancy and what is a persistent disease or cancer that would require treatment.

   How will this be treated? The treatment is through a simple procedure called suction evacuation. A small tube will be passed into the womb, and the abnormal cells sucked out. Sometimes some of the cells may be left behind, and further treatment may be needed to remove them, but in most cases they go away.

What happens after the treatment? While some of the abnormal cells which may be left in the womb after treatment usually go away on their own within a few months, further treatment may sometimes be needed to remove them in a few patients. In order to identify those women who will need this further treatment, there is a need to have regular blood or urine tests to measure the level of the hormone hCG (human chorionic gonadotrophin). The amount of this hormone in the body increases during pregnancy. If it does not go down after treatment for a molar pregnancy, it might mean some abnormal cells are left in your womb/body. For most women, having these regular blood or urine tests will only be for around 6 months after the surgical treatment and no further treatment will be needed.

There are three highly specialised centres in the UK (Dundee, Sheffield and Charing Cross) that follow up women with molar pregnancies and direct treatment if required. Women with this condition will be registered with one of these centres depending on where they are, and they will send these women the necessary containers for a follow-up urine test through the post on a regular basis. The results are sent to your doctor and consultant in the hospital to keep them informed. If there is need for further action, these will also be notified.

What happens if the hormone levels do not go down to normal? In a few cases, the abnormal cells left in the womb after treatment do not go away on their own. This is called persistent trophoblastic disease (PTD). The chances of this happening are about 1 in 7 (15%) following a complete mole and about 1 in 200 (0.5%) following a partial mole. Because these abnormal cells can remain and grow in the womb or spread and grow in other parts of the body similar to how cancer behaves if untreated, it is recommended for those women in whom the hormone levels are increasing (instead of falling) or fail to return to normal within a definite period, to have treatment known as chemotherapy to kill these cells . Instructions on when and how to start this treatment will come from the follow-up regional centres.

When can pregnancy occur after a molar pregnancy? You can usually get pregnant after treatment if you wish, but you will be advised not to try for at least 6 months if your hormone levels are back to normal within 56 days (8 weeks), but if they are not back to normal within 8 weeks, you should avoid pregnancy for at least a year from when they are back to normal because there's a chance (about 1 in 30) that PTD could come back during this time. You can have sex as soon as you feel physically and emotionally ready. If you have any bleeding after your treatment, you should avoid sex until it stops. Having a molar pregnancy does not affect your chances of getting pregnant again, and the risk of having another molar pregnancy is small (about 1 in 80). It is best not to try for a baby until after monitoring has finished, in case you need further treatment to remove any cells left in your womb/body. Apart from the intrauterine contraceptive device (the coil), most forms of contraception are acceptable. In the past, it used to be thought that the combined pill delays a return to normal of the hormones, but there is no evidence for this. Doctors say it's safe to get pregnant again. You can however use the coil once your hCG level has returned to normal.

What causes a molar pregnancy? A molar pregnancy is not caused by anything you or your partner have done. It happens if the amount of genetic material in a fertilised egg is not right – for example, if an egg containing no genetic information is fertilised by a sperm, or a normal egg is fertilised by two sperms. It is unclear as to why this happens, but the following things can increase the risk: (a) age – molar pregnancies are more common in teenage women and women aged >45 years; (b) ethnicity – molar pregnancies are about twice as common in women of Asian origin; and (c) previous pregnancy – if you've had a molar pregnancy before, your chance of having another one is about 1 in 80, compared with 1 in 600 for women who have not had one before. If you have had two or more molar pregnancies, your risk of having another is around 1 in 5.

You may contact a support group, such as the *Molar Pregnancy Support Group* or *MyMolarPregnancy.com*. They may be able to put you in touch with other people in a similar situation.

5. **Endometriosis.** This is a condition in which tissue similar to that which lines your womb (uterus), called the endometrium, is present and grows outside of the uterus and attaches to other parts of your body.

6. **Adenomyosis.** This is a condition in which cells similar to those that make up the lining of your womb (uterus), called the endometrium, grow into the muscles of the uterus.

7. **Fibroids.** These are benign tumours (abnormal growths) of the muscles and fibrous tissue (tissue between the muscles) of the womb. They vary in size and commonly occur during the reproductive years of women. Most women with fibroids do not have any symptoms. Of the approximately 1:3 who have symptoms, these may include (a) heaving periods which may or may not be painful, (b) tummy (abdominal) swelling and/or pain, (c) lower backache, (d) a frequent need to pass urine (or spend a penny), (e) constipation, (f) pain or discomfort during sexual intercourse and (f) in rare cases, further complications caused by fibroids can affect pregnancy or cause infertility.

8. **Detrusor overactivity (overactive bladder).** Normally when urine collects in the bladder, we are able to control when to empty the bladder. That control comes from the brain. In cases of an overactive bladder, the bladder does not respond to the message the brain sends to it not to empty itself but does so when there is urine in it. It therefore acts out of control of the brain and is said to be overactive.

9. **Borderline ovarian cyst (BOC).** Borderline ovarian tumours are abnormal cells that form in the tissue covering the ovary. They are not cancerous and are treated by surgery, which is usually a complete cure. Approximately 15 in 100 cases (15%) of ovarian tumours are borderline tumours. These tumours are different from ovarian cancer because their growth is limited, and they never invade the supportive tissue of the ovary, called the stroma. They are also called low malignant potential (the possibility to become cancerous) tumours as they tend to grow slowly and in a more controlled manner when compared to cancer cells. Most ovarian tumours are either benign (not cancerous) or malignant (cancerous). Ovarian cancer develops when cells grow uncontrollably on the surface of the ovary and are able to spread to other organs. Borderline tumours arise from the same type of cells, but their growth is much more controlled, and they are usually not able to spread. These abnormal cells are also from the same area as cancer cells, but they are not cancerous.

Borderline ovarian tumours are classified as serous (covered in serum) or mucinous (covered in mucus), depending on their appearance under the microscope. They are also classified by the stage (development) according to their size or how far they have spread. Serous tumours are more common in 65 of 100 cases (65%) of patients treated.

A small number of women who have been diagnosed with a borderline ovarian tumour will be diagnosed at a more advanced stage, where the disease has spread. When borderline ovarian tumours spread, they attach small seedlings onto the peritoneum (a layer covering the organs in the abdomen). These seedlings can be successfully removed surgically, but occasionally they may remain on this surface layer, for which you will be closely monitored by your consultant and team.

Most cases of ordinary ovarian cancer are found at an advanced stage (stage 3 or 4). This is when cancer has spread beyond the ovary. Because BOC behaves in a much less aggressive way, in most people the condition has not spread beyond the ovary when it is diagnosed (stage 1 disease). This means that for those who have had surgery to remove early disease, the risk of it coming back is very small, at less than 5% (5 in a 100). Most experts recommend that no special follow-up is needed after surgery for stage 1 BOC.

There are three situations which can cause greater concern or uncertainty: (1) borderline ovarian tumours which have spread beyond the ovary; (2) mucinous borderline tumours involving the ovary, when tests suggest these could originate from a tumour in the appendix; (3) stage 1 borderline ovarian tumours in young people treated with limited surgery to keep an ovary. There could be an increased risk of the disease coming back in the ovary you have kept.

How are borderline tumours treated? Most of the time, the diagnosis is made from an examination of a cyst that has been removed during surgery. If the whole ovary has been removed, then all that would be needed is a follow-up.

If, however, a borderline ovarian tumour is suspected prior to surgery, a thorough examination of the abdomen (tummy) should be undertaken by the expert and an internal (vaginal) examination undertaken if necessary. This is to make sure that there are no other features that may make this diagnosis unlikely. An ultrasound scan should be performed if not already done. Further investigations including computerised tomography (CT) scans and blood tests may also be arranged.

As borderline ovarian tumours are slow growing, many of them are diagnosed at an early stage and can be cured by surgery. Many women are treated by surgical removal of only the affected ovary and fallopian tube, with the womb and the other ovary left in place. In about 1 in 20 cases (5%), the tumour will come back in the remaining ovary if only the affected ovary is removed and the disease is at an early stage. For those at high risk of developing further tumours, it may be recommended that both ovaries and both tubes are removed, to avoid further surgery. This surgery is called bilateral salpingoophorectomy, with or without a total abdominal hysterectomy. If the borderline tumour is of the mucinous type, the appendix may also be removed as it is suspected that the tumour may have started in the appendix and spread to the ovary.

Will treatment prevent me from having babies? If the borderline ovarian tumour is only within one ovary, and there is the wish to have more children, fertility-conserving surgery (i.e. surgery which will allow you to have children), in which the ovary, fallopian tube and womb are saved, should be discussed and offered.

How will follow-up be undertaken? Currently there is no clear evidence on what the best follow-up is for patients who have had a borderline ovarian tumour. However, regular follow-up is required. This is usually at 6 monthly intervals at the hospital with clinical examination and occasional scans for 2 years and then yearly. Occasionally, the borderline tumour cells can change to cancerous cells. It is for this reason that regular close follow-up is very important. Later it may be appropriate for those who have completed their family to have the remaining ovary removed. This removes the risk of problems in the future and means they will not have to go for follow-ups.

10. **Endometrial hyperplasia.** The cells that line the womb (called the endometrium) have over divided. This is likely to be because of overstimulation by estrogen. If not checked, this may progress to cancer.

11. **Abnormal cervical smears.** Your smear test has come back as abnormal. An abnormal smear test is graded into borderline, low grade and high grade. This depends on the degree of abnormal cells found in the smear. The most severe type of abnormal smear is the high-grade dyskaryosis. A test like this is an indication for an examination of the cervix (neck of the womb) under the microscope – an examination called colposcopy. In this examination, you will have your legs up in stirrups. A special solution (acetic acid and Lugol's iodine) will then be applied to the cervix and the top of the vagina and inspected under the colposcope, which magnifies these. Treatment may be performed at this test or a biopsy taken, and treatment offered later if it is necessary.

12. **Polycystic ovary syndrome.** This is a condition in which you have several tiny cysts in your ovaries and the ovaries produce hormones in a fashion that is different from that in most women. The hormones that your ovaries produce have more male type hormones compared to what women without this condition produce. The symptoms you have are as a result of this abnormal hormone production. They include weight gain, thickening at the back of your neck, irregular periods and excessive hair growth on your legs, tummy and around your breast. Although you have multiple cysts (called follicles) in your ovaries, you are ovulating (producing an egg) infrequently and therefore may not be able to get pregnant easily. This condition is very common, and depending on which symptom is bringing you to the hospital today, the treatment varies. You may be given hormones to regulate your periods, to help with the hair growth and also to help you ovulate and get pregnant.

This condition is associated with an increased risk of various medical complications including diabetes (also in pregnancy), high blood pressure, heart diseases and cancer of the womb. It is therefore important that you take the necessary steps to reduce your risk of these complications and also make sure that you are followed up regularly.

Explanation of Some Gynaecological Surgical Procedures

1. **Minimally invasive surgery.** Minimally invasive surgery is also known as keyhole surgery. In this type of surgery, very tiny cuts are made on the tummy, and through these cuts, a camera and instruments are inserted into the tummy to perform surgery. The number of cuts and their size will depend on the type of surgery being performed. The advantages include small cuts on the tummy, shorter hospital stay, less pain after surgery and quick recovery and return to work. It is also more cosmetic.

2. **Hysterectomy.** This is an operation to remove the womb (uterus). This can be done either through (a) a cut on your tummy (called an abdominal hysterectomy or open hysterectomy), (b) through keyhole surgery (where we make small cuts on your tummy and with the help of a camera remove the womb and then bring it out through the vagina or in small pieces (using a process called morcellation) inside a small bag through one of the cuts on your tummy) or (c) through the vagina without making any cut on your tummy (called a vaginal hysterectomy).

Furthermore, a hysterectomy can be total where the uterus as well as the cervix (neck of the womb), or subtotal where only the body (and the cervix is left behind), are removed. The medical terms for these are total abdominal hysterectomy (removing the uterus and the cervix through the tummy), subtotal abdominal hysterectomy (again through the tummy), total laparoscopic hysterectomy (keyhole but with removal from the vagina), laparoscopic-assisted vaginal hysterectomy (combined vaginal and keyhole surgery but removal from the vagina) or robotic (where a robot performs the surgery). The different types of hysterectomy are explained in detail below:

a. **Abdominal hysterectomy:** This is a hysterectomy through a cut on the tummy. The cut is commonly on the bikini line (what is called a 'bikini cut') – just above the public hairline. Occasionally, this may be done through an 'up and down cut' (called a vertical incision). This is typically an approach where the womb is very large and the surgery is anticipated to be very difficult and good exposure is required to make it safe. This is not as cosmetic as that through the 'bikini cut', and the pain from surgery is greater than that through the 'bikini cut'.

b. **Vaginal hysterectomy:** This is the operation in which your womb is removed through the vagina. In some cases, one or both ovaries and fallopian tubes may also be removed. This surgical approach avoids giving you a visible scar on your tummy, and it also allows for a quicker recovery, as well as less post-operative pain and complications as compared with other types of hysterectomy. There is a small risk that it may not be possible to remove your womb this way or you may bleed and require being opened up to complete the procedure.

c. **Laparoscopic-assisted vaginal hysterectomy (LAVH):** This is the operation which combines keyhole surgery (which uses video technology) to provide the surgeon with greater visibility when removing the uterus through the vagina. The laparoscopic-assisted approach entails small external cuts on the tummy – one commonly just below or in the navel, through which the laparoscope (small video camera) is inserted, and two others in the lower abdomen for the use of surgical instruments. This procedure may be preferred because of the rapid healing time, a less noticeable scar and less pain, although actual surgery time is longer than the abdominal approach. Because of the longer time in the operation room and the use of extra electronic equipment, this procedure is also costlier and other risks associated with the laparoscopic-assisted vaginal approach include a slight risk of bladder injury and urinary tract infection.

d. **Robotic-assisted laparoscopic hysterectomy:** This is hysterectomy in which a robot is used. It requires three to four incisions near the belly button. A laparoscope is inserted, and the surgeon performs the procedure from a remote area. This procedure results in smaller scars, but the procedure has not been shown to have better surgical outcomes. Rates of discharge from the hospital have been shown to be similar to those of other surgical options for hysterectomies. It is also significantly more costly than the other types of hysterectomies.

3. **Wertheim's (radical) hysterectomy.** This is also called a radical hysterectomy. This is a surgery in which the womb, neck of the womb, the upper part of the vagina and the tissues around the upper part of the vagina and the neck of the womb are removed. It is a surgical treatment for cancer of the cervix. Part of this surgery involves removing the lymph nodes that drain from the cervix to check whether the cancer cells have not spread to them.

4. **Pelvic floor repair for prolapse.** This is an operation to correct prolapse of the pelvic organs through the vagina. There are different types depending on the type of prolapse. If it is a prolapse of the bladder (coming through the front of the vagina), then the operation is called an anterior repair. If it is to correct the prolapse of the back of the vagina, it is called a posterior repair. Where the prolapse is coming from the top, especially after a hysterectomy, the repair may be done through a cut on the tummy (this is called a sacrocolpopexy) or from below (this is called a vault repair) or an enterocele repair (if the prolapse is of small bowel coming down the top of the vagina).

5. **Sacrocolpopexy.** This is an operation through a cut on the tummy to correct prolapse of the top of the vagina. In this operation, the top of the vagina is attached to the cover of your backbone, just at the entrance to your pelvis using a mesh, which remains inside and is not absorbed or does not melt away. This mesh does not cause any reaction to your body.

6. **Colposuspension.** This is an operation to treat urinary incontinence, which is due to the weakness of the bladder neck. This operation is undertaken through a cut on the tummy – a bikini-line cut. The neck of the bladder is exposed, and stitches are inserted to both sides and then attached to the back of the pelvic bone to the front of the pelvis. These stitches will dissolve (melt away) after some time.

7. **Uterine artery embolisation.** This is a type of treatment in which a special catheter (very fine tube) is passed through a blood vessel (usually on your thigh) into the blood vessels that go to your womb. A special chemical (special particles) is then put into this blood vessel to block the blood going to fibroids that you have. Because the blood to the fibroids is blocked, the fibroids are starved of blood and therefore oxygen, and therefore shrink.

    The procedure is done by experts called interventional radiologists under sedation and as a day procedure (in which case you will go home after). Although it is commonly used to treat fibroids, it can also be used to treat adenomyosis, and in emergency situations, to stop bleeding after delivery and adenomyosis.

8. **Large loop excision of the transformation zone of the cervix.** This is an operation in which abnormal cells on the inner lips of the cervix (neck of the womb) are removed using a wire loop that cuts through the cervix very quickly. This is done in most cases as an outpatient procedure and usually at the time of colposcopy (examination of the cervix, vagina and sometimes the vulva with a colposcope).

9. **Tension-free vaginal tape.** This is an operation to treat stress urinary incontinence (that is, leakage of urine when you cough, sneeze, jump or do your exercises). It is a very simple operation in which two small cuts are made in the lower part of your tummy, and a tape is passed through them to the neck of your bladder in the vagina. You will therefore have a small cut on your vagina. This tape that is inserted does not get absorbed and therefore remains inside your body. Very occasionally it may cause problems and have to be removed.

10. **Burch colposuspension.** This is an operation to treat stress urinary incontinence (that is, leakage of urine when you cough, sneeze, jump or do exercise such as in aerobic classes). In this operation, you will have a cut on your tummy, usually in the bikini line after which the neck of the bladder will be exposed. Stitches will then be placed on both sides of the neck of the bladder and then attached to the back of your pelvic bone in front. This lifts up the bladder neck and increases the resistance in it and therefore corrects any weakness that may be causing you to leak urine. Following the surgery you will have a catheter in your bladder for a few days

before you are allowed to pass urine on your own. Some people put this catheter through your tummy, while others put in from below.

11. **Salpingectomy/salpingotomy.** This is an operation in which your tube is either removed (salpingectomy) or an opening is made in your tube and whatever is inside is removed (salpingotomy). This is typically done when you have an ectopic pregnancy (pregnancy in the tube).

12. **Cone biopsy.** A cone biopsy is an operation to treat an abnormality (which if not treated can progress to cancer) in the cervix (neck of the womb), following an abnormal smear test and colposcopy. In this operation, part of the cervix is removed in the form of a cone. A surgical blade or laser or diathermy loop can be used for this operation. It can be done as an outpatient procedure at the time of colposcopy or in the theatre, depending on the type of cone biopsy. Those with a loop are often done in the colposcopy clinic, while those with a knife (surgical blade) are typically done in the operating theatre under general anaesthesia.

13. **Ovarian cystectomy.** This is an operation to remove a cyst on your ovary. It is typically done through keyhole surgery, although it can also be done by open surgery.

14. **Trachelectomy.** This is an operation done for very early-stage cancer of the cervix or neck of the womb for women who wish to have children. In this operation, the lower part of the cervix is removed as well as the tissues around it to ensure that most of the cancer cells are removed. Sometimes this is called a radical trachelectomy, in which case, apart from removing the cervix and the tissues around it, the lymph nodes are also removed. These nodes are usually removed by keyhole surgery through cuts on the tummy.

Explaining Investigations

1. **Urinalysis and urine culture**. When we collect urine from you, we do a point-of-care test called urinalysis. This is where we put a highly sensitive special paper (called a strip) into the urine to tell whether the urine is normal or not. Most importantly, it tells us whether we should send the urine to the lab to check for infections. We also look for protein in urine, which, if present in significant quantities, will require further investigations. The presence of some of the things we look for in urine does not mean something is wrong, as in most people it may be contamination at the time urine is being collected.

2. **Full blood count and the elements in the count**. This blood test checks what your iron level is. It helps determine whether you have anaemia or not. It also checks for the levels of the different types of cells that are in your blood, especially white cells and platelets. White cells are useful when there is a suspicion of an infection while platelets are useful if there is a risk of bleeding.

3. **Liver function test (*refers to the specific reason for the test)**. This is a test to check how well your liver is working. This test measures the levels of some important enzymes that your liver produces, the level of bilirubin (which causes jaundice) and the levels of proteins in your blood. This particular test is done for various conditions* as well as in preparation for some specialised treatments*.

4. **Urea and electrolytes (kidney function test) (*refers to the specific reason for the test)**. This test checks how well your kidneys are working. It measures several things, the most important of which are urea and potassium levels. This particular test is done for various conditions* as well as in preparation for some specialised treatments*.

5. **Coagulation screen**. This test checks the factors in your blood that are involved in blood clotting. It tells us how well your blood is clotting.

6. **Thrombophilia screen**. This is a test to check the factors that control blood clotting. Some of these are inherited while others are acquired. Some of the ones that are inherited include Protein C and S, anti-thrombin III and factor V. Acquired factors include antiphospholipid antibodies and lupus anticoagulant.

7. **Oral glucose tolerance test (OGTT)**. This is a test for diabetes. It requires you to fast overnight (from 12 midnight i.e. 8 hours without eating) and have a blood test in the morning, after which you will be given a drink. This drink will contain about 75 g of glucose. Some units use Lucozade. Blood will then be collected from you on two occasions – 1 hour and 2 hours after you drink this glucose load. The levels of glucose in your blood will be measured from these blood samples to determine whether you have diabetes or not.

8. **Screening for aneuploidy**. This is a test which allows us to calculate the risk of you having a baby with a chromosome abnormality. Chromosomes are the things that carry genes. Each person has 46 or 23 pairs, one pair (23) comes from each of our parents.

9. **Hormone assays**. A series of hormones are produced in the body that we often measure in the blood as part of investigations for various problems. These hormones are produced in different parts of the body such as the brain, the thyroid gland (which is in the front of the neck), the ovaries and the adrenals – which sit just above the kidneys. The hormones produced by the brain control how your ovaries work, and these include follicle-stimulating hormone (FSH) and luteinising hormone (LH). We also measure prolactin (which is involved in milk production). The hormones produced by the ovaries are estrogen, progesterone and testosterone (which is also produced in the testes). We measure progesterone in the middle of the second half of your menstrual cycle, which helps us determine whether you are producing an egg or not. This test is called 21-day progesterone.

10. **Hysterosalpingogram (HSG)**. This is a test to check if your womb is normal and also whether your tubes are normal and also open. In this test, a small chemical (contrast), which an X-ray can see, is pushed up your womb through a small tube inserted into your cervix (neck of the womb) and then X-rays are taken. This is done in the X-ray department. You will have a speculum inserted into your vagina as if you are having a smear test. A small instrument will then pick up the lip of your cervix to allow the tube to be inserted into it. This may be uncomfortable or painful, but most women describe it as a discomfort. The dye will then be pushed up into your womb through the tubes, and X-rays are taken. Some women may react to this dye.

11. **Serum CA125 and other tumour markers**. This is a test to measure the levels of certain 'chemicals in the blood', which we call tumour markers. These include CA125, hCG and lactate dehydrogenase (LDH). Some of these may be raised in women who do not have cancer, but we will need to perform more tests if it's abnormal, as it is only a screening test. We measure them not only in women we suspect may have cancer but also in those with a variety of benign conditions such as endometriosis.

12. **Cervical cytology**. This is a screening test for cervical cancer. Every woman who is sexually active should have this test done from the age of 25 and on a regular basis. It is a test in which we take cells from the inside of the neck of your womb (cervix) and send to the lab to examine these cells to make sure that there are no changes that could eventually lead to cancer. If the

cells are abnormal, you may either be asked to have a colposcopy (see below) or be tested for a viral infection called human papilloma virus (HPV), depending on the degree of abnormality.

13. **Colposcopy**. This is a special procedure in which your cervix (otherwise known as the neck of the womb), the vaginal walls and in some cases the vulva are examined with a special instrument called the colposcope. It allows the cells in these areas to be examined under magnification. It is done as a day case procedure, and you do not need any anaesthesia for this. It is very similar to you having a smear test, except that you will have your legs put up in either stirrups or something similar to allow this examination to take place. In most cases, a special solution will be applied to the areas being examined and the doctor may take a biopsy if the area being examined looks abnormal and the doctor wants it to be examined under the microscope.

   The commonest reason for doing this procedure is a follow-up of an abnormal smear test. In most women, an area of the cervix that looks abnormal can be removed using a small wire (called a loop). If this is to be done, you will be given a local anaesthetic to numb the area so that you do not feel pain. As this is a day procedure, you will not stay in the hospital. If any treatment is done, you will be advised not to do douching or use a tampon for a few weeks. You may have a discharge for a few days after this procedure, especially if a biopsy or treatment was performed at the same time

14. **Cystoscopy**. This is a test in which a camera is inserted into the bladder to examine it. During this, the bladder is filled up with fluid so that the camera is able to thoroughly examine it.

15. **Diagnostic laparoscopy**. This is a test in which a camera is passed through a small cut on your tummy to inspect the inside of your tummy. At the beginning of this procedure, gas will be introduced into your tummy to make it easier to insert the camera and reduce the risk of injury to the bowel.

16. **Hysteroscopy**. This is a test in which a camera is inserted into your womb to examine it.

17. **Urodynamics**. This is a test to check how well your waterworks are working (functioning). Prior to (3 days before) this test, you will be asked to keep a diary of how much you drink and how much and often you pass urine with associated symptoms. At the test, a tube will be passed into the bladder, and also into your back passage. The bladder will be filled with fluid, and you will be asked to jump to see whether you wet yourself. This test is important in that it will help differentiate one type of incontinence from the other and therefore help with the planning of treatment.

18. **MRI of the pelvis and abdomen**. This is an investigation in which you will go through a tube which is dark to have a scan of your body. This could be of the pelvis or your tummy. This test uses a magnet, and so if you have any metal on your body, you must let us know as you will not be able to have it. Furthermore, if you do not like to be in closed/dark spaces (that is, you suffer from claustrophobia), then this is not a suitable test for you. You may also have this test because your baby has an abnormality, and we want to define the nature of the abnormality. This test will give us more information that a typical ultrasound scan will not.

19. **Follicular tracking**. As you are having an induction of ovulation, we need to see how you are responding to the drugs you are taking to make you ovulate. The reason we do this is to follow how the eggs (follicles) grow in your ovaries by doing regular ultrasound scans. This is known as follicular tracking.

12
Paper I

Task 1: Instrumental Delivery (Forceps Delivery). Module 1 – Teaching

Candidate's Instructions

This is a teaching task (both forceps and ventouse, but in the exams, only one will be a task at a time) assessing the following:

- Information gathering
- Communication with patients and families
- Communication with colleagues
- Patient safety
- Applied clinical knowledge

You have 10 minutes in which you should:

- Give an overview of the theory of instrumental delivery
- Teach a specialist training in her first year to conduct an instrumental delivery
- Demonstrate that the teaching has been successful

A good candidate will cover the following (note that the details here will not necessarily be covered in 10 minutes, but it is important to know them and the sequence in which they occur so as to apply appropriately):

A. **Introduction and state role**
   - Introduction – e.g. Hello Dr **Z** I am Dr **XY**, an ST5 who will be teaching you how to conduct a forceps delivery
   - Firstly, establish what the trainee knows and any previous experience with instrumental delivery

B. **State the objectives of the teaching session**
   By the end of this session, you would be able to:
   a. Identify the indications for assisting/expediting vaginal delivery
   b. Understand the conditions that have to be fulfilled before conducting an operative vaginal delivery
   c. Perform an operative vaginal delivery (ventouse/forceps, depending on which one you are teaching)
   d. Recognise and manage complications that arise from the procedure
   e. Understand how operative vaginal deliveries are classified

C. **The indications for an instrumental delivery include:**
   - Presumed fetal compromise in the second stage of labour

- Shortening and reducing the effects of the second stage of labour on medical conditions (e.g. cardiac disease Class III or IV, hypertensive crises, myasthenia gravis, spinal cord injury patients at risk of autonomic dysreflexia and proliferative retinopathy)
- Inadequate progress – in nulliparous women – lack of continuing progress for 3 hours (total of active and passive second-stage labour with regional anaesthesia) or 2 hours without regional anaesthesia; in multiparous women – lack of continuing progress for 2 hours (total of active and passive second-stage labour with regional anaesthesia) or 1 hour without regional anaesthesia. Maternal fatigue/exhaustion

D. **Brief overview of the instrument**
- Shows the trainee the instrument and its parts
  - Forceps – blades (with two curves – pelvic and cephalic), shanks, handle and locks
  - If it's a ventouse, briefly explain the instrument

E. **Classification of operative vaginal delivery**
- *Outlet* – Fetal scalp visible without separating the labia; fetal skull has reached the pelvic floor. Sagittal suture is in the anteroposterior diameter or right or left occiput anterior or posterior position (rotation does not exceed 45°). Fetal head is at or on the perineum
- *Mid* – Fetal head is no more than 1/5th palpable per abdomen, and the leading point of the skull is above station plus 2 cm but not above the ischial spines; two subdivisions:
  i. Rotation of 45° or less from an occipitoanterior position
  ii. Rotation of more than 45° including from an occipitoposterior position
- Note that *High* operative vaginal delivery, where the head is 2/5th or more palpable abdominally and the presenting part is above the level of the ischial spines, is not advisable

F. **Conditions to be fulfilled (prerequisites) for operative vaginal delivery**
- Head is ≤ 1/5th palpable per abdomen
- Vaginal examination – vertex presentation
- Cervix is fully dilated and membranes ruptured
- The exact position of the head can be determined so proper placement of the instrument can be achieved
- Caput and moulding are assessed
- The pelvis is deemed adequate
- Irreducible moulding may indicate cephalo-pelvic disproportion
- Adequate analgesia

G. **Preparation of mother**
- A clear explanation should be given and informed consent obtained
- Appropriate analgesia is in place for mid-cavity rotational deliveries; regional block is preferable but pudendal block may be appropriate, particularly in the context of urgent delivery
- Maternal bladder emptied. Indwelling catheter should be removed or balloon deflated
- Aseptic technique

H. **Application of the instruments**
Forceps
- First, assemble instruments on the trolley to ensure that they fit snugly
- Dismantle and take the right blade with your left hand (this sequence can be reversed)
- Lubricate the blade with an appropriate lubricant
- Place your right hand inside the vagina and insert blade holding it with the left hand between the hand and the fetal head. Gently push the instrument into position

- Repeat the above with the next blade (holding it with your right hand and with the left hand in the vagina)
- Lock blades and ensure that there is not too much pressure in doing so (they should lock with ease) and check for their correct placement and safety (e.g. the sagittal suture is in the midline, the blades are equidistant from the sagittal and occipital sutures and you should be able to insert a fingertip between the fenestrations and the fetal head)
- Gently apply traction to assess the fit and anticipated degree of force required and also chances of success
- Await contraction and ask the woman to push and at the same time gently pull– the direction of pull (usually downwards and forwards – following the axis of Carus or pelvic curve) will depend on the station of the presenting part. Stop pulling between contractions
- When the head is crowning, ask the woman to stop pushing
- Just before delivering the head, determine if an episiotomy is needed, and, if so, give one
- Once the head is delivered, dismantle the forceps and conduct the rest of the second stage having administered syntocinon with the delivery of the anterior shoulder
- Examine perineum and cervix for tears after the delivery of the placenta
- Make sure paired blood samples are obtained for cord pH and lactate
- Abandon the procedure if after three pulls the baby is not delivered and call your senior

Ventouse – if it requires a suction pump
- Check that the pressure pump is working
- Select the correct size cup
- Connect to the suction machine
- Lubricate the cup
- Apply the cup to the posterior vertex and check to make sure that it does not include the vagina
- Increase pressure initially to 0.2 kg/M^2 and then check to make sure the cup is not catching vagina
- Increase pressure to 0.8 kg/M^2 and then await contractions
- With each contraction, ask the woman to push and, at the same time, pull (direction of pull depends on the station and whether it's a rotation or not)
- Once crowned, either administer an episiotomy, if needed, or continue pulling until delivery of the head
- Once the head is delivered, disconnect the pump, dismount the cup and conduct the rest of the second stage having administered syntocinon with the delivery of the anterior shoulder
- Examine the perineum and the cervix for tears after the delivery of the placenta
- Make sure paired samples are obtained for cord pH and lactate

Ventouse – Kiwi cup
- Principles are the same except you will increase to the various colour levels
  - Green and orange, and then once delivery is complete, deflate and remove

Postscript

Although not part of the teaching, these should be understood by the candidate preparing for the examination in case this is a discussion task, as questions can be asked on these.

Preparation of Staff

- The operator must have the knowledge, experience and skill necessary
- Adequate facilities are available (appropriate equipment, bed and lighting)

- Backup plan in place in case of failure to deliver. When conducting mid-cavity deliveries, theatre staff should be immediately available to allow a caesarean section to be performed without delay (less than 30 minutes)
- A senior obstetrician, competent in performing mid-cavity deliveries, should be present if a junior trainee is performing the delivery. Anticipate complications that may arise (e.g. shoulder dystocia and postpartum haemorrhage)
- Personnel present who are trained in neonatal resuscitation

Delivery of the Baby

- There is insufficient evidence to favour either a rapid (over 2 minutes) or a stepwise increment in negative pressure with vacuum extraction
- Paired cord blood samples should be processed and recorded following all operative vaginal deliveries
- Is there a place for sequential instruments?
- Use of sequential instruments is associated with an increased risk of trauma to the infant and should therefore be discouraged
- The operator must balance the risks of a caesarean section following failed vacuum extraction with the risks of forceps delivery following failed vacuum extraction
- Obstetricians should be aware of increased neonatal morbidity with failed operative vaginal delivery and/or sequential use of instruments and should inform the neonatologist when this occurs to ensure appropriate management of the baby. In the absence of robust evidence to support the routine use of episiotomy in operative vaginal delivery, restrictive use of episiotomy, using the operator's individual judgement, is supported

Examiner score sheet		
Information gathering		
Standard not met	Standard partly met	Standard met
0	1	2
Communication with patients and families		
Standard not met	Standard partly met	Standard met
0	1	2
Communication with colleagues		
Standard not met	Standard partly met	Standard met
0	1	2
Patient safety		
Standard not met	Standard partly met	Standard met
0	1	2
Applied clinical knowledge		
Standard not met	Standard partly met	Standard met
0	1	2

Examiner Expectations and Basis for Assessment

Information gathering

- Understands the need to first determine the skills of the tutee – what are the skills
- The expectations of the tutee – state clearly the expectations at the end of the teaching

---

Communication with patients and families

- Appropriately introduces the patient and partner
- Explains the role of the tutee and the nature of the interaction to the patient
- Obtains informed consent for teaching from the patient
- Debriefs the patient and partner (if available) after the procedure

---

Communication with colleagues

- Introduces self and role to trainee
- Understands the principles of adult learning and giving feedback
- Takes appropriate steps to increase clinical and technical skills of the learner (tutee)
- Able to use appropriate language as well as non-verbal language to encourage learning
- Invites questions and encourages dialogue
- Shows a logical approach to building the pre-existing skills of the learner
- Gives feedback to tutee at the end of the procedure
- Notifies midwife and neonatologist of the instrumental delivery, and if necessary, the anaesthetist

---

Patient safety

- Maintains patient safety and dignity when teaching a practical skill, showing an understanding of when to continue teaching and when to intervene to halt the teaching session
- Undertakes appropriate checks to ensure that the procedure has been appropriately undertaken

---

Applied clinical knowledge

- Understands the steps in the tasks being undertaken (teaching task)
- Understands the learning objectives and outcomes in relation to the tasks being taught
- Able to conduct and give feedback on using a work-based assessment tool in this task
- Demonstrates knowledge of the current RCOG/NICE guidelines on operative vaginal delivery and contemporary literature on this

Reference: *Assisted vaginal birth. The Royal College of Obstetricians and Gynaecologist Green-top Guideline No. 26. 29 April 2020*

Task 2: Diabetes in Pregnancy. Module 5 – Maternal Medicine

Candidate's Instructions

This is a simulated patient task assessing:

- Information gathering
- Communication with patients and families
- Communication with colleagues
- Patient safety
- Applied clinical knowledge

You are an ST5, who is working with a consultant, with interest in medical disorders in pregnancy. You are about to see Mrs Deborah Stone for her visit to the clinic. The referral letter from her General Practitioner is given below.

The Windfield Surgery
London Road
Windfield, WB1 5TU

Dear Dr,
Re: Deborah Stone
I would be grateful if you could see Mrs Deborah Stone, who is 37 years old and is currently about 10 weeks pregnant. The reason for referring her to you rather than sending her to the midwife is because of her medical problems. She was diagnosed with diabetes 7 years ago and has been on metformin since then. She is currently on 1 g twice a day, but the control has been poor. This was an unplanned pregnancy.
This is her second pregnancy – the first was 8 years ago, and that was uncomplicated. She has a daughter who is otherwise healthy.
She does not have any other medical or surgical problems although she has problems with her weight. Her BMI is 36 kg/M².
She smokes 10–15 cigarettes per day.

I placed her on folic acid 400 µg and have advised that she continues with this until she is 12 weeks.

I have done a full blood count, and the results are attached.

Yours sincerely

Dr John Fothergill MBChB, MRCP, DRCOG

You have 10 minutes in which you should:

- Take relevant clinical history
- Counsel the patient about the implications of her diabetes on pregnancy and vice versa
- Outline the management of her pregnancy
- Answer any questions that she may ask

Simulated Patient's Information

You are Mrs Deborah Stone, a 37-year-old housewife. This is your second marriage. You have an 8-year-old daughter from your first marriage. She was delivered normally, and the pregnancy was uncomplicated.

You were smoking 20–25 cigarettes per day, but since finding that you are pregnant, you have cut down to 10–15. You have a problem with your weight and have been trying very hard to lose weight as you know it does not help diabetes. You drink alcohol occasionally.

Seven years ago, you were diagnosed with type II diabetes, and you have since been on Glucophage – currently taking 1 g twice a day. You had started with 500 mg twice a day, but this has been going up as the control for diabetes has not been very good.

This is an unplanned pregnancy as you had not been expecting to be pregnant. You and your husband had been having unprotected sexual intercourse for more than 4 years without pregnancy, and so you both had given up on the idea of having a child of your own.

You think your last menstrual period was about 8–9 weeks ago. You are not very sure as your periods are not very regular.

Your mother and father are both diabetic, as well as your senior brother, who is 42 years old. It was for this reason that the GP decided to test you 7 years ago.

You have never had surgery before and do not suffer from any other medical problems. You are not aware of any allergies.

The candidate will ask you questions about your history and then discuss issues around the investigations that will be performed on you now and later, on how your pregnancy will be managed and what should happen at different stages of your pregnancy.

If not covered by the candidate, you should ask the following questions:

1. Will my diabetes get worse in pregnancy?
2. Will diabetes affect my baby – will it be deformed or too big (you hear that babies of women with diabetes tend to be big and you are worried)
3. I am a bit old – what does this mean for my pregnancy? Will any test be performed for this?
4. Will I have to have a caesarean section?

Lay Examiner's Instructions

Familiarise yourself with the candidate's and simulated patient's instructions. You should score the candidate's performance on the result sheet. The competent candidate will:

- Quickly obtain a good history and establish the problems
- Explain the medical issues and how these will be dealt with
- Explain the social issues (smoking and alcohol) sensitively and provide a rationale for the advice being given
- Give a detailed explanation of the monitoring and care to be provided
- Advice on options for prenatal diagnosis
- Advice on what the patient should take to reduce the risk of spina bifida in the baby, high blood pressure and blood clots in herself
- Explain the need for combined medical care with the physician
- Explain the monitoring of the woman and the baby throughout the pregnancy and the timing of delivery and care postpartum
- Establish that the woman is happy with the agreed management plan and ensure that all questions have been answered

Examiner score sheet		
Information gathering		
Standard not met	Standard partly met	Standard met
0	1	2
Communication with patients and families		
Standard not met	Standard partly met	Standard met
0	1	2
Communication with colleagues		
Standard not met	Standard partly met	Standard met
0	1	2
Patient safety		
Standard not met	Standard partly met	Standard met
0	1	2
Applied clinical knowledge		
Standard not met	Standard partly met	Standard met
0	1	2

Examiner Expectations and Basis for Assessment

Information gathering

- Able to take a concise and relevant medical history
- Skilled in signposting and guiding the consultation
- Able to ensure that the patient understands and encourages questions
- Initiates appropriate investigations (offer and explain why in the course of pregnancy)

Communication with patients and families

- Introduces self
- Able to give information to the patient with diabetes in pregnancy on both the impact of the pregnancy on her diabetes and the impact of diabetes on the pregnancy and the fetus
- Able to discuss management of the pregnancy – from booking investigations, screening for aneuploidy, follow-up, diabetic control and planned delivery
- Provides information in stages, ensuring that the patient understands, and encourages and answers all questions

---

Communication with colleagues

- Multidisciplinary team (obstetrician with interest in medical disorders in pregnancy, endocrinologist or physician involved in the management of pregnant women with medical disorders, specialised midwife/diabetic midwife, anaesthetist, dietician and GP)
- Timely involvement of members of the team

Patient safety

- Confirms patients identify (name etc)
- Awareness of safety of investigations and therapeutics during pregnancy and in the postnatal period, including safe prescribing. Assures that metformin is safe and insulin may be required if blood sugars are controlled
- Understands the impact of pregnancy on pre-existing diabetes (increases medication) and the impact of diabetes on the pregnancy (maternal and fetal complications)

- Ascertains drug allergy history and safe prescription – aspirin to reduce the risk of hypertensive disorders of pregnancy
- Able to discuss the risk of venous thromboembolism in this patient – four risk factors: age, smoking, diabetic and high BMI – should be offered antenatal Fragmin

Applied clinical knowledge

- Demonstrates knowledge of the current approach to antenatal and postnatal care of women with co-morbidities in pregnancy (in this case, obesity and diabetes)
- Demonstrates knowledge of NICE guidelines on diabetes in pregnancy and RCOG Green-top guidelines on obesity and pregnancy and prevention of venous thromboembolism in pregnancy

Reference: Diabetes in pregnancy: Management from preconception to postnatal period. NICE guideline [NG3] 25 February 2015. Last updated 25 July 2018

Task 3: Monochorionic Twin Pregnancy. Module 4 – Antenatal Care

Candidate's Instructions

This is a simulated patient task assessing:

- Information gathering
- Communication with patients and families
- Communication with colleagues
- Patient safety
- Applied clinical knowledge

You are an ST5 in the antenatal clinic with your consultant. You are about to see one of the women who has just had her first ultrasound scan. A summary of the ultrasound scan report is given below.

You have 10 minutes in which you should:

- Obtain relevant history from the woman
- Explain the ultrasound scan findings and implications
- Explain the complications that you will recommend monitoring for during her antenatal care
- Ascertain and address the patients concerns
- Agree a plan for her care and the timing of delivery

Summary of Ultrasound Findings

Name: Saadia Mustafa. **Age**: 26 years
Transabdominal ultrasound scan with the patient's verbal consent
Uterus contains two gestational sacs – image attached

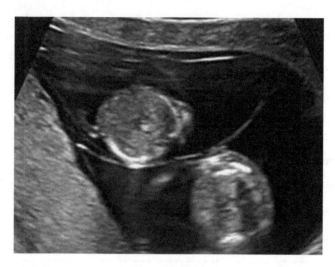

The CRL of twin 1 is 57 mm = 12 weeks, FHR – 156 bpm, with an NT of 1.8 mm = 12
The CRL of twin 2 is 60 mm = 12 + 6 weeks, FHR – 160 bpm, with an NT of 2.0 mm
No obvious abnormality is present at this gestational age
The uterine wall is normal, and there are no adnexal masses
The cervix is long and closed

Simulated Patient's Information

You are a 26-year-old lawyer who is just happy to be pregnant. This is your first pregnancy, and it was conceived after three years of trying. Your periods have always been regular, and the last one was 3 months ago. You have been very sick ever since you missed your period. You had to be admitted twice with excessive vomiting. On both occasions, you were given fluids through a drip and some injections to stop you from vomiting. The vomiting is getting better now. You feel that you have lost some weight since pregnancy. The last time you weighed yourself (which is only a week ago), you were 60 kg. You are 5′6″ tall.

You have been married for 3 years and work in a law firm in the City Center. Your job is not too demanding physically, but you work long hours sitting down. Your husband is also a lawyer but does not work in the same firm. You have been trying for a baby since you got married, and this has caused so much stress in your relationship and the family, and so this has been a very welcoming change. You are both very pleased with the pregnancy.

Your periods are regular, and the last one was 12 weeks ago.

You are one of three children (a sister and a brother). Your aunt has twins, and your sister has identical twins as well. Your brother is still single. Your mother has type II diabetes, and your father has high blood pressure. Both are taking tablets for their illnesses but are otherwise well.

You have nothing of relevance in your past medical or surgical history. You do not smoke and also do not drink alcohol. You were very active prior to pregnancy but have stopped all your exercises because of fear of losing the pregnancy. When you were admitted the second time, you had an ultrasound scan which suspected you might be having twins. This was a quick scan on the ward by the junior doctor who was not very sure.

You have been taking folic acid, which you bought from the chemist, long before you became pregnant and are still taking it. You are not on any other medication and are not aware of any allergies.

If not covered by the candidate, you could ask the following questions:

- What type of twin pregnancy do I have?
- What complications may I have during the pregnancy?
- How will I be monitored?
- I would like to have a test for Down syndrome
- When and how will I be delivered?

A good candidate will cover the following:

Information gathering

- That this was a spontaneous twin pregnancy and there is a family history of multiple pregnancies, family history of diabetes and hypertension
- Previous admissions and treatment for hyperemesis/nausea and vomiting in pregnancy
- Her anxiety about the pregnancy and desire to have aneuploidy screening
- Plans and offers to obtain admission records for review

Communication with patients and family

- Explains the ultrasound report
- Explains the complications associated with monochorionic diamniotic twin pregnancy
- Explains the details of her antenatal care (regular fetal monitoring and the rationale for this – risks of twin-to-twin transfusion, selective FGR, TRAP and TAP sequence and IUD of one twin)

Communication with colleagues

- Demonstrates when to refer to colleagues, e.g. fetal medicine
- Involves specialised clinics, e.g. multiple pregnancy clinics

Patient safety

- Confirms patients identify
- Minimisation of maternal risks (e.g. hypertension and anaemia) and fetal (see above)
- Increased risk of VTE and precautions (patient is now not active, and the job involves sitting down all day)
- Medication – assurance and safety
- Screens for gestational diabetes
- Ascertains drug allergy

Applied clinical knowledge

- Screening for aneuploidy in MC/DA twins
- Details of complications – twin-to-twin transfusion syndrome (TTTS), sIUGR, TRAP, TAPs and PET
- Timing of delivery – will be determined by the presence or the absence of complications
- Place of delivery – should be in a consultant unit with neonatal and anaesthetic facilities
- Evidence of using Green-Top Guideline for the management of MC twin pregnancies

Examiner score sheet		
Information gathering		
Standard not met	Standard partly met	Standard met
0	1	2
Communication with patients and families		
Standard not met	Standard partly met	Standard met
0	1	2
Communication with colleagues		
Standard not met	Standard partly met	Standard met
0	1	2
Patient safety		
Standard not met	Standard partly met	Standard met
0	1	2
Applied clinical knowledge		
Standard not met	Standard partly met	Standard met
0	1	2

Examiner Expectations and Basis for Assessment

Information gathering

- Able to take a concise and relevant antenatal history
- Skilled in signposting and guiding the antenatal consultation
- Able to ensure that the patient understands and encourages questions
- Able to describe to the antenatal patient a clear action plan and the rationale for follow-up based on the discussion

Communication with patients and families

- Able to discuss investigations, monitoring and follow-up and plan for antenatal care monochorionic twin pregnancy
- Able to succinctly summarise discussions with antenatal patients
- Provides information clearly and at a sensible rate, ensuring that the patient/couple understands, and encourages and addresses all questions

---

Communication with colleagues

- Able to communicate with colleagues in other specialties, e.g. fetal medicine (for aneuploidy screening and to monitor the twins), twin pregnancy services, obstetric anaesthetics and midwifery colleagues, including specialist midwives and paediatricians, especially in view of the risk of preterm delivery and if complications arise

---

Patient safety

- Confirms patients identify at the start of the task
- Able to triage the patient to different patterns of antenatal care according to the risk factors, in this case, a high-risk woman with MC/DC twins
- Awareness of safety of investigations and therapeutics during pregnancy, including safe prescribing
- Demonstrates safe prescription after ensuring no drug allergy

---

Applied clinical knowledge

- Knowledge of antenatal care of women with multiple pregnancies
- Knowledgeable of the RCOG Green-top Guidelines on the management of multiple pregnancies and NICE guideline on antenatal care
- Aware of the current literature on antenatal care of multiple pregnancies, including the role of NIPT/NIPD and the timing of delivery

---

Reference: *Management of monochorionic twin pregnancy. The Royal College of Obstetricians and Gynaecologists Green-Top Guideline No. 51. November 2016*

Task 4: Previous Fourth-Degree Perineal Tear. Module 7 – Management of Delivery

Candidate's Instructions

This is a simulated patient task assessing:

- Information gathering
- Communication with patients and family
- Communication with colleagues
- Patient safety
- Applied clinical knowledge

You are an ST5, working with a consultant in the general obstetrics clinic of your hospital. You are in the antenatal clinic and have been called by the midwife to see a patient who has been referred by her GP for counselling at 36 weeks of gestation.

Stanhope Surgery
Stanhope
Basebrough
BS11 8RE

Dear Dr,
Re: Ms Bola Akintunde
I will be grateful if you would be kind enough to see Ms Bola Akintunde, a 33-year-old staff nurse in her second pregnancy, for counselling about the mode of delivery. She had her first child 3 years ago in London and sustained a fourth-degree perineal tear. She will like to review her options for this pregnancy.

Yours sincerely

Dr Hasan Ghassan MBBS, MRCP

You have 10 minutes in which you should:

- Take a focused history
- Counsel the patient
- Answer any questions she may have

Simulated Patient's Information

You are Ms Bola Akintunde, a 33-year-old staff nurse, who works on the Male Adult Ward. You have a 3-year-old daughter, who is very well. You live with your partner Biodun, who is a 40-year-old GP in your own house.

You came today to discuss the birth of your pregnancy. You are now 34 weeks, and the pregnancy has so far been uncomplicated. Your last delivery, which was in another hospital, was, however, very difficult, which is why you are here today.

You went past your due dates and were induced with prostaglandin pessaries. You think you laboured for more than a day, but your records show that you were in labour only for 10 hours. You had three pessaries after which the baby's waters were broken, and then a drip of oxytocin was put up 4 hours later. You then progressed to fully 6 hours later, having had an epidural. The baby was all the time in good condition as she was monitored continuously. When you were fully, you were told to wait until the baby's head was down enough for you to start pushing. After 3 hours, you started pushing. You did your very best, and eventually your daughter was delivered. She weighed 3,500 g.

After the placenta was delivered, the midwife examined you and then called the doctor. He examined you and said you had a tear which needed to be repaired in the theatre. As you had a working epidural, it was repaired without any additional pain killers. This took a very long time and after, you were informed that you had sustained a fourth-degree tear. You were then given some antibiotics and something to soften your stools. You went home after 4 days and came back for a follow-up after 6 weeks.

When you came for follow-up, you were examined and given the all-clear. You have not had any problems, and sexual intercourse is not painful or uncomfortable. You do not suffer from any leakage of flatus (gas), urine or faeces. You are well and not on any medication. You do not have any known allergies.

You are, however, very frightened of a repeat experience although you have been told to go for another vaginal birth and would therefore like to discuss your options.

If not covered, you may wish to ask the candidate the following questions:

- What are the chances of this type of tear happening again?
- This baby seems bigger than my daughter, and I am not sure it would be wise for me to have a vaginal delivery.
- Would you recommend a CS?
- What steps will be taken to reduce the chances of this happening again if I were to try for a vaginal delivery?

A good candidate will cover the following:

Information gathering

- Takes a good history about the events that led to the tear
- Obtains information about the asymptomatic repaired fourth-degree tear
- Requests delivery record from previous hospital and review to appreciate the difficulties experienced with the delivery
- Be able to appreciate the concerns of the patient and doubts about the mode of delivery

Communication with patients and families

- Demonstrates an understanding of the anxieties of the patient
- Discusses the pros and cons of vaginal versus CS – counsel in an unbiased way using evidence, e.g. that there is no evidence for not allowing women like her to undergo either a vaginal delivery or a CS
- Allows the woman to use the information provided in an unbiased manner to make an informed decision

Communication with colleagues

- Discusses referral to expert for review if she needs more reassurance and plan of care
- Involves consultant in counselling and conformation of the decision on management
- Involves one of the most skilled midwives in planned intrapartum care

Patient safety

- Confirms patients identity
- Listens to the concerns with empathy and ensures the woman feels she is the one making choices
- Empowers the woman to make choices
- Discusses the risks of CS versus vaginal delivery
- Delivery to be conducted by a skilled midwife
- Ascertains drug allergy and demonstrates safe prescription

Applied clinical knowledge

- Risk factors do not allow for accurate prediction of OASIS
- Baby's size will be reviewed after an ultrasound scan at 37–38 weeks to gauge fetal size
- No convincing evidence that episiotomy offers protection
- Warm compression during the second stage reduces the risk of OASIS
- Perineal protection at crowning can be protective
- Instrumental delivery is associated with an increased risk
- If had endo-anal ultrasonography with abnormality or symptomatic, CS would be considered as an option

Examiner score sheet		
Information gathering		
Standard not met	Standard partly met	Standard met
0	1	2
Communication with patients and families		
Standard not met	Standard partly met	Standard met
0	1	2
Communication with colleagues		
Standard not met	Standard partly met	Standard met
0	1	2
Patient safety		
Standard not met	Standard partly met	Standard met
0	1	2
Applied clinical knowledge		
Standard not met	Standard partly met	Standard met
0	1	2

Examiner Expectations and Basis for Assessment

Information gathering

- Obtains information from patients or clinical notes (including the partogram, CTG and maternal vital signs), and uses these to formulate a clear clinical picture of the patient
- Able to describe a clear action plan and rationale for decisions made based on discussions with the patient

Communication with patients and families

- Able to communicate to the woman and her partner and/or the family the interventions for abnormal labour and instrumental or operative delivery
- Able to explain the risks and benefits of interventions for both the mother and the fetus

Communication with colleagues

- Understands the limits of one's own competence and thus knows when to call for senior help or involve other specialties
- Provides appropriate amount of details (a clear and agreed plan of intrapartum care) is documented in notes to ensure management plans are clear and easily understood by the colleagues
- Considers referring to specialised antenatal clinic for women with perineal injuries if there is one

Patient safety

- Confirms the patients identify at the beginning of the task
- Awareness of patient safety in labour in different environments, e.g. water birth and birthing outside the hospital – may have to discuss if the patient asks
- Understanding the risks from interventions such as regional analgesia and operative deliveries (if indicated) on the perineum
- Ability to critically appraise adverse events

Applied clinical knowledge

- Knowledge of the current literature on intrapartum care, including the induction of labour, management of normal and abnormal labour and obstetric interventions in relation to the prevention of severe perineal trauma during labour
- Familiar with the RCOG and NICE guidelines on intrapartum care and care of the perineum

Reference: The Management of Third-and Fourth-Degree Perineal Tears. The Royal College of Obstetricians and Gynaecologists Green-Top Guideline No. 29. June 2015

Task 5: Urinary Retention Postpartum. Module 8 – Postpartum Problems (the Puerperium)

Candidate's Instructions

This is a simulated patient task covering:

- Information gathering
- Communication with patients and families
- Patient safety
- Communication with colleagues
- Applied clinical knowledge

You are the ST5 running a postnatal clinic in the hospital. The patient you are about to see next was referred by the GP. The letter from the GP is given below.

Sterling Road Surgery
Drubridge
West Midlands
DR7 9LB

Dear Dr,
I would be grateful if you could see Mrs Kitty Simonds, a 30-year-old housewife, who had a ventouse delivery 6 weeks ago for failure to progress in the second stage. She saw the midwife at the surgery today and complained of dribbling urine and not feeling any sensation to void. When I examined her, I found a mass in the lower abdomen.
Her infant is doing very well, and she is breastfeeding.

Yours sincerely

Dr James Scraft MBBS, MRCGP, DCH

You have 10 minutes in which you should:

- Obtain relevant history
- Discuss investigations
- Explain the possible causes of the problems
- Discuss an agreed management plan
- Answer any questions the patient may have

Simulated Patient's Information

You are Mrs Kitty Simonds, a 30-year-old housewife. You delivered your daughter 6 weeks ago and were discharged home 2 days after delivery. You had an uncomplicated pregnancy and went into spontaneous labour at 41 weeks. You had an epidural, and after labouring for 10 hours, you were asked to push. You had been fully for 2 hours. You pushed for 30 minutes, and your daughter was not coming out. You were very tired, and the doctor came and helped with a forceps. You had a cut which was repaired. You were a bit swollen down below and struggled to walk straight for a few days. You were encouraged to mobilise, and every time you passed urine it was painful. Once you got home, the pain gradually got better, and you are now completely pain free. You realised that you could only pass small amounts of wee (urine) every time you went and, over the last week, you have been wetting yourself. You also feel that your tummy has not gone down; if anything it's getting bigger. The midwife asked the doctor to see you, and he asked you to come to the hospital clinic today.

You do not have any temperature, and there are no pains when you pass urine. You do not have any abnormal vaginal discharge or bleeding. You are breastfeeding exclusively.

You have had no problems with your waterworks in the past.

You live with your husband, who is an accountant, and although you are also an accountant, you are on maternity leave. You do not smoke but drink occasionally.

You have no other medical or surgical problems and have no known allergies.

If not covered by the candidate, you should ask the following:

- Why am I dribbling urine?
- What tests will you undertake to find out?
- How will you treat me?
- Do I have to stay in the hospital?
- Will this affect my chances of having another baby?
- Is there a permanent injury to my waterworks?
- Should I not have a caesarean section next time?
- Are there any drugs I can take, and will these affect breastfeeding or my baby?

A good candidate will cover the following:

Information gathering

- What form of analgesia did she have – epidural or not?
- Was she catheterised after delivery, and if so, for how long?
- Any perineal trauma and repair?
- Previous bladder problems?
- History of pelvic pathology – USS in pregnancy etc.
- Examination – abdominal and pelvic
- Investigations
  - Catheter specimen of urine/MSU for urinalysis
  - MSU – culture and sensitivity – if positive urinalysis
  - Ultrasound scan of the bladder and pelvis

Communication with patients and families

- Discusses the possible causes of the leakage of urine
- Explains the investigations and management plans
- Discusses the long-term implications
- Ascertains her anxieties and addresses them
- Offers pelvic floor exercises
- Counsels on early symptoms of infections
- Educates patient on catheter care if she is to go home with one

Communication with colleagues

- Liaising with other specialties, e.g. physiotherapy and urogynaecologist
- Referral to seniors for management
- Feedback to the GP

Patient safety

- Establishes patient's identity at start of task
- Chaperones at examination
- Assures her of the implications for the next pregnancy
- Allays anxieties about delivery and CS
- If any drugs used, assures of safety with regard to breastfeeding and the baby

Applied clinical knowledge

- Empty the bladder at initial assessment
- Indwell catheter for at least 24–48 hours
- Remove only when residual is <150 ml (some guidelines/units may use 100 mls rather than 150ml)
- If residual >150, keep indwelling and allow home or offer intermittent catheterisation
- Consider drugs to improve bladder tone, e.g. cholinergics
- Offer physiotherapy and training by incontinence adviser
- Loss of bladder compliance
- Increased frequency of micturition

Examiner score sheet		
Information gathering		
Standard not met	Standard partly met	Standard met
0	1	2
Communication with patients and families		
Standard not met	Standard partly met	Standard met
0	1	2
Communication with colleagues		
Standard not met	Standard partly met	Standard met
0	1	2
Patient safety		
Standard not met	Standard partly met	Standard met
0	1	2
Applied clinical knowledge		
Standard not met	Standard partly met	Standard met
0	1	2

Examiner Expectations and Basis for Assessment

Information gathering

- Able to take concise and relevant postnatal history
- Skilled in signposting and building the postnatal consultation
- Ensure patient understanding and encouraging questions
- Able to succinctly summarise discussions with the postnatal patient

---

Communication with patients and families

- Able to describe to the postnatal patient a clear action plan and the rationale for follow-up based on the discussion
- Able to educate the patient on bladder and catheter care if the patient is to go home on a catheter

---

Communication with colleagues

- Able to communicate with colleagues in primary care and other specialties, e.g. General Practitioner and community nurse, urogynaecologists and physiotherapists
- Clear agreed management pathway detailed in her notes and in communication to GP

Patient safety

- Confirms patients identify at the start of the task
- Awareness of safety investigations and therapeutics during the postnatal period
- Able to discuss the risks of chronic urinary retention on bladder function, including the risk of infections
- Understanding the psychological impact of managing chronic retention on the mother and possibly on her baby
- Ensuring that adequate support is available, including the provision of information leaflets

Task 6: Labour Ward Prioritisation. Module 6 – Management of Labour

Candidate's Instructions

This is a structured discussion task assessing:

- Information gathering
- Communication with patients and families
- Communication with colleagues
- Patient safety
- Applied clinical knowledge

You are the Specialist Trainee 5 on call on the delivery suite. You have just arrived for handover at 0830.

Attached, you will find a brief resume of the eight women on the delivery suite, as shown on the board.

The staff who are available today are as follows – an obstetrics ST1 (Specialist Trainee 1) in her fourth month of GP training, a fifth-year Specialist Anaesthetic Trainee and a consultant on call, who is not yet available on the unit.

Six midwives: MD in charge; BK, ON & NN can suture episiotomies; AR, PK & LM can insert IV lines; and MW is a midwife in the Alongside Midwifery Unit.

You have 10 minutes to study the board carefully and decide and discuss with the examiner what tasks need to be done, in which order they should be done and who should be allocated to each task.

Delivery Suite Board

Room No	Name	Parity	Gestation	Liquor	Epidural	Oxytocinon	Comments	Staff/ MW
1	PNM	1^{+1}	32^{+3}	-	Yes	Yes	LSCS@0100 for PET. EBL 800 ml. Baby in NICU	BK
2	CO	2^{+0}	T^{+9}	Meconium	Yes	Yes	7 cm@0300/ Low-risk midwifery care	MW
3	JB	0^{+0}	39^{+0}	Intact M	No	No	Undiagnosed breech, spontaneous labour, 4 cm@0730	PK
4	RT	0^{+0}	28^{+4}	-			Dr to See. Abdominal pain. CTG Normal	NN

5	AAB	0+0	41+0	Meconium	Yes		Fully @0700	AR
6	STB	1+0	T+2	Clear	No	No	Trial of labour after CS. ARM@0300. FBS@0600, pH 7.29, BE-3 mEQ/L, 6 cm	AR
7	MR	2+0	39+0	Intact	No	No	Routine admission for ELLSCS	ON
8	JSB	0+0	39+6				Delivered, awaiting suturing	LM

A good candidate will cover the tasks that are detailed in the table below.

Room No	Task	Delegate	Order
1	Review – blood pressure pulse, urine output and pain control. Check blood for platelets, liver function test, urea and electrolytes and coagulation	Specialist anaesthetist	4
2	Review CTG; needs vaginal examination	ST5/midwife	3
3	Review and counsel about the mode of delivery – place on CTG, offer CS and consent, IV line, group and safe and the anaesthetist to review	ST5	2
4	History and examination; review notes, especially with reference to the location of the placenta and blood group; if bleeding significant, FBC (full blood count), group and safe and IV line and CTG	ST1 to take history and take blood	5
5	Review CTG, and if ther is any urge to push, inform the paediatrician (if not already informed)	Midwife	6
6	Review CTG – fetal heart rate contractions and exclude any pains	ST5	1
7	Admit, check consent and appropriate investigations, has she been reviewed by the anaesthetist?	ST1	8
8	Check if there is bleeding, and review the vital signs	Midwife	7

Tips for the Candidate at This Station

1. Do not read the information for each room loud to the examiner
2. Where the action is urgent, if the consultant is around, it should be either yourself or the consultant
3. For each room, think thoroughly and logically – history, examination, investigations (including CTG and FBS) and the decision of delivery
4. Cannulation for high-risk women (e.g. VBAC, grand multipara, obese, twins, previous PPH, polyhydramnios and anaemia, for CS)
5. Dr to see – is either the junior trainee, yourself or the consultant
6. Inform the paediatrician if meconium, preterm or abnormal CTG or emergency CS occurs
7. Prepare the patient for CS is by the midwife

Examiner score sheet		
Information gathering		
Standard not met	Standard partly met	Standard met
0	1	2
Communication with patients and families		
Standard not met	Standard partly met	Standard met
0	1	2
Communication with colleagues		
Standard not met	Standard partly met	Standard met
0	1	2
Patient safety		
Standard not met	Standard partly met	Standard met
0	1	2
Applied clinical knowledge		
Standard not met	Standard partly met	Standard met
0	1	2

Examiner Expectations and Basis for Assessment

Information gathering

- Obtains information from patients or clinical notes (including the partogram, CTG and maternal vital signs) and use these to formulate a clear clinical picture of the patient
- Able to describe a clear action plan and rationale for decisions made based on discussions with the patient

Communication with patients and families

- Able to communicate to the woman and her partner and/or family the interventions for abnormal labour and instrumental or operative delivery
- Able to explain the risks and benefits of interventions, for both the mother and the fetus

Communication with colleagues

- The ability to give a clear reason for the interaction with colleagues, e.g. handover
- Able to prioritise cases appropriately as urgent, semi-urgent and non-urgent cases
- Able to delegate tasks appropriately
- Understands the limits of one's own competence and knows when to call for senior help or involve other specialties
- Able to form a logical differential diagnosis for intrapartum complication and to be able to convey that to colleagues, including when the consultant is off-site
- Provide an appropriate amount of details to ensure management plans are clear and easily understood by colleagues
- Team working to support colleagues during peaks of activities on the labour ward
- Able to teach appropriate skills to other colleagues in a logical and coherent manner, with recognition of the learner's environment and resources available

Patient safety

- Aware of patient safety in labour in different environments, e.g. water birth and birthing outside hospital
- Understands the risks from interventions such as regional analgesia, therapeutics in labour and invasive procedures
- Appropriate use of chaperone for intimate examinations
- Able to maintain patient dignity at all times
- Accurately prescribes during labour including management of intravenous infusions
- Acknowledges medical errors, poor care or omissions and apologises as appropriate
- Understands risk management and clinical governance processes in relation to intrapartum care
- Able to critically appraise adverse events

Applied clinical knowledge

- Knowledge of intrapartum care, including induction of labour, management of normal and abnormal labour and obstetric interventions the interpretation of CTG
- Able to critically appraise the literature including guidelines, protocols and scientific papers
- Able to think and work under pressure, with competing priorities, when the workload on the labour ward is heavy
- Has working knowledge of the roles of other members of the multidisciplinary team

---

Task 7: Contraception in an 18-Year-Old with Learning Disabilities. Module 11 – Sexual and Reproductive Health

Candidate's Instructions

This is a structured discussion assessing:

- Information gathering
- Communication with patients and families
- Communication with colleagues
- Patient safety
- Applied clinical knowledge

You are an ST5 with your consultant in the clinic. He has asked you to review a letter from the GP and come and discuss the patient with him. The examiner has four questions to structure the discussion around the management of the patient.

The letter from the GP is given below.

The Hillton-on-Lyme Surgery
Hillton-on-Lyme
Sutherfield Road
HL8P34

Dear Mr Staycliffe,
Re: Miss Yvonne Sutherland aged 18 years
I would be grateful if you could see this 18-year-old who came to see me with her caregiver requesting contraception. She has learning disabilities, and the caregiver was very insistent that I prescribe contraception for her. I did not feel competent to deal with this and hope that you would be able to provide appropriate advice and recommendation.

Yours sincerely

Dr Claire Thorpe MBBS, MRCGP, DRCOG

You have 10 minutes in which you should:

- Take a focused history
- Discuss her contraceptive needs
- Answer any questions that may arise from the consultation

Examiner's Instructions

Familiarise yourself with the candidate's instructions and use the questions below to structure a discussion on the management of the patient. You should guide the candidate with respect to time management.

1. What information will you seek prior to initiating discussions on contraception?
2. What would be the basis for offering contraception to this patient?
3. What steps will you take to ensure that you are able to offer contraception to her?
4. What options will you consider?

A good candidate should cover the following:

What information will you seek prior to initiating a discussion on contraception?

- What is the learning disability, and what is the severity of this? Who is in the position of *locus parentis* (parent or relative or another person – e.g. parent and foster carer)
- Establish a level of understanding by the patient (capacity)
- Why the request for contraception – from herself or caregiver?
- Is she in a relationship, has been in one before, or has the potential to be in one?
- Menstrual cycle including LMP
- Sexual history – sexually active in a relationship? Any previous pregnancies
- Previous contraceptive use
- Current medication and allergy
- Medical and surgical history, especially related to contraindications
- Examination – weight, assess the level of understanding and check BP

What would be the basis for offering contraception?

- There is an obvious indication – it should be in the interest of the patient
- To regulate menstrual problems or prevent unwanted pregnancies
- If her health is at risk or if she gets pregnant
- If she is at risk of STIs as well as unwanted pregnancy

What steps will you take to ensure that you are able to offer her contraception?

- Ascertain ability to consent and ensure compliance with the Mental Capacity Act, which states that 'doctors have a legal duty to consult a range of people when determining the best interest of a person who lacks capacity'
- If not, seek legal support for decision/refer for assessment of mental ability to consent (e.g. by a psychiatrist)
- Refer to a senior colleague and possibly a Family Planning consultant
- Multidisciplinary team (physician, GP, social worker and carer including Mental Health Team)

What options will you consider?

- Explanation of the types of contraception and complications to both the patient and the mother (caregiver)
- Choice will depend on the ability to comply – LARC most suitable
- Choice has to be determined by several factors from her history, including her level of disability (ease of administration and ability to remember – compliance and side effects)
- LARC – best option – levonorgestrel (if period problems), subdermal implants or copper IUD
- Depot preparation need three monthly injections and may not be easy to administer

Examiner score sheet		
Information gathering		
Standard not met	Standard partly met	Standard met
0	1	2
Communication with patients and families		
Standard not met	Standard partly met	Standard met
0	1	2
Communication with colleagues		
Standard not met	Standard partly met	Standard met
0	1	2
Patient safety		
Standard not met	Standard partly met	Standard met
0	1	2
Applied clinical knowledge		
Standard not met	Standard partly met	Standard met
0	1	2

Examiner Expectations and Basis for Assessment

Information gathering

- Takes good history on the rationale for the request, menstrual history, previous contraception use, sexual history and previous pregnancies
- Defines the degree of learning disability
- Ascertains who is making the request for contraception
- Excludes contraindications to the various options
- Offers to examine and undertake any appropriate investigations, including the involvement of experts to assess mental capacity

---

Communication with patients and families

- Liaises with a caretaker or the family on the reason behind the request
- Demonstrates empathy, concern and respect for the caregiver/parent as well as the patient
- Clearly explains the process of deciding the choice of contraception to patient and caregiver/parent

---

Communication with colleagues

- Able to liaise with a consultant for a decision where appropriate
- Links up with the Mental Health Team to evaluate and assess the mental capacity of the patient
- Involves multidisciplinary team (consultant, social worker, General Practitioner, caregiver/parents, Mental Health Team)

Patient safety

- Discusses the side effects of the various options
- Ensures no contraindications to a chosen method
- Demonstrates an understanding of safe prescription in relation to drug interactions (interactions of drugs patient is with chosen contraception)
- Ascertains drug allergy and how this allows for safe prescription

---

Applied clinical knowledge

- Demonstrates an understanding of the UKMEC for contraception
- Familiar with NICE guidelines on LARC
- Familiar with the Mental Health Act and capacity for treatment (informed consent)
- Demonstrates familiarity with current literature on the treatment of women with learning disabilities

Task 8: Missed Miscarriage and Recurrent Pregnancy Loss. Module 12 – Early Pregnancy Care

Candidate's Instructions

This is a patient simulated task covering:

- Information gathering
- Communication with patients and families
- Communication with colleagues
- Patient safety
- Applied clinical knowledge

You are an ST5 covering the Early Pregnancy Assessment Unit. You are about to see your next patient, who was referred by the GP for evaluation in the Early Pregnancy Assessment Unit of your hospital. The details of the referral are given below.

The Blasfield Surgery
Cutton
Soutfield
SF16 7PB

Dear Dr,
Re: Gemma Splitz – Age 25 years
Please kindly see Gemma Splitz, a 25-year-old, who called in today complaining of a brownish vaginal discharge and not feeling pregnancy symptoms again. A urine pregnancy test taken today has come positive.

Yours sincerely

Dr Gabriel Ntumfon MD, MRCGP

You have 10 minutes in which you should:

- Take a focused history
- Discuss management
- Answer any questions the patient may have

Simulated Patient's Information

You are Gemma Splitz, a 25-year-old support worker, living with your boyfriend in a rented apartment in the city. You smoke about three to five cigarettes per day and drink alcohol socially.

Your last menstrual period was 8 weeks ago. You were not planning to become pregnant but were very thrilled when you found out about the pregnancy. Your partner is unsure at this time, but you feel that he will come round. You were feeling very sick, and your breasts were very sensitive; however, over the last 1 week, the sickness has stopped, and your breasts are no longer sore and tender. You were not worried until this morning when you had a brownish discharge. You panicked and went to the doctor who sent you in. You have neither had any bright red vaginal loss nor pain in your tummy. You are still having sexual intercourse with your partner. Since finding out that you are pregnant, you have been taking folic acid and have cut down on your smoking and alcohol.

Your last period was 8 weeks ago. Your periods were very regular, and you have never used any form of contraception. Your partner used condoms from time to time when it felt unsafe.

You have been pregnant twice and lost both at 7 and 10 weeks respectively. The first was called a missed miscarriage (you had no symptoms and was told this when you came for your first scan). You were told the baby had died around 6 weeks. For the second one, you started with bleeding associated with severe pains and then everything just came out. You were seen in the hospital, and a scan was done, which showed that you had had a complete miscarriage. This was 4 years ago with another partner. Your current partner does not know about these miscarriages.

You have no other medical problems and are not on any medications other than folic acid. You have no known allergies.

If not asked, you should consider asking the following questions:

- Why did I have the brownish discharge?
- What investigations will you order on me, especially that this is my third miscarriage?
- How will you treat me?
- Will this happen again?
- Is there anything I can do to minimise the recurrence of this condition?
- What treatment should I have?

A good candidate should cover the following:

Information gathering

- Obtains good history, highlighting the nature of the miscarriage – recurrent
- Requests for notes to be reviewed
- Starts investigations, including pregnancy test, ultrasound scan and full blood count (FBC)

Figure 12.1 will be shown to the candidate by the examiner when he/she mentions an ultrasound scan as an investigation.

There is an irregular gestational sac measuring 25 × 29 mm, with no obvious fetal pole or yolk sac.

Communication with patients and families

- Informs the patient of the ultrasound findings – breaking bad news (follows the principles)
- Explains the management options (expectant, medical and surgical) – pros and cons including details, how long it will take to complete and the complications (will it require inpatient care or outpatient?); what is the follow-up associated with each option
- Discusses the investigations for recurrent miscarriages
- Offers follow-up in an appropriate clinic for investigations

Communication with colleagues

- Liaises with an anaesthetist for surgical management
- Involves other disciplines for investigations – histopathology/cytogenetics of products of conception
- Referral to a specialist clinic such as the Recurrent Miscarriage Clinic
- Writing to the GP after the discharge from the hospital

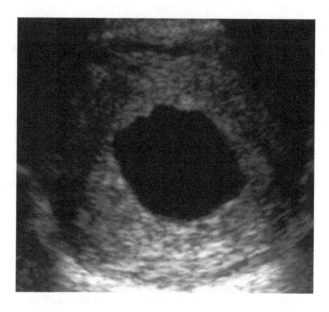

Figure 12.1   Ultrasound scan image

Patient safety

- Confirms patients identify prior to starting the task and ensures the report belongs to the patient
- Empowers patient to make an informed choice
- Safe prescription and follow-up depending on the management option
- Establishes no allergies to medications
- Ensures confidentiality of the information disclosed about the miscarriages (assures the patient that these will be confidential)

Applied clinical knowledge

- Using NICE and RCOG guidelines to make decisions about the management

Examiner score sheet		
Information gathering		
Standard not met	Standard partly met	Standard met
0	1	2
Communication with patients and families		
Standard not met	Standard partly met	Standard met
0	1	2

Communication with colleagues		
Standard not met	Standard partly met	Standard met
0	1	2
Patient safety		
Standard not met	Standard partly met	Standard met
0	1	2
Applied clinical knowledge		
Standard not met	Standard partly met	Standard met
0	1	2

Examiner Expectations and Basis for Assessment

Information gathering

• Takes a comprehensive history about the pregnancy
• Requests appropriate investigations and interpret results – ultrasound findings

Communication with patients and families

• Breaks bad news appropriately
• Demonstrates an empathic approach to counsel the patient about the failed pregnancy
• Demonstrates an empathic approach to describing clearly the logical approach to different management options (pros and cons), including complications and rationale for care and follow-up
• Maintains (assures) confidentiality of information given
• Summarises discussions about diagnosis succinctly, and checks patient's understanding at appropriate intervals
• Provides contact numbers of support groups/associations and Early Pregnancy Assessment Unit and counsellor

Communication with colleagues

• Able to prioritise cases appropriately – the ability to link up with colleagues
• Able to describe the differential diagnosis and formulate an appropriate management plan, including referral to a specialised clinic, e.g. the Recurrent Miscarriage Clinic
• Feedback to the GP after the discharge from the hospital

Patient safety

- Confirms patients identify at the start of the task
- Safe prescription of medical options for managing miscarriage – asking about allergies and medical disorders that could be considered contraindications to the medications for medical management of miscarriage
- Knowledge of the principles of safe surgery if surgery is the chosen option for the patient
- Informs the risks of various management options and mitigation
- Appropriate recognition and dealing with special circumstances, e.g. Jehovah Witnesses

---

Applied clinical knowledge

- Has an understanding of the knowledge and complications of early pregnancy in terms of explaining diagnosis and management options
- Use of various information leaflets, e.g. RCOG and Miscarriage Association
- An understanding of the contents of NICE/RCOG guidelines, with regard to management, follow-up and recurrence rate, including management in subsequent pregnancies following a miscarriage

---

Reference: Ectopic pregnancy and miscarriage: diagnosis and initial management. NICE Clinical Guideline CG154 December 2012

Task 9: Primary Amenorrhoea. Module 9 – Gynaecological Problems

Candidate's Instructions

This is a simulated patient task covering:

- Information gathering
- Communication with patient and family
- Communication with colleagues
- Patient safety
- Applied clinical knowledge

You are the ST5 in the gynaecology clinic, working alongside your consultant Mr Thompson. Your next patient is coming for her first appointment, having been referred by the GP. The referral letter is given below.

Grange Farm Surgery
Tamford Heath
Salford
SF2 9TT

Dear Mr Thompson FRCOG,
Would you be kind enough to see Miss Gail Swanson, who is 18 years old and complains that she is yet to have periods? She has a sister who had periods at a much younger age. I did a hormone

profile as well as karyotype and the results are TSH = 1.73 mIU/L, FT4 = 14.5 pmol/L, FSH = 22.7 IU/L, LH = 28.6 IU/L, SHBG <55 mmol/L, Testosterone = 1.2 nmol/L; karyotype = 46XY.

Yours sincerely

Dr Joythi Kaur MBBS, MRCGP, DRCOG, DFFP

You have 10 minutes in which you will:

- Obtain a relevant and focused history
- Discuss the investigations you will order
- Explain the results of any investigations (the examiner will show you some)
- Discuss the management of the patient having explained what the diagnosis is

Simulated Patient's Information

You are Miss Gail Swanson, an 18-year-old university student studying biochemistry. This is your first year at the university. You live in university accommodation with other students that you met on the day of registration. You are in the first term of the year. You do not smoke but drink with your friends.

You have a boyfriend who also studies in the same university. You have known him for 1 year, and you are sexually active. He uses the condom as you do not want to get pregnant.

Your breast started developing when you were 10 years old, and shortly after you started growing hair under your armpit and also in your pubis. You were surprised not to have had a period up to now. Your mother said you ought to have had a period by now though her sister had the same problem and has never had a child although she is married.

You do not suffer from excessive hair growth, and your voice is normal. You do not have any discharge from your breasts. Your weight has remained stable over the last few years. You consciously try to keep your weight to around 63 kg. You are 1.6 m tall.

You do not suffer from headaches or problems with your eyesight.

You have no other problems, and your friends are the ones that made you go to your GP.

You have a sister who is 16 years old. She started having periods when she was 12 years old. Your auntie says that she has never had periods, and she is married but has never been pregnant.

You have no allergies, no medical problems and have not been on any medication for as long as you remember.

If not covered, you should ask the following questions:

- What do you think may be wrong with me?
- Are there any tests you will like me to do?
- What will you do to make me have periods?
- Will I be able to have children?
- Does this problem have any long-term effects on my health?

A good candidate will cover the following:

Information gathering

- Obtains detailed history about her symptoms – to exclude possible causes; sexual history, especially asking after dyspareunia
- Explains that a physical examination will have to be performed (the examiner will provide information on the physical examination findings – phenotypically female, well-developed breast, pubic hair – scanty or not – and normal vulva and vagina which ends blindly)
- Discusses the investigations to be undertaken (biochemical and imaging)
- Ascertains family history
- Obtains history about anxieties with periods and children

Communication with patients and family

- Explains the examination – general, breast, abdomen and pelvis/vaginal
- Investigations – biochemical and ultrasound/MRI
- Explains the diagnosis of androgen insensitivity syndrome (AIS)
- Discusses the management
- Explains the long-term implications – menstruation, fertility and HRT following surgery

Patient safety

- Confirms patients identify at the start of the task
- Empowers the patient to make informed choices about treatment options
- Explains why gonads have to be removed
- Ascertains drug allergy

Communication with colleagues

- Referral to an expert on paediatric and adolescent gynaecology or malformations of the genital tract
- Referral to geneticists and clinical psychologist
- MDT meeting

Applied clinical knowledge

- Discusses treatment options – gonadectomy and HRT
- Explains genetic basis of diagnosis and possible family history
- Offers family screening – patterns of inheritable
- Explains the rationale for the removal of gonads and why amenorrhoeic

Examiner score sheet		
Information gathering		
Standard not met	Standard partly met	Standard met
0	1	2
Communication with patients and families		
Standard not met	Standard partly met	Standard met
0	1	2

Communication with colleagues		
Standard not met	Standard partly met	Standard met
0	1	2
Patient safety		
Standard not met	Standard partly met	Standard met
0	1	2
Applied clinical knowledge		
Standard not met	Standard partly met	Standard met
0	1	2

Examiner Expectations and Basis for Assessment

Information gathering

- Able to obtain a detailed history of the presenting symptom of amenorrhoea
- A logical approach to a clear, reasoned style of questioning
- Able to present appropriate investigations and interpret results in order to develop a clear management plan and rationale for follow-up
- Able to summarise discussions succinctly and checks the patient's understanding at appropriate intervals

Communication with patients and families

- Gives information sensitively at appropriate intervals, ensuring understanding regarding investigations, diagnosis and management of primary amenorrhoea
- Describes a clear and logical action and rationale for follow-up
- Explains hormone results clearly

Communication with colleagues

- Demonstrates an ability to involve other specialties (clinical genetics, clinical psychologist, paediatric and adolescent gynaecologist)
- Describes the differential diagnoses and formulates an appropriate management plan
- Provides feedback to the GP after consultation about investigations, diagnosis and recommended treatment

---

Patient safety

- Confirms patients identify at the start of the task
- Understands the limits of their clinical abilities and when to call for help and involve senior colleagues and other disciplines
- Understands safe prescription, having established allergy in this woman with primary amenorrhoea

---

Applied clinical knowledge

- Knowledge of causes, investigations and treatment of primary amenorrhoea
- Able to critically appraise current medical literature on treatment options for primary amenorrhoea with structural abnormalities
- Understands the role of imaging in the investigation/management of primary amenorrhoea
- Understands referral pathways – reproductive medicine, counsellors, geneticists, clinical psychologist, paediatric and adolescent gynaecology in managing androgen insensitivity
- Able to present management options and their risks and benefits using non-directional counselling

---

Task 10: Anovulatory Infertility. Module 10 – Subfertility

Candidate's Instructions

This is a stimulated patient task assessing the following clinical skills:

- Information gathering
- Communication with patients and families
- Communication with colleagues
- Patient safety
- Applied clinical knowledge

You are an ST5 who is about to see Ms Adegoke, a 30-year-old engineer, attending the gynaecology clinic with a 3-year history of failure to conceive. Ms Adegoke had been to the clinic before with her partner John (a 28-year-old teacher), and various investigations were ordered. She is coming back to discuss the results and management. You have been informed that her notes are not available for the clinic, but the clerks were able to print copies of the results of the investigations for you.

Results of investigations

Semen analysis of John Wigglesworth, Age 28 years (partner of Ms Bola Adegoke)
Produced at 0900 and received at 0945
Volume = 3 ml
Concentration = 25 × 10^6/ml
Total count = 75 × 10^6
Motility = 40%
Normal morphology = 25%
White cell count = 0.5 × 10^6/ml
Progression
1 – 10%
2 – 10%
3 – 30%
4 – 60%
pH = 7.46
Investigations on Ms Adegoke
Follicular phase biochemistry
FSH = 8.7 iu/L (normal 3–10 iu/L)
LH = 10.5 iu/L 10 (normal 2–8 iu/L)
Testosterone – 1.4 nmol/L
Prolactin = 654 miu/L (normal 0–400 miu/L)
Sex hormone–binding globulin = 46 nmol/L (normal 40–120 nmol/L)
21-day progesterone 15 iu/L (non-ovulatory <10 nmol/L, pre-ovulatory 10–30 nmol/L, and ovulatory >30 nmol/L)
Free androgen index (FAI) = 3.1% (normal 5–25%)

You have 10 minutes to:

1. Obtain a brief, targeted clinical and fertility history
2. Explain the likely cause of the couple's subfertility
3. Establish the issues involved in the management of this couple and discuss them sensitively

Simulated Patient's Information

Ms Bola Adegoke, Age: 30 years
No 5b Haven Gardens
Stafford ST2 6BD

You are Ms Bola Adegoke, a 30-year-old engineer who has been living with your partner John Wigglesworth (a 28-year-old secondary school teacher) for the past 4 years. You have not been using any form of contraception but have failed to conceive. You have struggled to control your weight and suffer from facial spots. Your weight is 86 kg.

You have sexual intercourse 1–2 times per week and especially around the middle of your irregular cycles, which occur every 26–36 days. You are aware of your fertile period. Your periods started when you were 12 years old and have been irregular since. You do not have any other gynaecological problems.

You have never been pregnant.

You suffer from migraines and intermittent headaches, and from time to time, you have a milky discharge from your breast. Apart from these, you are otherwise well.

You live in a rented terrace two-bed-room house with John. You neither drink alcohol nor smoke, but John drinks alcohol mainly over the weekends and smokes about 10 cigarettes per day. You are not very active but walk to work – about half a mile away from the house. You eat healthy, and your BMI is $30/M^2$ (weight = 86 kg).

Two years ago, you were admitted to the hospital and treated with antibiotics for a chest infection.

Your parents are in Nigeria – your mother is healthy, but your father suffers from high blood pressure. You have four siblings – three brothers and one sister. Your sister has been married for 4 years and has a son. She took about 2 years to get pregnant. None of your brothers is married. John is adopted.

You are currently taking folic acid and are allergic to penicillin (you had breathing difficulties when you had penicillin in the hospital).

If not covered by the candidate, you could ask the following questions:

1. Why do you think I am struggling to get pregnant?
2. What are our options?
3. Of these options, which one would you recommend and why?
4. What should I be doing now?

Acting Requirements

You understand what is being told to you, and you are very obviously disappointed that you need further tests as time is ticking away.

You are worried about your age and worried that you are wasting time with more investigations.

A good candidate will cover the following:

Information gathering

- Obtains appropriate fertility-focused history
- Obtains specific information relevant to possible causes of infertility
- Correctly interprets and explains clearly the investigation results and their implications
- Offers additional investigations (tubal patency test and explains why this is needed)
- Reassures patient that management will not be unnecessarily delayed

Communication with patients and family

- Explains possible reasons for the failure to conceive
- Explores the women's fears and concerns
- Expresses empathy for the situation and the patient's bitter disappointment at the need for further investigations
- Explains the rationale for recommending treatment options
- Conveys suggested management plan and offers hope: recommend weight loss followed by ovulation induction after HSG or laparoscopy if patent tubes are shown. IVF may be an option as the last alternative (estimated costs £3–4K per cycle, less for subsequent cycles if embryos frozen); entitled to one IVF cycle on the NHS
- Encourages and welcomes her partner to attend a consultation in the future

Patient safety

- Confirms patient's identity at the start of the task
- Demonstrates an understanding of the processes and procedures to keep individual patients safe
- Presents the pros and cons of proposed management in a balanced way
- Recognises the limits of their clinical abilities and refers appropriately
- Highlights all governance issues and necessary actions to reduce risks and mishaps in future
- Does not discuss semen analysis results with patient without the express consent of the husband
- Identifies any allergies and demonstrates safe and accurate prescribing techniques

Applied clinical knowledge

- Appreciates how the diagnosis of anovulatory infertility is made, based on family history, history and investigation results
- Demonstrates a sound and comprehensive evidence-based clinical knowledge
- Interprets and explains the clinical findings accurately
- Justifies investigations and management options, and demonstrates a rationale for each
- Synthesises a comprehensive and well-organised management plan, based on the history and investigations and taking into consideration the various factors

---

Task Synopsis

- Most likely anovulatory infertility with PCOS is the likely culprit although hyperprolactinaemia cannot be excluded
- Breaking bad news in the context of having to do more investigations
- Explain possible options – but these are less likely to be successful (NICE recommends IVF)

The competent ST5 candidate will discuss and mention many of the following:

- Pathway for managing couples with anovulatory infertility, based on NICE recommendations
- Understands that although this is a cause, a tubal factor also has to be excluded before treatment is initiated – hence the need for an HSG or diagnostic laparoscopy, depending on the assessment of pros and cons of one versus the other – in this obese woman, an HSG would be better
- May need a referral to a specialist fertility clinic for further treatment/advice
- Comment on the need to lose weight, as this is likely to improve her chances of spontaneous conception
- Check the patient's identity details and allergy status

Examiner score sheet		
Information gathering		
Standard not met	Standard partly met	Standard met
0	1	2
Communication with patients and families		
Standard not met	Standard partly met	Standard met
0	1	2
Communication with colleagues		
Standard not met	Standard partly met	Standard met
0	1	2
Patient safety		
Standard not met	Standard partly met	Standard met
0	1	2
Applied clinical knowledge		
Standard not met	Standard partly met	Standard met
0	1	2

Examiner Expectations and Basis for Assessment

Information gathering

- Takes a comprehensive and focused infertility history from the patient and also ask her about her husband
- Interprets results from both female and male partners and requests appropriate investigations in order to develop a clear and rationale management plan
- Summarises discussions succinctly and checks that the patient understands at appropriate intervals

Communication with patients and families

- Able to sensitively give information about infertility, investigations and treatment options and in manageable amounts using patient-friendly language and avoiding jargon
- Honesty around benefits, side effects, complications and outcomes of fertility treatments
- Understands the psychological needs of the woman as well as the infertile woman
- Understands the psychological issues and sensitivities surrounding infertility

Communication with colleagues

- Able to describe the differential diagnosis and formulate an appropriate management plan
- Able to know when to refer and who to refer to for further management – involving a dietician (weight loss) and reproductive medicine to manage anovulation

Patient safety

- Confirms patients details/identify at start of task
- Demonstrates an understanding of the risk management and clinical governance and regulatory processes in relation to infertility, including issues of confidentiality with regard to discussing partner's results in his absence without his permission
- The need to consider the welfare of the child in providing fertility treatment
- The risks of ovulation induction, especially multiple pregnancies associated with fertility treatment

Applied clinical knowledge

- Knowledge of the treatment of infertility, including surgical management of tubal disease, endometriosis and male infertility
- Sound evidence-based clinical knowledge of ovulation induction, assisted conception and gamete donation, including the risks and limitations of these treatments
- Able to critically appraise medical literature in relation to infertility treatment
- Understands the role of HEFA and the NHS funding restrictions and rationing of assisted conceptions
- Understands the role of counselling for the infertile couple
- Knowledgeable of the current NICE guidelines on the management of the infertile couple

Reference: Fertility problems: assessment and treatment. NICE Clinical Guideline CG156 20 February 2013. Last updated 06 September 2017.

Task 11: Stress Incontinence. Module 14 – Urogynaecology and Pelvic Floor Problems

Candidate's Instructions

This is a simulated patient task covering:

- Information gathering
- Communication with patients and families
- Communication with colleagues
- Patient safety
- Applied clinical knowledge

You are an ST5 in the clinic and are about to see your next patient who has been referred by the GP with urinary incontinence. The letter from the GP is given below.

> *Sporeland Surgery*
> *Greenfield*
> *Stoke ST9 3TR*

Dear Dr,
I would be grateful if you could see Ms Samantha Scriven, 45-year-old who has been complaining of leaking urine on coughing for the past 1 year. The symptoms have got worse over the last 6 months. She is a mother of three and generally very healthy.

Yours sincerely

Dr Pomptous Siddeon MBChB, MRCGP, DRCOG

You have 10 minutes in which you should:

- Take focused history
- Discuss any investigations considered appropriate
- Discuss management
- Answer any questions that the patient may have

Simulated Patient's Information

You are Ms Samantha Scriven, 45 years old, and work as a nurse assistant in the geriatrics ward of the hospital. You have been working there for the past 10 years. You live on your own and smoke 15 cigarettes per day and drink alcohol regularly but never have more than a glass of wine a day.

You have a boyfriend who lives in his own house.

Over the last 1 year, you have had problems with your 'waterworks'. You wet yourself every time you cough or sneeze. When it started, you thought it was associated with the change, but it's got worse. You now have to wear a sanitary towel before you go out. You can no longer go to your aerobic classes because you are scared someone will smell the wee. You tend to go more often now than before, mainly for fear of wetting yourself when you cough. You do not suffer from cough or constipation. You do not wake up at night to pass urine, and when you feel like going, you do not have to rush to avoid an accident (wetting yourself). The only time you wet yourself is when you cough, sneeze or jump. You drink about four cups of coffee daily – usually one in the morning and then three others when you have a break at work. You drink diet coke but no energy drinks. When you pass urine, there is no burning sensation. You do not have any dragging sensation below, and there is no vaginal discharge. You do not suffer from constipation or diarrhoea.

You have had three normal vaginal deliveries. The first was 20 years ago. It was a normal pregnancy, and your labour lasted for 12 hours. The baby weighed 2,890 g. Your second was 2 years later, and again the pregnancy was problem free. He weighed 3,600 g at birth, and your labour lasted 8 hours. The third was problematic as you had diabetes during pregnancy and delivered 2 weeks early. She weighed 4 kg, and it was a forceps delivery as she did not want to come out. You had a bad tear, which was repaired without problems.

You have yearly tests for diabetes, and so far you are fine. You do not suffer from any other medical problems and have had no surgery in the past. You have, however, been experiencing hot flushes and night sweats for the last 18 months. You are not on HRT though. You are not taking any medications and have no known allergies.

You are overweight and have been unsuccessfully struggling to lose weight.

You are very worried about the embarrassment this is causing you.

If not discussed, you should ask the following questions:

- What is wrong with me?
- How will you investigate my problem?
- What treatment will I receive? What if I do not want surgery? Will the surgery guarantee cure, and will there be a chance of recurrence?
- What are the risks of surgery?
- Is this because of my weight. I am a bit on the big side with a BMI of 36 kg/M^2?

Examiner's Instructions

Familiarise yourself with the candidate's instructions and also study the simulated patient's information. Score the candidate on the domains highlighted in the instructions.

A good candidate should cover the following:

Information gathering

- Obtains a good history which demonstrates an understanding of the clinical problem
- Initiates appropriate investigations to help make a diagnosis
  - Fluid diary
  - Urinalysis
  - Blood glucose
  - Urodynamics if necessary

Communication with patients and families

- Explains the diagnosis of stress urinary incontinence
- Explains the need for investigations
- Discusses the treatment options, including lifestyle changes, physiotherapy and drugs
- Ultimate treatment is surgery – sling procedures are those of choice
- Discusses menopause and the symptoms
- Discusses weight sensitively and emphasises on the benefit of losing weight

Communication with colleagues

- Discusses referral to urogynaecology team (specialist nurse, incontinence adviser and urogynaecologist)
- Involves MDT in treatment where appropriate, for example, before surgery

Patient safety

- Confirms patients identify at start of task
- Outlines the safety issues with tapes for sling surgery
- Empowers patient to make informed choices
- Discusses the safety of drugs prescribed for control of symptoms
- Offers safe prescription for menopause symptoms having excluded allergies

Applied clinical knowledge

- Explain the pathophysiology of stress incontinence
- Discuss the basis of treatment – physiotherapy, lifestyle changes, drugs and surgery – surgery can be performed without urodynamics
- Explain the type of surgery and benefits plus complications – overactive bladder, failure rate (10–15%) and problems with bladder control
  - Discuss the details of surgical options, the type of anaesthesia and post-operative course (length of hospital stay, success rates, benefits and complications)
- Demonstrate the use of current NICE guidelines to form the basis of the management

Examiner score sheet		
Information gathering		
Standard not met	Standard partly met	Standard met
0	1	2
Communication with patients and families		
Standard not met	Standard partly met	Standard met
0	1	2
Communication with colleagues		
Standard not met	Standard partly met	Standard met
0	1	2
Patient safety		
Standard not met	Standard partly met	Standard met
0	1	2
Applied clinical knowledge		
Standard not met	Standard partly met	Standard met
0	1	2

Examiner Expectations and Basis for Assessment

Information gathering

- Takes comprehensive urogynaecology history and undertakes a urogynaecological examination
- Initiates appropriate investigations (urinalysis and voiding diary) and cystometry if required
- Interprets investigations (microbiological and urine microscopy results)
- Interprets cystometry, imaging and fluid balance charts in order to reach a diagnosis and develop a management plan

Communication with patients and families

- Able to give information about urogynaecological examination, investigations and treatment in a manageable amount, using patient-friendly language and avoiding jargon
- Discusses honestly the pros and cons of treatment options, including clinical uncertainty about long-term outcomes of urogynaecological treatment options
- Demonstrates an understanding of the psychological issues and sensitivities surrounding urogynaecological disorders and incontinence

Communication with colleagues

- Describes the differential diagnoses and formulates management plans with senior colleagues
- Clearly communicates requirements and situation with theatre staff, assistants and anaesthetists
- Determines when and who to refer to (urogynaecologist, urodynamics, physiotherapy etc.)
- Communicates with the GP after consultation

Patient safety

- Confirms patients identify at start of task
- Understands the principles of safe surgery, including the WHO safe surgery checklist
- Understands safe prescription in relation to urogynaecological therapeutics
- Understands the contraindications and interactions of urogynaecological drugs and common medical co-morbidities
- Ascertains drug allergy and demonstrates safe prescription
- Discusses the complications of the various surgical options

Applied clinical knowledge

- Knowledgeable of the surgical, non-surgical and medical management options of urogynaecological disorders including pelvic organ prolapse, acute voiding disorders, overactive bladder and stress urinary incontinence
- Able to critically appraise the literature/evidence in relation to urogynaecological treatment options
- Knowledgeable of NICE and RCOG Guidelines on urinary incontinence and pelvic floor prolapse

Reference: Urinary incontinence and pelvic organ prolapse in women: management. NICE Clinical Guideline NG123 02 April 2019. Last updated 24 June 2019

Task 12: Endometrial Cancer. Module 13 – Gynaecological Oncology

Candidates Instructions

This is a simulated patient task assessing:

- Information gathering
- Communication with patients and families
- Communication with colleagues
- Patient safety
- Applied clinical knowledge

You are an ST5 working with Mr Spencefield. You are about to see a 52-year-old woman, who presented 2 weeks ago with irregular vaginal bleeding and had an endometrial biopsy. The histology report of the biopsy is given below.

Histopathology Report

Name: **Helen Preston**
Hospital number: **S01673521N**
Specimen: **Pipelle endometrial biopsy**
The specimen received contained fragments of tissue, the largest of which measured 0.5 mm. The fragments consist of endometrial tissue and mucus mixed with blood. There is generalised glandular hyperplasia with areas of atypia interspersed within areas of well-differentiated adenocarcinoma. There are foci of squamous metaplasia in some of the glandular structures.
Impression: Well-differentiated adenocarcinoma

You have 10 minutes in which you should:

- Obtain relevant history
- Explain the result to the patient

- Discuss and justify management options
- Ascertain her anxieties and deal with them appropriately

Simulated Patient's Information

You are Mrs Helen Preston, a 52-year-old secretary. You are married and have one child who is 25 years old. You wanted to have more but could not get pregnant. Your husband is age 50 years and is an engineer, running his own company.

Your periods have always been irregular, but over the last 6 months have become more irregular and heavy. You therefore went to the GP who referred you to the hospital. You are overweight and suffer from type II diabetes, but this is controlled on diet alone. Your last period was so heavy that you had to stay away from work for 3 days.

When you came to the clinic, a sample was taken with a small tube and sent to the lab. You have come back for the results. You were told that it should be easy to manage this with hormones.

You were on the contraceptive pill for 6 years before you got married but have not been on any hormonal treatment since then. Your son, who is 25 years old, was conceived naturally. You were investigated for failing to conceive for the second time and were told that you were not ovulating regularly. You and your husband were not prepared to take any treatment for that.

Your last weight was 83 kg. You do not smoke but drink alcohol socially. You are up to date with your smears – the last one was only 6 months ago and was clear. You do not suffer from blood pressure problems and have no known allergies.

You have had no surgical or medical problems in the past. Your sister suffers from PCOS.

You are attending today in the hope that you will be reassured and given some hormones to help with the bleeding and your hot flushes. You are fed up with periods as most of your age mates have gone through the change already. You have some fear, though, as the doctor who saw you last time mentioned that there was a little possibility of cancer, which is why he took the sample.

If not covered, you should ask the following questions:

- What causes cancer in the womb?
- What stage of cancer do I have?
- What treatment will I have?
- What is the outlook for me? Should I be preparing myself for the worse?
- How will you follow me up?
- If I have surgery, is there a guarantee that everything will be removed?

A good candidate should cover the following:

Information gathering

- Asks to review notes or states that you will review notes and then asks for more information to include risk factors for endometrial carcinoma
- Obtains from the history the pattern of menstruation, difficulties conceiving, family history of possible PCOS, diabetes, overweight and irregular periods

Communication with patients and families

- Explains the diagnosis in layman's language (follows the steps of breaking bad news – see communication tips)
- Explains the need for further investigations – to ensure fitness for surgery and help exclude the spread of cancer

- Explains treatment – surgery – laparoscopic total or laparoscopic-assisted hysterectomy and bilateral salpingoophorectomy
- Histological staging – so will require follow-up to review report on tissues removed
- Explains that prognosis in early cases – very good
- Refers to oncologist or cancer specialist for MDT
- Provides support – contact numbers of a hospital with cancer support team, information leaflets and support groups

Communication with colleagues

- Liaises with oncology MDT (oncologist, cancer nurse, counsellor and gynaecological oncologist)
- Liaises with the cancer support team
- Feedback to GP

Patient safety

- Confirms the patients details at start of task ensuring the names on the report belong to the patient
- Counsels about diagnosis
- Timing of surgery and fitness for surgery
- Provides appropriate empowerment to make informed choices on treatment
- Takes into consideration allergies with treatment
- Demonstrates an understanding of waiting times for oncology treatment

Applied clinical knowledge

- Explains the reason behind endometrial cancer
- Explain the types of endometrial cancer – well differentiated the best type
- Discusses prognosis – 5 year which depends on stage but in general very good for early stage disease
- Explains the need to review to determine adjuvant therapy after surgery
- Explains the follow-up and rationale for follow-up

Examiner score sheet		
Information gathering		
Standard not met	Standard partly met	Standard met
0	1	2
Communication with patients and families		
Standard not met	Standard partly met	Standard met
0	1	2
Communication with colleagues		
Standard not met	Standard partly met	Standard met
0	1	2

Patient safety		
Standard not met	Standard partly met	Standard met
0	1	2
Applied clinical knowledge		
Standard not met	Standard partly met	Standard met
0	1	2

Examiner Expectations and Basis for Assessment

Information gathering

- Takes comprehensive and relevant oncology history from patients
- Requests appropriate and timely investigations; interprets results and operative findings in order to develop a clear management plan and rationale for follow-up

Communication with patients and families

- Gives information in a sensitive way and in manageable amounts to the patient and family regarding investigations, diagnosis and management of endometrial cancer
- Deals sensitively with palliation and death – in advanced cases but unlikely in this case
- Describes a clear and logical action plan
- Summarises discussions succinctly and checks that the patient understands at appropriate intervals
- Provides contacts of national and local support groups

Communication with colleagues

- Prioritises cases appropriately in line with oncology waiting times
- Describes the differential diagnoses and formulates an appropriate management plan
- Discusses the case (endometrial cancer) with different specialties in an MDT (oncologist who will lead chemotherapy, oncologist nurse who will provide support and gynaecological oncology – who will lead the surgical team)

Patient safety

- Confirms the patients details at start of task ensuring the names on the report belong to the patient
- Able to apply referral pathways and targets for investigations in the treatment of gynaecological cancer
- Understands risk management and clinical governance in relation to gynaecological cancer
- Able to recognise limits of their clinical abilities and demonstrate an understanding of when to call for help and involve senior colleagues and other disciplines line radiotherapy and chemical oncology
- Understands safe prescription in gynaecological oncology, including recognition of drug interaction, allergies and special circumstances, e.g. renal and liver impairment
- Understands the principles of surgery, including the WHO safe surgery checklist

---

Applied clinical knowledge

- Knowledgeable of the epidemiology, presentation, investigation and treatment of gynaecological malignancies, including palliation
- Understands the roles and responsibilities of the members of the multidisciplinary team
- Able to critically appraise the literature/evidence in relation to gynaecological cancer
- Understands the role of screening and imaging in gynaecological malignancies
- Understands referral pathways in gynaecological malignancies
- Ability to present management options and their risks and benefits using non-directional counselling
- Demonstrates knowledge of current literature on endometrial cancer

Task 13: Bladder Injury at Hysterectomy. Module 3 – Post-Operative Care

Candidate's Instructions

This is a structured discussion task assessing:

- Communication with colleagues
- Patient safety
- Applied clinical knowledge
- Communication with patients and families

You are the ST5 in the unit and are performing a total abdominal hysterectomy on a 45-year-old woman with heavy menstrual bleeding that has failed to respond to medical treatment. You are being assisted by an obstetrics and gynaecology ST1. Your consultant is sitting in the coffee room doing his paperwork.

The patient whose BMI is 30 kg/M^2 has had two previous caesarean sections. She is otherwise well.

Having gone through the pre-operative routine, including the WHO safety checklist and pro-phylactic antibiotics, you open the abdomen through the previous caesarean section scar. You enter the peritoneal cavity, and there are adhesions onto the anterior abdominal wall which you manage to separate. You then try to push down the bladder and suspect that you may have made a hole in the bladder.

You have 10 minutes to have a structured discussion on how you will manage this patient from now on with the examiner.

Examiner's Instructions

Familiarise yourself with the candidate's instructions.

Use the following four questions to guide the discussion you will have with the candidate. Provide some guidance on how much time the candidate spends on each question.

1. What will be your immediate action?
2. How will you approach the rest of the surgery?
3. What will your post-operative management be?
4. What clinical governance issues will you deal with post-operatively?

A good candidate should cover the following:

What will be your immediate action?

- Stop further surgery or dissection
- Inform the theatre team (anaesthesia and scrub nurse and additional staff in theatre) of the suspected injury and that the procedure is likely to take longer
- Call for help (consultant) and may be a urologist
- May need to inform the ward that the list may be delayed with possible cancellations if not finished

How will you approach the rest of the surgery?

- Confirm injury with a consultant (may require filling bladder with methylene blue to confirm and localise injury)
- Define the extent of the injury and decide whether the consultant can deal with it or require input from a urologist
- Proceed with hysterectomy with the assistance of the consultant
- Repair bladder in two layers (to be done by consultant or urologist)
- As the injury is posterior, great care must be taken to avoid the ureters – may require ureteric catheterisation
- Check that repair is effective by filling bladder with methylene blue saline/Hartman's solution
- Indwell catheter and possibly a drain (intraperitoneal)

What will your post-operative management be?

- Antibiotics for 5 days
- Catheter for 7–10 days
- Debrief the patient
- Complete incident form (inform risk manager)
- On removing the catheter, check post-void residual and no leakage of urine
- Inform GP when discharged

What clinical governance issues will you deal with post-operatively?

- Inform risk manager (incident form/Datix)
- Perform root cause analysis – an unanticipated complication
- Reflect on one's own practice
- Inform the patient honestly (duty of candour) about the results of investigations and putting in place processes of how to minimise the recurrence of this complication (may require defining cases for ST5 etc.)
- Follow-up with the consultant to discuss the complication and ensure no residual effects

Examiner score sheet		
Information gathering		
Standard not met	Standard partly met	Standard met
0	1	2
Communication with patients and families		
Standard not met	Standard partly met	Standard met
0	1	2
Communication with colleagues		
Standard not met	Standard partly met	Standard met
0	1	2
Patient safety		
Standard not met	Standard partly met	Standard met
0	1	2
Applied clinical knowledge		
Standard not met	Standard partly met	Standard met
0	1	2

Examiner Expectations and Basis for Assessment

Communication with colleagues

- Able to communicate with colleagues in theatre – anaesthetist nursing team and others (runners etc.)
- Involves consultant when suspects complication
- Involves urologist
- Communicates with GP on the complication and treatment

Patient safety

- WHO safety surgery checklist
- Recognizes complication and appropriately dealing with it
- Intraoperative confirmation of injury and effectiveness of repair
- Post-operative care – catheter and antibiotics
- Ascertains allergy and safe prescription

Applied clinical knowledge

- Demonstrates an understanding of the current literature on managing bladder injuries at the surgery
- Familiar with contemporary complications of gynaecological surgery

Communication with patients and families

- Offers to debrief the patient immediately after surgery (when the patient is able to understand)
- Communicates with the patient on the after-risk management report and shares the report with the patient (duty of candour)
- Invites the patient to follow-up and discuss the complication with consultant/ST5

Task 14: Abdominal Hysterectomy. Module 2 – Core Surgical Skills

Candidate's Instructions

This task is a structured discussion covering:

- Information gathering*
- Communication with patients and families*
- Communication with colleagues
- Patient safety
- Applied clinical knowledge

You are the ST5 who is working with a consultant, and you are preparing to assist her on the theatre list. The next case is an abdominal hysterectomy. The details of the patient are as follows:

You are about to perform an abdominal hysterectomy and bilateral salpingoophorectomy on a 53-year-old, with uterine fibroids and endometrial hyperplasia. She was placed on the waiting list for surgery after being seen and investigated for postmenopausal bleeding of 4 months duration. Her BMI is 30 kg/M², and she had two caesarean sections, the last one 15 years ago.

You have 10 minutes to discuss the procedure of abdominal hysterectomy with the examiner. The examiner has four questions to help guide the discussions.

Examiner's Instructions

Familiarise yourself with the candidate's instructions. Use the four questions to structure the discussion with the candidate. Direct the candidate to the use of time.

1. Explain what preparation you will undertake prior to performing a hysterectomy on this patient once she has been put to sleep?
2. Describe in detail the various steps you will take in performing a hysterectomy
3. If you suspect that the bladder has been damaged, what steps will you take?
4. How will you manage the patient, if her bladder was indeed damaged?

A good candidate will cover the following under each question:

1. *Explain what preparation you will undertake prior to performing a hysterectomy on this patient once she has been put to sleep?*
    - As this is a high-risk patient, I will ensure that I am assisted by a senior colleague, preferably my consultant
    - Discuss WHO checklist with the team (patient identify, procedure, site, staff, allergies, antibiotics, etc.)
    - Position the patient on her back
    - Clean the vulva and vagina with an antiseptic solution (may paint vagina with methylene blue)
    - Empty the bladder with an 'in and out' catheter (may leave catheter *in-situ*)
    - Perform a pelvic examination (why – to determine the size of the uterus, mobility and any adnexal masses – this will influence the type of incision and also provide an idea on how difficult the surgery may be)
    - Clean abdomen and drape

2. *Describe in detail the various steps you will take in performing a hysterectomy*
    - Low transverse skin incision
    - Transverse incision on rectus sheath
    - Separate rectus muscle centrally
    - Enter peritoneal cavity taking extra care to avoid bowel or bladder injury
    - Explore cavity
    - Insert pack to push away bowel from pelvis
    - Insert a self-retaining retractor (Balfour or an alternative)
    - Identify the round ligaments and attach clamps (Kocher/long artery forceps)
    - Lift up uterus
    - Apply two clamps to round ligament and divide between clamps – close to the uterus
    - Separate broad ligament and then isolate the ovary and infundibulo-pelvic ligament and apply two clamps to this ligament
    - Divide between clamps and transfix
    - Repeat the procedure on the other side
    - Divide the uterovesical peritoneum transversely and push down the bladder
    - Apply a clamp to the uterine artery and divide it close to the uterus and transfix (if possible, palpate for the ureters, but the clamps must be applied as close to the uterus as possible)
    - Clamp the uterosacral, divide and transfix
    - Perform the same on the transverse cervical ligament and transfix
    - Push the bladder to expose the anterior vagina wall. Open this and dissect the vagina off the cervix

- Apply a clamp to the lateral angles of the vagina and detach it from the uterus. Transfix the lateral angles of the vagina
- Close the vagina with a continuous stitch, and once haemostasis is secured, remove the pack and close the abdomen after ensuring that instruments and swabs have been counted and are correct

3. *If you suspect that the bladder has been damaged, what steps will you take?*
   - Stop all surgical procedures and inform the anaesthetist and scrub nurse and the rest of the team
   - Call the consultant or at least inform her (if not in theatre at the time)
   - Inspect to see if the damage is obvious
   - If not, instil methylene blue in the bladder – if damaged, the dye will spill
   - Call a urologist or senior consultant to close the damage in two layers, check that this is tight by distending it with saline and methylene blue. If no leakage, empty bladder and leave an indwelling catheter
   - Close abdomen in layers with either subcuticular skin or interrupted skin stitches
   - Arrange a team debrief and undertake a reflection on the case and consider adding it to your e-portfolio

4. *How will you manage the patient if her bladder was indeed damaged?*
   - Indwell catheter for 7–10 days
   - Prescribe antibiotics for 5–7 days, having excluded allergy
   - Inform patient after (debrief patient) – be honest with the patient and family (duty of candour)
   - Complete incident form – Datix form which ensures risk manager is notified and risk management undertaken
   - On discharge, arrange a follow-up and also inform her GP

Examiner score sheet		
Information gathering		
Standard not met	Standard partly met	Standard met
0	1	2
Communication with patients and families		
Standard not met	Standard partly met	Standard met
0	1	2
Communication with colleagues		
Standard not met	Standard partly met	Standard met
0	1	2
Patient safety		
Standard not met	Standard partly met	Standard met
0	1	2
Applied clinical knowledge		
Standard not met	Standard partly met	Standard met
0	1	2

Examiner Expectations and Basis for Assessment

Information gathering

- Able to review the clinical information provided in order to assign patient as high risk for visceral (bladder, bowel and ureteric injuries) and take appropriate steps to minimise these

---

Communication with patients and families

- Be honest about the complication of bladder injury and management plans, including risk management, and communication of findings to patient
- Arrange a follow-up to review progress and addresses any issues or queries

---

Communication with colleagues

- Able to communicate legibly and with an ordered approach (date, time, etc.), e.g. clinical and operation notes
- Able to communicate with assistant and members of the team – anaesthesia and nursing at appropriate stages during surgery, including the WHO safety checklist
- Liaises with senior colleague/urologist when bladder injury occurs
- Communication with risk management team following a serious complication
- Communicates with GP

Patient safety

- Understands the principles of safe surgery, including the WHO safe surgery checklist
- Understands the positioning of the patient for abdominal hysterectomy and the unconscious and recovering patient
- Able to logically talk through the steps of safety during surgery (ensuring the minimisation of complications – bowel, bladder and ureters)
- Recognize limitations of abilities and demonstrates an understanding of when to call for help and involve senior colleagues and other disciplines

---

Applied clinical knowledge

- Appropriate knowledge of gynaecological surgery (abdominal hysterectomy), including techniques and the risks and minimising these
- Knowledgeable of the current literature and guidelines on perioperative care and management of bladder injuries

13
Paper II

Task 1: Conduction of a Twin Delivery. Module 1 – Teaching

Candidate's Instructions

This is a simulated trainee task assessing:

- Information gathering
- Communication with patients and families
- Communication with colleagues
- Applied clinical knowledge
- Patient safety

You are an ST5, who is working on the labour ward with an ST1. On the labour ward is a multiparous woman with twins in labour. Your task is to teach the ST1 how to conduct a twin delivery. You will be assessed on your ability to teach a Specialist Trainee in her first year to conduct the vaginal delivery of twins. You will be assessed on the conduct of the teaching and your ability to successfully guide the trainee to undertake this procedure.

You have 10 minutes in which you should:

- Explain to the ST1 what is essential in preparing for a twin delivery
- Teach the ST1 how to conduct a twin delivery
- Demonstrate how you have been successful in the tasks of teaching

Simulated Trainee's Instructions

You are an ST1 who is on call with an ST5. You spent the first 3 months doing gynaecology and this is your second month in obstetrics. You know that there is a woman with twins in labour. You are yet to see a twin delivery. You have, however, read about how to conduct a twin delivery.

If not covered, you should ask:

- Do I need to perform an episiotomy for all twin deliveries?
- Is an ultrasound scan always necessary for the second twin?
- When are you allowed to perform a breech extraction?

The candidate should:

- State very clearly, from the outset, the objectives of the teaching
- Compliment you on your knowledge and having read about twin delivery
- Explain the principles of twin delivery, including the preparation for it

- Outline the correct steps in twin delivery
- Encourage reflection and self-directed learning

A good candidate will cover the following:

a. *State the objectives of the teaching session and find out what the trainee knows – complimenting where appropriate*
   - At the end of this session, you should understand how to conduct a twin delivery and the various steps to take to minimise risk to the babies and the mother
   - What do you know about conducting twin deliveries? Have you read this up? Compliment the trainee for reading about this

b. *Preparation for a twin vaginal delivery*
   - Make sure that there are no contraindications to a vaginal delivery
   - Ensure that the first twin is cephalic – may need to check and confirm by USS. Monitoring is for both twins and ensure there is no fetal distress (use a dual CTG machine)
   - Intravenous line *in-situ*
   - Make sure two skilled midwives, paediatrician and anaesthetist are around
   - Make sure adequate analgesia is provided or can be provided
   - Make sure intravenous syntocinon is available to be commenced with the delivery of the first twin
   - Ensure ultrasound scan machine is available in the room
   - Ensure two cots available for resuscitation

c. *Conduct of the delivery*
   - Delivery of the first twin is as normal and is probably conducted by a midwife
   - After delivery of the first twin, quickly examine the abdomen to check for the lie of the second twin – use ultrasound to confirm the lie
   - Commence syntocinon (10 iu in 500 ml of normal saline) drip to augment or initiate uterine contractions and ensure monitoring is continuing
   - Once contractions have started, await descent of the presenting part
   - Rupture membranes once the presenting part is engaged or enters the pelvis (rupture prior to this may result cord prolapse)
   - Conduct the rest of the delivery as expected (if breech, conduct an assisted breech delivery)
   - Syntocinon drip (10 iu in 500 ml of normal saline over 4 hours) with the management of the third stage – increased risk of primary PPH
   - Examine the perineum for trauma and manage accordingly
   - Note that the interval between the delivery of the twins should in general not exceed 30 minutes

d. *Abnormal lie*
   - External version and allow labour to progress
   - Fetal distress – internal podalic version and/or breech extraction
     i. Explain this procedure to the trainees (prerequisites for this include informed consent and appropriate anaesthesia, undertaken by a very experienced clinician). The details of the procedure will vary depending on how much time you have. If there is time, locate the feet with ultrasound and then insert the dominant hand with a long glove into the uterus to grasp the feet of the baby using the external hand to stabilise the baby. Bring down the feet through the cervix, and in the process, the baby will rotate.

Perform a breech extraction (i.e. do not wait for maternal effort to push the baby out). Continue to monitor the baby during the process
ii. Caesarean section

Examiner score sheet		
Information gathering		
Standard not met	Standard partly met	Standard met
0	1	2
Communication with patients and families		
Standard not met	Standard partly met	Standard met
0	1	2
Communication with colleagues		
Standard not met	Standard partly met	Standard met
0	1	2
Patient safety		
Standard not met	Standard partly met	Standard met
0	1	2
Applied clinical knowledge		
Standard not met	Standard partly met	Standard met
0	1	2

Examiner Expectations and Basis for Assessment

Information gathering

- Understands the need to first determine the skills of the tutee
- Identifies the gaps in knowledge and skills of the tutee that have to be addressed in the session
- Understands the timing during twin deliveries (especially the interval between the first and the second twin)
- Excludes all contraindications to a vaginal delivery, e.g. abnormal presentation of twin I, placenta praevia and fetal compromise

Communication with patients and families

- Appropriate introduction of the tutee and the task to the patient and their partner
- Explanation of the role of the tutee and the nature of the interaction to the patient
- Informed consent obtained for teaching from the patient

Communication with colleagues

- Introduces self and role in the teaching
- Understands the principles of adult learning and giving feedback with regard to twin delivery
- Knows the appropriate steps in increasing the clinical and technical skills of the learner (tutee)
- Ability to use appropriate language and non-verbal clues to encourage learning
- Invites questions and encourages dialogue
- Show a logical approach to building the pre-existing skills of the leaner

---

Patient safety

- Patient safety is maintained when teaching conduction of a twin delivery, showing an understanding of when to continue teaching and when to intervene to halt the teaching session
- Appropriate safety checks are in place and knows when to abandon vaginal delivery for emergency CS (e.g. IV fluids, CTG abnormality, availability of anaesthetist and neonatologist)
- Appropriate checks are undertaken to ensure procedure has been appropriately undertaken

---

Applied clinical knowledge

- Understands the steps of the tasks being undertaken (teaching task)
- Understands the learning objectives and outcomes in relation to the tasks being taught
- Able to conduct and give feedback on using a work-based assessment tool in this task
- Knowledgeable of the principles of twin delivery as detailed in standard Operative Obstetrics and RCOG – Green-top Guidelines

---

Task 2: Systemic Lupus Erythematosus. Module 5 – Maternal Medicine

Candidate's Instructions

This is a simulated patient task assessing:

- Information gathering
- Communication with patients and families
- Communication with colleagues

- Patient safety
- Applied clinical knowledge

You are an ST5, who is running the clinic with the consultant. You are about to see Ms Pam Stephen, a 29-year-old referred by the GP. The referral letter is given below.

The Mulbium Surgery
Old Hill Estate
Brompton
BR12 8YT

Dear Dr,
Re: Ms Pam Stephen
Thank you for seeing this 29-year-old who is 8 weeks pregnant. She suffers from systemic lupus erythematosus (SLE) and was taking methotrexate and aspirin when I saw her last week. I asked her to stop the methotrexate but to continue with the aspirin. She is very well informed about her condition and should provide you with more information on investigations that were performed prior to the diagnosis being made.

Yours sincerely

Dr Jane Smith MBBS (Bristol) MRCP

You have 10 minutes in which you should:

- Take focused history
- Discuss the antenatal management of this patient
- Explain the complications that should be screened for and why
- Discuss and agree the management of her pregnancy and labour including puerperal care

Simulated Patient's Information

You are Ms Pam Stephen, a 29-year-old postdoc in the university. You suffer from systemic lupus erythematosus (SLE), which was diagnosed 5 years ago. You were place on steroids and aspirin but last year methotrexate was added as the flares were too frequent, affecting your joints and making it difficult for you to walk.

The first symptoms you had were rashes on your face and joint pains. Your GP suspected and took some blood samples that were sent to the hospital. You were told that you were lupus anti-coagulant positive and also had anti-rho antibodies. You regularly have a blood test to check your kidneys, and so far, all the tests have been normal.

This is not a planned pregnancy. You do not have a steady boyfriend and have been having casual relationships for the last 1 year. Unfortunately, you had sexual intercourse without protection and find yourself pregnant. You are thrilled but worried as you were taking methotrexate at the time of pregnancy. You have since stopped.

You have problems with your joints, especially at the wrist, but these have been better for the last few months. You do not have any other medical problem and have never had surgery.

You are allergic to egg yolk so you keep away from egg.

You used to smoke 5–10 cigarettes per day and also drink. You have cut down (one to two per day) on your smoking since you found out that you are pregnant and stopped drinking alcohol completely. Your weight is well controlled, and you regularly exercise (only as much as your joints can tolerate).

Your last period was 8 weeks ago and prior to that your periods were regular.

Your BMI is 24 kg/M².

If not covered by the candidate, you could ask the following questions:

- What will be the effect of the methotrexate on my baby – will it be deformed?
- Will my SLE get worse during pregnancy?
- What problems may my baby have and how will you screen and monitor for these?
- Will the SLE affect my pregnancy?
- What will happen to my SLE after delivery?

A good candidate will cover the following:

Information gathering

- History and review of notes, bringing out points on recent investigations, medications and time of initiation and dose (e.g. methotrexate)
- Blood test – implication for SLE (anticardiolipin and anti-rho antibodies) – heart block, FGR, VTE etc.
- Obtains history on concerns about methotrexate and the fetus

Communication with patients and families

- Explanation of diagnosis and implications
- Likely association with – pregnancy loss complication – demonstrating sensitivity in discussing this
- Discussion of treatment options
- Implications for the fetus and newborn

Communication with colleagues

- Involvement of multidisciplinary team in care (obstetrician with interest in connective tissue disorders, fetal medicine, midwife, GP and internist/rheumatologist)
- Liaison with rheumatologist antenatally and postnatally
- Liaison with anaesthetist to discuss pain relief during labour and/or operative delivery

Patient safety

- Ensure patient's identity is confirmed at the start of the task
- Establish/identify drug and other allergies
- Safe prescription for the mother and considerations for the fetus
- Prescription of low-dose aspirin and fragmin – counselling about implications for labour and delivery
- Empowering to make informed choices about management

Applied clinical knowledge

- Using evidence to support discussions and management plans
- Showing evidence of familiarity with current literature, including Green-top Guidelines and protocols, on managing and counselling patient with connective tissue disorders

Examiner score sheet		
Information gathering		
Standard not met	Standard partly met	Standard met
0	1	2
Communication with patients and families		
Standard not met	Standard partly met	Standard met
0	1	2
Communication with colleagues		
Standard not met	Standard partly met	Standard met
0	1	2
Patient safety		
Standard not met	Standard partly met	Standard met
0	1	2
Applied clinical knowledge		
Standard not met	Standard partly met	Standard met
0	1	2

Examiner Expectations and Basis for Assessment

Information gathering

- Able to take a concise and relevant medical history about SLE (timing, symptoms, diagnostic tests and treatments)
- Skilled in signposting and guiding the consultation (able to show logic in history)
- Able to obtain information about past management, including investigations for complications, especially renal

Communication with patients and families

- Able to tackle difficult or sensitive topics, including the risk of miscarriage, complications during pregnancy and flare up after delivery
- Able to give information to the patient about SLE in terms of both the impact of pregnancy on SLE and SLE on the pregnancy and the fetus and possible effects of methotrexate on the fetus
- Able to explain the management of SLE in pregnancy and screening both the fetus and the mother
- Able to ensure that the patient understands and encourages questions – provide information in a step-wise manner in appropriate quantities, checking to ensure understanding

---

Communication with colleagues

- A clear and logical approach to management plan for patients with SLE, including the need to exclude renal complications involvement of rheumatologist or internist
- A clear plan of involvement of MDT – internist (rheumatologist, fetal medicine, specialist midwife, anaesthetist and neonatologist) and their role
- Ability to communicate with colleagues in primary care and within the multidisciplinary team

---

Patient safety

- Establishes the patients identify at the start of the task
- An understanding of both the impact of pregnancy on SLE and the impact of SLE on the pregnancy and the fetus
- Safe prescription and implications of especially methotrexate and corticosteroids in pregnancy
- Safety with regard to allergy

Applied clinical knowledge

- Knowledge of pre-conception and antenatal and postnatal care, including the risks of maternal morbidity and mortality related to SLE
- Awareness of contemporary literature on SLE in pregnancy and the puerperium

---

Task 3: Pregnant Patient with Renal Transplant. Module 4 – Antenatal Care

Candidate's Instructions

This is a structured discussion task assessing:

- Information gathering
- Communication with patients and families (*this is not applicable in this station as its structured, but if it's a simulated patient, this will be applicable*)
- Communication with colleagues
- Patient safety
- Applied clinical knowledge

You are an ST5, who is in the clinic with your consultant. You have just seen a 37-year-old who had a kidney transplant 4 years ago. She is now 12 weeks, and her pregnancy has been uncomplicated so far. You have presented the case to your consultant who has asked to review the case with you. He will lead the discussion using four questions.

You have 10 minutes in which you should discuss the management of this patient with the examiner who has four questions to guide the discussions.

Examiner's Instructions

Familiarise yourself with the candidate's information, and use the following four questions to form the basis of discussion on the management of the patient. Provide the candidate some guidance on time management.

1. If this woman had come to see you pre-pregnancy, what would your management/advice be?
2. What was your management of this woman at this gestation?
3. What complications may she have and can you justify the investigations you will be offering her?
4. She comes in spontaneous labour, how will you manage her?

A good candidate should cover the following:

1. *Pre-pregnancy*
   - How long was the transplant? It's best to wait for 12–18 months after transplant before pregnancy
   - Review medication to ensure that she is not on teratogenic drugs such as an ACE (angiotensin receptor antagonist) inhibitor, and if she is, recommend review by nephrologist and changing to a less teratogenic option
   - Ensure that blood pressure is well controlled
   - Ensure that immunosuppressants and steroids are stable – i.e. minimum dose required for stability
   - Check renal function test to make sure its normal – proteinuria is minimal (pregnancy outcome is better with minimal proteinuria)
   - Check immunisation and screen for opportunistic infection
   - Appropriate contraception, if not generally fit for pregnancy, and counsel about pre-pregnancy folic acid (5 mg)
   - Involve nephrologist in her care where appropriate

2. *Management now*
   - Weigh patient and measure BP
   - Check renal function and other investigations – routine pregnancy investigations
   - Ultrasound scan to date pregnancy
   - Counsel about screening for diabetes mellitus
   - Screen for infections such as cytomegalovirus (CMV)
   - Consider commencing on aspirin for pre-eclampsia prevention from 12 weeks of gestation
   - Commence on folic acid 5 mg daily
   - Discuss aneuploidy screening – first trimester (biochemistry and nuchal translucency – combined)
   - MDT (nephrologist, transplant physician, obstetrician with interest in medical disorders/renal disorders in pregnancy and specialist midwife) review – medication and plan of care (antenatal, intrapartum and postpartum)
   - Venous thrombosis risk assessment

3. *Justification of investigations*
   - Renal function test
   - Full blood count
   - Routine booking investigations (blood group and antibodies, rubella immunity, syphilis, HIV and hepatitis serology)
   - Urinalysis and culture if indicated

- Dating ultrasound scan and NT measurements at 11–14 weeks
- Serial fetal growth ultrasound scans from 24 weeks

4. *Complications that may arise*
   - Fetal
     - i. Miscarriages
     - ii. Fetal growth restriction
     - iii. Preterm labour (spontaneous and iatrogenic)
   - Maternal
     - i. Gestational diabetes mellitus
     - ii. Pre-eclampsia
     - iii. Urinary tract infection
     - iv. Deterioration in renal function (in a small number, renal function will deteriorate)

5. *Presents in labour*
   - Monitor fetus as high risk – continuous electronic fetal monitoring (EFM)
   - Cephalic presentation – no additional precautions – allow vaginal delivery
   - Abnormal presentation or requiring CS – be aware of the position of the kidney which tends to be the pelvic brim
   - Watch out for infection risk
   - May consider IV corticosteroids (hydrocortisone: 50–100 mg every 6–8 hourly) if on steroids throughout pregnancy or on at least 5 mg of prednisolone per day for at least 2 weeks
   - Follow-up renal function test and appropriate contraception

Examiner score sheet		
Information gathering		
Standard not met	Standard partly met	Standard met
0	1	2
Communication with patients and families		
Standard not met	Standard partly met	Standard met
0	1	2
Communication with colleagues		
Standard not met	Standard partly met	Standard met
0	1	2
Patient safety		
Standard not met	Standard partly met	Standard met
0	1	2
Applied clinical knowledge		
Standard not met	Standard partly met	Standard met
0	1	2

Examiner Expectations and Basis for Assessment

Information gathering

- Able to take a concise and relevant history about transplant – timing and renal function status
- Drug history – ACE inhibitors, corticosteroids, immunosuppressants and immunisation
- Skills in signposting and guiding the consultation – pre-pregnancy
- Able to obtain information about past management, including investigations pre-pregnancy (including last renal function test), screening for diabetes, immunisation and contraception

Communication with patients and families (for this particular discussion task this does not apply, but if it's a simulated patient task, this would be appropriate)

- Able to tackle difficult or sensitive issues of pregnancy after renal transplant (e.g. deterioration in renal function) and the possibility of transplant being affected
- Able to give information to the patient about transplant in terms of both the impact of pregnancy on it and vice versa, especially drugs
- Able to signpost management of renal transplant in pregnancy and screening both the fetus and the mother

Communication with colleagues

- Has a clear and logical management plan for patients with renal transplant, including the need to exclude hypertension and involvement by renal physician/transplant physician
- Has a clear plan for an MDT – internist (nephrologist/transplant team, fetal medicine, specialist midwife, anaesthetist and neonatologist) and their roles
- Able to communicate with colleagues in primary care and within the multidisciplinary team

Patient safety

- Awareness of safety of investigations and therapeutics in early pregnancy, during late pregnancy and in the postnatal period, including safe prescription (e.g. ACE inhibitors, steroids and immunosuppressants)
- An understanding of both the impact of pregnancy on transplant and the impact of immunosuppressants on the pregnancy and the fetus
- Safe prescription and implications of antihypertensives and immunosuppressants in pregnancy
- Safety with regard to allergy

Applied clinical knowledge

- Knowledge of pre-conception and antenatal and postnatal care, including the risks of maternal morbidity and mortality related to renal transplant
- Knowledge of the issues surrounding transplant and pregnancy, including approaches to CS
- An understanding of contraception post delivery
- Familiarity with contemporary literature on transplants and pregnancy

Task 4: Management of Primary Postpartum Haemorrhage. Module 7 – Management of Delivery

Candidate's Instructions

This task is a structured discussion assessing:

- Information gathering
- Communication with colleagues
- Communication with patients and families
- Patient safety
- Applied clinical knowledge

You are the Specialist Trainee on a busy labour ward in your hospital, and the sister on the unit has fast bleeped you to come to one of the rooms because a 30-year-old primigravida who has just delivered is having severe postpartum haemorrhage. The placenta has been delivered.

The examiner will have a conversation with you based on a series of questions and will provide you with further relevant information as the conversation progresses. The examiner will guide you on timings.

You have 10 minutes in which you should:

- Read the information provided
- Answer the questions asked by the examiner

Examiner's Instructions

Please spend some time familiarising yourself with the candidates' instructions.

You should use the following questions as a basis for a discussion with the candidate about the management of this patient. Before question 3 (below), show the candidate the full blood count results and ask how he/she will deal with them.

1. What will be your initial management of this patient on arrival in the room?
2. You have undertaken the initial resuscitative steps in the management of PPH, talk me through the various steps you will take after this.
3. All the medical methods have failed to stem the bleeding. What will be your next step?
4. What will be your post-operative management of this patient?

A good candidate should be able to discuss the following (following the algorithm in the Green-top Guideline No. 52, 2016, on Prevention and Management of Postpartum Haemorrhage):

1. *What will be your initial management of this patient on arrival in the room?*
   - Call for help
     - i. Senior midwife, senior trainee/consultant and anaesthetist on call
     - ii. Alert haematologist
     - iii. Alert blood transfusion laboratory (blood bank)
     - iv. Alert consultant obstetrician on call
   - Commence resuscitation
     - i. Airway, breathing and circulation
     - ii. Oxygen face mask (15 L/min)
     - iii. Fluid balance (e.g. 2 L of isotonic crystalloid and 1.5 L colloid) and then blood transfusion (Group O Rh negative K negative or group specific)
     - iv. Keep patient warm
   - Monitoring/investigations
     - v. Insert two 14-gauge cannulae
     - vi. Obtain blood for FBC, coagulation, U&E, LFTs and fibrinogen levels
     - vii. Cross-match four units of red blood cells, FFP, platelets and cryoprecipitate
     - viii. Pulse oximetry and commence ECG
     - ix. Foley's catheter to record urine output (fluid balance)
2. *Medical treatment of the bleeding – step-wise approach*
   - i. Rub uterine fundus
   - ii. Oxytocin 5 iu slowly IV (repeat) and start infusion – 40 iu/500 ml isotonic crystalloid to run at 125 ml/hour
   - iii. Ergometrine 0.5 mg IV slowly or IM
   - iv. Carboprost – IM 250 µg every 15 minutes up to 8 doses (within 2 hours) – ensuring that there are no contraindications like asthma. Once the third dose is being administered, start preparing for theatre if no response after this
   - v. Misoprostol 800 µg (PR or sublingual) may be considered
   - vi. Consider tranexamic acid 1 g IV
3. *Theatre – management in theatre*
   - i. Obtain consent for if uterus is not contracting for examination under anaesthesia and repair any tissue trauma

    ii. WHO safe surgery checklist

    iii. If coagulation problem develops as a result of massive haemorrhage, correct as soon as possible prior to surgery

    iv. Call consultant/senior obstetrician if not already around

    v. Uterus not contracting – balloon tamponade – Bakri Balloon or Rusch Balloon

    vi. Brace suture

    vii. Hysterectomy – decision to be made by consultant and another colleague

4. *Post-surgical management*

    i. Transfer to a high-dependency unit – monitor using Modified Early Obstetrics Warning Score (MEOWS) chart

    ii. Commence on thromboprophylaxis (involve haematologist if possible)

    iii. Debrief husband/family

    iv. Debrief patient

    v. Complete incident form (enter onto Datix) and organise a formal clinical incident review and follow-up appointment

    vi. Debrief team

Results of blood investigations

1. Hb – 65 g/L
2. WCC – 12 × 10^9/L
3. Platelets – 78 × 10^9/L
4. Fibrinogen – 1.0 g/L
5. APTT – 1.5 times normal

In view of these results, the candidate has to discuss the following:

1. Ensure adequate transfusion
2. Administration of FFP at a rate of 15 ml/kg
3. Administration of fibrinogen products or cryoprecipitate

Examiner score sheet		
Information gathering		
Standard not met	Standard partly met	Standard met
0	1	2
Communication with patients and families		
Standard not met	Standard partly met	Standard met
0	1	2
Communication with colleagues		
Standard not met	Standard partly met	Standard met
0	1	2

Patient safety		
Standard not met	Standard partly met	Standard met
0	1	2
Applied clinical knowledge		
Standard not met	Standard partly met	Standard met
0	1	2

Examiner Expectations and Basis for Assessment

Information gathering

- Obtains information from patients, staff (midwives) and clinical notes (antenatal, the partogram, CTG and maternal vital signs) and use these to formulate a clear clinical picture of the cause of the PPH
- Examines – looking for causes of PPH – 4Ts (tone, trauma, tissues [placenta, uterus, vulva and vagina] and thrombin)
- Initiates appropriate investigations (FBC, cross-match, coagulation screen, urea and electrolytes and liver function test) to rule out thrombin and help map out the management, including fluid replacement

Communication with patients and families

- Able to communicate to the woman and her partner and/or family the interventions for the PPH, including investigations and management steps
- Able to explain the risks and benefits of interventions to both the mother and her partner
- Communicating clearly and appropriately the management plans at appropriate intervals with the patient/family

Communication with colleagues

- Ability to prioritise appropriately the steps to take with senior colleagues in a logical sequence
- Ability to delegate tasks appropriately – involvement of anaesthetists, blood bank and junior colleague
- Understands the limits of one's own competence and when to call for senior help or involve other specialties
- Ability to form a logical differential diagnosis for the causes of the PPH and to be able to convey that to colleagues on- and off-site
- Communicating appropriately and succinctly the management plans at appropriate intervals with colleagues

---

Patient safety

- Ensures allergy profile is ascertained to ensure safe prescription
- Understands risks from interventions such as IV oxytocin, fluid overload and carboprost (especially in asthmatic patients)
- Accurate prescription to stimulate uterine contractions, including management of intravenous infusions
- Understands risk management and clinical governance processes in relation to massive PPH
- Understands fluid management, including blood and blood components transfusion

---

Applied clinical knowledge

- Knowledgeable of causes (4Ts) and management of postpartum haemorrhage
- Ability to think and work under pressure within an MDT
- Understands the roles of members of the multidisciplinary team in the management of PPH
- Knowledgeable and able to critically appraise the current literature, including guidelines (Green-top Guideline on PPH and NICE Intrapartum Care)

Reference: Prevention and management of postpartum haemorrhage. The Royal College of Obstetricians and Gynaecologists. Green-top Guideline No. 52 16 December 2016

Task 5: Fourth-Degree Perineal Tear – Follow-up. Module 8 – Postpartum Problems (The Puerperium)

Candidate's Instructions

This task is a structured discussion assessing:

- Information gathering
- Communication with patients and families
- Communication with colleagues
- Patient safety
- Applied clinical knowledge

You are the ST5 covering the postnatal ward and are conducting your ward round. Your next patient is Mrs Stephanie Pensford, a 34-year-old who had a forceps delivery and sustained a fourth-degree perineal tear that was successfully repaired in theatre under regional anaesthesia (epidural). This was 3 days ago, and she is ready to go home.

You have 10 minutes in which you should:

- Read the information provided
- Answer the questions the examiner will ask

Examiner's Instructions

Familiarise yourself with the candidate's instructions. Use the following four questions as the basis for a discussion with the candidate about the management of Mrs Pensford. Provide some guidance to the candidate about the use of their time. You should suggest they move to the next questions after about 2.5 minutes.

a. What will you like to check before discharging the patient home?
b. What instructions will you give her on discharge?
c. She is seen in the postnatal perineal clinic at 6 weeks, what would be your approach to her management?
d. How will you manage her next pregnancy?

A good candidate should cover the following:

a. *What will you like to check before discharging her home?*
   - Check notes to make sure that all documented swabs were documented as removed
   - Has she opened her bowels?
   - Has she been given enough antibiotics to complete the 7 days course?
   - Examine her perineum to make sure that the repair has not broken down
   - Make sure she does not have a temperature and there is no unusual pain
   - Ensure the summary of her care and complication to be sent to the GP has been completed

b. *What instructions will you give her on her discharge?*
   - To ensure she is not constipated for a few weeks – to continue with stool softeners
   - Not to resume sexual intercourse until at least 4 weeks post surgery
   - To undertake regular pelvic floor exercises
   - To keep a symptom diary – bowel – flatus and faecal incontinence if any
   - Avoid tampons
   - Encourage eating high-fibre diet and drinking fluid to avoid constipation
   - Perineal hygiene
   - Arrange a follow-up visit with the perineal clinic
   - Educate on when to call the GP or report to the hospital – safety net

c. *She is seen in the postnatal perineal clinic at 6 weeks, what will your approach be to her management?*
   - Review her symptom diary
   - Ask about sexual intercourse and contraception
   - Examine the vagina and do a PR
   - Arrange an anal manometry and ultrasound scan if symptomatic
   - If normal and asymptomatic – discharge
   - If abnormal and symptomatic arrange a referral to MDT

d. *How will you manage her next pregnancy?*
   - Depends on whether she is symptomatic or not and whether the manometry and ultrasound scan are normal or not
   - If manometry and ultrasound normal and asymptomatic – vaginal delivery
   - Minor symptoms and manometry/ultrasound normal – offer conservative management (dietary advice, regulate bowel action, PFE and biofeedback) – offer CS
   - Abnormal and symptomatic (e.g. faecal incontinence) – vaginal delivery and secondary sphincter repair when family is complete

Examiner score sheet		
Information gathering		
Standard not met	Standard partly met	Standard met
0	1	2
Communication with patients and families		
Standard not met	Standard partly met	Standard met
0	1	2
Communication with colleagues		
Standard not met	Standard partly met	Standard met
0	1	2
Patient safety		
Standard not met	Standard partly met	Standard met
0	1	2
Applied clinical knowledge		
Standard not met	Standard partly met	Standard met
0	1	2

Examiner Expectations and Basis for Assessment

Information gathering

- Ability to obtain information prior to discharge and on follow-up
- Ability to obtain/use information (history, examination and investigations) to help signpost management plans and follow-up
- Ability to obtain information about plans for subsequent pregnancies

Communication with patients and families

- An ability to communicate with the woman and her partner the details of the complication and management from now and in the community
- Communicates the details of follow-up and symptoms, for which help from GP or hospital will be sought
- Provides information at a rate which allows for understanding and encourages and answers all questions

Communication with colleagues

- Understands the limits of one's own competence and when to involve the perineal trauma team (or consultant with expertise in this area) in the management of this patient
- Ability to communicate appropriate amount of detail to colleagues and ensure that management plans are clear and easily understood by colleagues
- Team working to support – MDT (physiotherapy, imaging and perineal trauma team/ expert)
- Communicates with GP and community midwife, detailing complication and management including follow-up plans

Patient safety

- Understands risk management and clinical governance processes in relation to investigations of women who develop 3/4th degree perineal tears intrapartum
- Demonstrates safe prescription after ensuring allergies, if any, are as established

Applied clinical knowledge

- Knowledgeable of postpartum care of 3/4th degree perineal tears
- Has a working knowledge of the roles of other members of the multidisciplinary team
- Ability to critically appraise the literature, including guidelines (Green-top Guideline on perineal tears and NICE guideline on urinary incontinence) and contemporary literature

References

Lone F, Sultan A and Thakar R. Obstetric pelvic floor and anal sphincter injuries. *The Obstetrician and Gynaecologist*, 2012; 14:257–266.
The Management of Third- and Fourth-Degree Perineal Tears. RCOG Green-top Guideline No. 29. June 2015

Task 6: Labour Ward Prioritisation. Module 6w – Management of Labour

Candidate's Instructions

This is a structured discussion task assessing:

- Information gathering
- Communication with patients and families
- Communication with colleagues
- Patient safety
- Applied clinical knowledge

You are the Specialist Trainee 5 on call on the delivery suite. You have just arrived for handover at 0830.

Attached, you will find a brief resume of the 8 women on the delivery suite as shown on the board.

The staff that are available today are as follows – an obstetrics ST1 in her fourth month of GP training, a fifth year Specialist Anaesthetic Trainee and a consultant on call, but not yet available on the unit.

Eight midwifes: MD in charge; BK, ON and NN can suture episiotomies; AR, PK and LM can insert IV lines and MW is a midwife in the Alongside Midwifery Unit.

You have 10 minutes to study the board carefully and then decide what tasks need to be done, in which order they should be done and who should be allocated to each task.

Delivery Suite Board

Room Number	Name	Parity	Gestation	Liquor/ membranes	Epidural	Oxytocinon	Comments
1	JJM	0^{+2}	33^{+2}	Membranes intact	No	No	DC/DA twins contracting ceph/ceph admitted @0700 and on CTG. Dr to see
2	SK	2^{+0}	T^{+6}	Membranes intact	No	No	Spontaneous labour, 4 cm @0650
3	PV	0^{+2}	36^{+2}	-	No	No	Emergency CS @0630 for fulminating pre-eclampsia
4	DA	1^{+0}	34^{+0}	Membranes intact	No	No	Admitted with significant PV loss @0630. CTG normal. Dr to see
5	OK	0^{+3}	39^{+2}	Meconium	Yes	No	FBS@0700 – pH 7.25, BE-5 mEq/L, 6 cm. Repeat @0800, pH-7.23, BE-6 mEq/L
6	JR	0^{+0}	42^{+1}	Clear	Yes	Yes	Fully @0530
7	FN	2^{+1} (CS × 2)	38^{+3}	Membranes intact	No	No	Admitted with pain @0730. Dr to see
8	VC	5^{+0}	40^{+4}	Membranes intact	No	No	Spontaneous labour @0500. 5 cm @0600. Dr to see

A good candidate will cover the tasks as detailed in the table below.

Room No	Task	Delegate	Order
1	Review – CTG and contraction frequency and duration, assess cervix, inform neonatologist to review and steroids possibly tocolysis. Urinalysis to rule out urinary tract infections (UTI)	ST5	4
2	Assess progress of labour @1050	Midwife	8
3	Review vital signs (including BP, pulse, respiratory rate and temperature), urine output and pain relief	Anaesthetist	5
4	History and examination (general and abdominal), review records, especially for USS localisation of the placenta; IV line, FBC, group and safe, steroids and neonatologist to review	ST5 – ST1 to take bloods and site IV	1
5	Review CTG and assess vaginally and decide if for delivery, anaesthetist to be informed	ST5	3
6	Review CTG and if active pushing had commenced. If not commenced or commenced, review progress	Sister in charge	7
7	Quick history and examination, especially if in labour; CTG. IV line and group and safe, consent for CS and alert OR and anaesthetist	ST5, MW to insert IV line and take blood	2
8	Grand multiparous; review previous deliveries if previous PPH; antenatal risk factors for PPH; IV line and active management of second stage	Midwife to take bloods and site an IV line ST5 to review	6

Examiner score sheet		
Information gathering		
Standard not met	Standard partly met	Standard met
0	1	2
Communication with patients and families		
Standard not met	Standard partly met	Standard met
0	1	2
Communication with colleagues		
Standard not met	Standard partly met	Standard met
0	1	2
Patient safety		
Standard not met	Standard partly met	Standard met
0	1	2

Applied clinical knowledge		
Standard not met	Standard partly met	Standard met
0	1	2

Examiner Expectations and Basis for Assessment

Information gathering

- Obtains information on patient at handover using the SBAR tool as well as from clinical notes (including the partogram, CTG and maternal vital signs where appropriate) and use these to formulate a clear clinical picture of each patient
- Ability to describe a clear action plan and rationale for decisions made based on discussions with colleagues

Communication with patients and families

- An ability to communicate to each woman and her partner and/or family the planned/scheduled interventions for the management of labour or post delivery
- An ability to explain the risks and benefits of interventions for both the mother and the fetus

Communication with colleagues

- The ability to justify the recommended interventions with colleagues at handover
- An ability to rationalise prioritisation with colleagues
- Ability to delegate tasks appropriately
- Has an understanding of the limits of one's own competence and when to call for senior help or involve other specialties

Patient safety

- Demonstrates safety in labour in various scenarios as present on the delivery suite
- Has an understanding of risks from interventions such as regional analgesia, emergency CS and therapeutics in labour and post delivery (e.g. after for severe pre-eclampsia)
- Accurate prescription in labour, including management of intravenous infusions and regional analgesia
- Has an understanding of risk management and clinical governance processes in relation to intrapartum care

- Ability to transfer patients from low- to high-risk maternity units and when to involve MDT care, including intensivists/anaesthetist
- Adequate delegation to minimise risk

Applied clinical knowledge

- Knowledgeable of intrapartum care, management of normal and abnormal labour, obstetric interventions and the interpretation of CTG
- An ability to think and work under pressure from competing priorities when the workload on the labour ward is heavy – prioritising appropriately
- A working knowledge of the roles of other members of the multidisciplinary team
- An ability to delegate tasks when the workload on the labour ward requires
- Ability to critically appraise the literature, including NICE Intrapartum Care and RCOG Green-top Guidelines, protocols and scientific papers

Task 7: Endometriosis. Module 9 – Gynaecological Problem

Candidate's Instructions

This is a simulated patient task assessing:

- Information gathering
- Communication with patients and families
- Communication with colleagues
- Patient safety
- Applied clinical knowledge

You are the ST5 in the gynaecology clinic today with your consultant. Below is a referral letter on your next patient.

Bridgewater Surgery
Prince Charles Way
Brigdewater
Somerset
TB15 6CS

Dear Mr Ojifor, FRCOG
Could you arrange to see Ms Susanne Graham, a 29-year-old hotel receptionist, who complains of painful periods and pain during sexual intercourse. She has had these symptoms for a long time, and they are gradually getting worse.

She is struggling to cope with work and has been to see me for sick leave three times in the last 4 months. I was able to persuade her to come and see you.

Thank you for seeing her.

Yours sincerely

Dr Christy Fowler MBBCh, MRCGP, DRCOG

You have 10 minutes in which you should:

- Obtain relevant history
- Discuss investigations
- Explain the treatment options
- Counsel on the impact of the condition on fertility
- Answer any questions

Simulated Patient's Information

You are Suzanne Graham, a 29-year-old hotel receptionist, who lives in Bridgewater and work in Taunton. You live with your partner Stuart James, a 41-year-old cricket coach. You have been together for 6 years.

Your problem started about 2 years after you started menstruating. You were having pains with your periods. At the beginning, the pain started a day before your periods, continued to the end of bleeding, sometimes persisting for a few days after. Over the years, this pain has gradually got worse, and in the last 1 year, you have been struggling to cope. You now have to take paracetamol and sometimes combine it with ibuprofen, as prescribed by the doctor. Over the last 6 months, the pain has become so severe that you had to take time off work three times. The pain no longer goes away and gets worse with your periods; it's most painful on the second and third days of your period.

Your periods are regular, occurring every 28–30 days and lasting for 3–5 days with the passage of clots on day 1. There is no intermenstrual bleeding and no bleeding after sexual intercourse.

You started going out with Stuart 6 years ago. Prior to that, you have had a few casual affairs but none lasted more than a few months. Although you had sexual intercourse with these boyfriends, it was never serious and you always had some pain with intercourse. You experience severe pain when Stuart is inside you. Sometimes you have to ask him to stop. On a few occasions, it was painful when he was trying to get inside but most often it is when he is inside. The pain is right inside your pelvis and tends to last for a few hours after. There have been a few occasions in which the pain has lasted more than a day after, but usually by the second day after intercourse, it's gone.

You have not had an infection or treatment for pelvic infections.

Your mother had painful periods and so does your sister. She is 32 years old and married with two kids.

You do suffer from bloating of the tummy and sometimes bad constipation.

You do not smoke but drink alcohol on a regular basis. Sometimes you have to drink in the hope that it will numb the pain!

You are not aware of any allergies. Your last period was 1 week ago.

You have been hoping to become pregnant but despite not using any protection you have failed to conceive. This is, however, not a priority at the moment, but if it did happen, you and Stuart will be thrilled.

If not covered, you should ask the following questions:

- What is the most likely cause of my symptoms?
- What investigations are going to help make a diagnosis?
- What are the treatment options?
- Will this affect my chances of getting pregnant?
- If the condition affects pregnancy, how can I remedy this?

A good candidate will cover the following:

Information gathering

- Chronic history – dating from soon after menarche
- Identifies relevant symptoms of endometriosis – family history, characteristic of pain, dyspareunia (deep) and occasionally superficial
- Identifies the impact of symptoms on work and sexual life
- Ascertains fears about fertility
- Outlines investigations, including diagnostic laparoscopy and ultrasound scan
- Enquires about symptoms of urinary tract infections (UTI), irritable bowel syndrome (IBS) and pelvic inflammatory disease (PID) – these are differentials diagnoses

Communication with patients and families

- Explains the suspected diagnosis and that it affects about 15–20% of women in the reproductive age group
- Discusses treatment options – medical (progestogens, combined hormonal contraception and GnRH agonist) and surgery – ablation/excision taking into consideration the fertility needs of the patient and the severity of symptoms
- Confirms that her priority here is the pain – treating this may actually allow her to conceive
- Addresses her fears – it may be associated with reduced fertility so it would be important for earlier referral to the infertility experts
- Communicates with colleagues
- Able to liaise with colleagues with expertise in endometriosis
- Involves an MDT where appropriate (pain specialist, anaesthetist, clinical psychologist and GP) – endometriosis support groups
- Offers the option of infertility investigations – this may be declined or delayed

Patient safety

- Confirms patients details at the start of the task
- Empowers the patient to make informed choices on treatment options
- Makes sure the patient is not pregnant (LMP, and if indicated, pregnancy test)
- Safe prescription, especially of GnRH agonist and hormonal options for and beyond 6 months
- Balances benefits versus risks of hormonal treatment for endometriosis

Applied clinical knowledge

- Discusses endometriosis – pathogenesis and genetics (positive family history)
- Explains the rationale for treatment options and how they work
- Outlines side effects and how to counter these
- Considers details of treatments

- Understands the impact on fertility
- Demonstrates knowledge of relevant literature and NICE and ESHRE Guidelines on endometriosis

Examiner score sheet		
Information gathering		
Standard not met	Standard partly met	Standard met
0	1	2
Communication with patients and families		
Standard not met	Standard partly met	Standard met
0	1	2
Communication with colleagues		
Standard not met	Standard partly met	Standard met
0	1	2
Patient safety		
Standard not met	Standard partly met	Standard met
0	1	2
Applied clinical knowledge		
Standard not met	Standard partly met	Standard met
0	1	2

Examiner Expectations and Basis for Assessment

Information gathering

- Takes comprehensive history about the painful period and sexual intercourse focusing on possible causes
- Requests appropriate investigations (abdominal and pelvic examination), diagnostic laparoscopy and biopsies and ultrasound, especially to rule out endometriomas and deep infiltrating endometriosis and adenomyosis

Communication with patients and families

- Summarises discussions about diagnosis, including differentials, succinctly and checks patient's understanding at appropriate intervals
- Counsels about the diagnosis and how these relate to symptoms
- Describes clearly the logical approach to different management options (pros and cons), including complications and rationale for care and follow-up
- Discusses that response to treatment may not be immediate and may involve trying more than one option

---

Communication with colleagues

- Refers appropriately to endometriosis expert or laparoscopist
- Understands the role of MDT in the management of endometriosis
- Understands the role of support groups (endometriosis society or help groups)

Patient safety

- Confirms patients details at the start of the task
- Safe prescribing medical options for managing endometriosis – asking about allergies and medical disorders that could be considered contraindications to the medications
- Knowledgeable of principles of safe surgery, if it is the chosen option of the patient

---

Applied clinical knowledge

- Good knowledge of implications of endometriosis as evidence from explaining diagnosis and management options
- Refers to patient educational materials on endometriosis (e.g. from the RCOG)
- Has an understanding of the contents of NICE/RCOG Guidelines on endometriosis with regard to management, follow-up and implications for fertility

Task 8: Unexplained Infertility. Module 10 – Subfertility

Candidate's Instructions

This is a simulated patient task assessing:

- Information gathering
- Communication with patients and families
- Communication with colleagues
- Patient safety
- Applied clinical knowledge

You are an ST5 who is about to see Mrs Patel attending the gynaecology clinic with a 2-year history of failure to conceive. Mrs Geeta Patel, a nurse, is 32 years old. Her husband Anish, who is a businessman, is 40 years old and is away today. They have been referred to the unit from a small district hospital, where they had a series of investigations. They first went to the hospital a year ago, after trying for 1 year unsuccessfully. Following investigations, they were simply asked to await a referral to your unit. A summary of the results of the investigations from the referring hospital are:

1. *Semen analysis – normal*
2. *Hormone profile – normal with an ovulatory 21-day progesterone*
3. *HSG – normal endometrial cavity, fallopian tubes and free spillage of contrast into the pelvis*

You have 10 minutes in which you should:

1. Obtain a brief, targeted clinical and fertility history
2. Explain the likely cause of the couple's subfertility
3. Establish the issues involved in the management of this couple and discuss them sensitively

Simulated Patient's Information

Mrs Geeta Patel, Age 32 years
No 5b Haven Gardens
Stafford ST2 6BD

You are Mrs Geeta Patel, a 32-year-old nurse, who has been married for the past 6 years. Your husband Anish is a 40-year-old businessman, who travels quite a lot. Although you got married 6 years ago, it has only been in the last 2 years that you have been trying for a baby. You used the contraceptive pill for 4 years and stopped 2 years ago.

Although your husband travels frequently, you have sexual intercourse two to three times per week when he is around. Your periods are regular, and he plans his trips around the timing of your periods so that you have the best chance to get pregnant. You are aware of your fertile period, and during this time, you try to have sexual intercourse thrice weekly.

About a year ago, your GP referred you to a local hospital; where after investigations, you were told you will be referred to a larger hospital. It has taken another year for this to happen.

Your periods started when you were 12 years old and have been regular since. You do not have any other gynaecological problems. You have never been pregnant.

You had your appendix removed through keyhole surgery 3 years ago. This was diagnosed soon after you developed severe pain in the lower abdomen, and as you were on duty, it was dealt with very quickly. You were discharged home the following day.

You live in your own detached house with Anish. You neither drink alcohol nor smoke but Anish drinks about a glass of wine daily and over the weekend, tends to have more than one. You are a member of a local gymnasium and walk about 1–2 miles every day. You eat healthily and watch your weight – your BMI is 26 kg/M^2.

Your mother and father suffer from diabetes and are on metformin and insulin. You have three siblings – a brother and two sisters. None of them have any children yet (you are the eldest). Your husband is one of three – his sister has two kids and his brother has three. His father died from stroke and his mother is alive and well. You are not on any medication but are allergic to eggs.

Acting requirements
You understand what is being told to you and you are very obviously disappointed that nothing has been found on the tests you did.

You are angry that it took the small hospital 1 year to refer you to this hospital. You are worried about your age and frustrated that you have wasted 1 year.

If not covered by the candidate, you could ask the following questions:

1. Why do you think we are struggling to get pregnant?
2. What are our options?
3. If we need IVF, what does it entail?

A good candidate should cover the following:

Information gathering

- Obtains appropriate fertility-focused history
- Obtains specific information relevant to possible causes of infertility
- Interprets correctly and explains clearly the investigation's results and their implications
- Ascertains anger and frustration at the delay in referral to the larger unit
- Ensures that the couple will provide a safe environment for a child (safeguarding child safety)

Communication with patients and families

- Explains possible reasons for the failure to conceive – unexplained infertility
- Explores the women's fears and concerns
- Expresses empathy for the situation and the patient's bitter disappointment at the delay in referral
- Reassures patient that the management will not be unnecessarily delayed
- Explains the rationale for recommending treatment options
- Conveys suggested management plan and offers hope: recommends IVF as per NICE guidelines – encouraging them to continue to try while awaiting for IVF
- Informs that they are entitled to one IVF cycle on the NHS
- Demonstrates understanding of the sensitivity in discussing partners results in his absence (this should only happen with his consent – implied or otherwise)
- Encourages and welcomes her partner to attend consultation in the future

Patient safety

- Confirm patients details at the start of the task
- Demonstrates an understanding of the processes and procedures to keep individual patients safe
- Presents the pros and cons of a proposed management in a balanced way
- Recognises the limits of their clinical abilities and refers appropriately
- Identifies any allergies and demonstrates safe and accurate prescription techniques

Applied clinical knowledge

- Demonstrates a sound and comprehensive evidence-based clinical knowledge on unexplained infertility
- Interprets and explains clinical findings accurately
- Justifies investigations and management options and demonstrates a rationale for each
- Synthesises a comprehensive and well-organised management plan, based on the history and investigations and taking into consideration the various factors
- Appreciates how the diagnosis of unexplained infertility is made based on exclusion of various causes – ovulatory, anatomical and male factor

Examiner score sheet		
Information gathering		
Standard not met	Standard partly met	Standard met
0	1	2
Communication with patients and families		
Standard not met	Standard partly met	Standard met
0	1	2
Communication with colleagues		
Standard not met	Standard partly met	Standard met
0	1	2
Patient safety		
Standard not met	Standard partly met	Standard met
0	1	2
Applied clinical knowledge		
Standard not met	Standard partly met	Standard met
0	1	2

Examiner Expectations and Basis for Assessment

Information gathering

- Takes comprehensive and focused history from both partners of an infertile couple
- Interprets results from the referring hospital in order to develop a clear and rationale management plan
- Sensitively obtains assurance about the suitability of the couple for ART – safeguarding child safety

Communication with patients and families

- Able to give information about infertility investigations and treatment options in incremental steps, using patient-friendly language and avoiding jargon
- Honest about benefits, side effects, complications and outcomes of fertility treatments
- Understands the psychological needs of the partner as well as the infertile woman
- Understands the psychological issues and sensitivities surrounding infertility
- Able to explain to the couple that they have unexplained infertility
- Summarises discussions succinctly at an appropriate level and at regular intervals and checks that the patient/couple understands

---

Communication with colleagues

- Knows when to refer and who to refer to for further management – in this case, referral to the reproductive medicine team for IVF
- Involvement of multidisciplinary team – counsellor and andrologist/embryologist in management

---

Patient safety

- Confirms details of patient at start of task
- Knowledgeable of risk management (delay in referral) and clinical governance and regulatory processes in relation to infertility, including issues of confidentiality
- Acknowledges the need to consider the welfare of the child in providing fertility treatment
- Knowledgeable of the risks of multiple pregnancies associated with fertility treatment

---

Applied clinical knowledge

- Knowledgeable of the treatment of infertility, especially unexplained infertility based on NICE guidelines
- Has sound evidence-based clinical knowledge of ovulation induction and assisted conception, including the risks and limitations of these treatments
- Able to critically appraise medical literature in relation to infertility treatment
- Has an understanding of the role of HEFA and the NHS in funding restrictions and rationing of assisted conceptions
- Has an understanding of the role of counselling for the infertile couple

Reference: Fertility problems: assessment and treatment. NICE Clinical guideline [CG156] 20 February 2013. Last updated 06 September 2017

Task 9: Follow-up after Sacrocolpopexy. Module 14 – Urogynaecology and Pelvic Floor Problems

Candidate's Instructions

This is a stimulated patient task assessing:

- Information gathering
- Communication with patients and families

- Communication with colleagues
- Patient safety
- Applied clinical knowledge

You are the ST5 in your unit and are in the clinic with your consultant (a generalist). You have been passed a set of notes for your next patient, and all you have in the notes is the discharge summary below. The notes are temporary as the clerks could not locate the notes. These are likely to be somewhere in transit from the records to the consultant's secretary.

Discharge Summary

Re: Fanny Brim, Age: 60 years
Diagnosis: vault prolapse
Operation: abdominal sacrocolpopexy
Clinical course: unremarkable
Fit note: no heavy lifting for 8 weeks
Analgesia: paracetamol

Signed:

Dr Kevin Dooremat

ST1

A brief history for the patient is given below.

Ms Brim has done very well since her surgery. She, however, complains of frequency and urgency but no incontinence. She is still experiencing backache, but this is getting better. She is not back to work yet but looks forward to doing so if she is discharged from the clinic today.

You have 10 minutes in which you should:

- Complete the history
- Make a management plan
- Answer the patient's questions

Simulated Patient's Information

You are Ms Fanny Brim, a 60-year-old cashier at Tesco. You had surgery for vault prolapse 8 weeks ago. The surgery went well although the catheter was only taken out after you had gone home. They tried to take it out in the hospital but you could not wee so it was left inside while you went home. The community nurse came to remove it after 7 days and since then you have been weeing okay. You, however, have been rushing to wee although you do not have any accidents. Your back remains a concern as it has continued to be painful although not as bad as before. You have been eating and opening your bowels without any problems. Your partner has not been near you yet as you are a bit worried.

You have four children – three were delivered vaginally without any help but the fourth one was a forceps delivery. Their weights varied from 3.2 kg to 3.6 kg.

When you were 50 years, you had irregular bleeding, and following investigations that included taking a sample from your womb with a small tube, you were offered a hysterectomy. You were told that you had something which if not treated could progress to cancer. As you had completed your family, you really did not hesitate. The surgery was done from below, and you were happy as you did not have to have a cut on my tummy. Three years ago, you started suffering from a dragging sensation in your vagina, and this got worse and worse until you could feel a bulge at the opening of your vagina. This was very uncomfortable, and you had on many occasions pushed it back to completely empty your back passage. It has not been possible for you and your partner to have sexual intercourse. You presented to the same doctor who removed your womb, and he offered to do this surgery.

You are very happy that you do not have this dragging sensation again but worried about your waterworks.

You are taking paracetamol for the backache but no other medication. You are allergic to voltarol.

If not covered, you should ask the following questions:

1. Why am I still having backache?
2. Why do I have bladder symptoms and when will they disappear?
3. Can I have sexual intercourse now?
4. Are there any tests that will say that I am okay and that my waterworks are also okay?
5. What do I need to do to make things better?

A good candidate should cover the following:

Information gathering

- Obtains complete history to help understand what was done
- Assesses progress of surgery and fitness to go back to work
- Elicits the concerns about urinary frequency
- Ascertains anxieties about sexual intercourse
- Enquires after symptoms (incontinence, hesitancy, urgency) of voiding dysfunction
- Enquires what fluid intake is like
- Offers to review notes to glean more information about the medical history

Communication with patients and families

- Apologises for the missing notes
- Explains the reasons behind the backache and urinary symptoms
- Counsels about sexual activity
- Encourages physiotherapy if urinary symptoms (incontinence) found, as this may improve them
- If symptoms of urgency and urge incontinence – consider bladder training
- Offers a fluid diary

Communication with colleagues

- Involvement of senior colleagues (consultant) – discusses the case with consultant
- Involvement of other disciplines – physiotherapy
- Considers referral to urogynaecology (as your consultant is not a urogynaecologist)

Patient safety

- Recognises the implications of missing notes
- Empowers the patient to make informed choices
- Ascertains drug allergy and prescribes safely if appropriate

Applied clinical knowledge

- Discusses the course of recovery following sacrocolpopexy
- Discusses the complications of this procedure – backache and a 10–15% risk of detrusor overactivity
- Discusses investigations and treatment of overactive bladder

Examiner score sheet		
Information gathering		
Standard not met	Standard partly met	Standard met
0	1	2
Communication with patients and families		
Standard not met	Standard partly met	Standard met
0	1	2
Communication with colleagues		
Standard not met	Standard partly met	Standard met
0	1	2
Patient safety		
Standard not met	Standard partly met	Standard met
0	1	2
Applied clinical knowledge		
Standard not met	Standard partly met	Standard met
0	1	2

Examiner Expectations and Basis for Assessment

Information gathering

- Takes comprehensive urogynaecology history focusing on symptoms of incontinence, relating these to the surgery and excluding co-morbidities (diabetes and hypertension)
- Requests notes for review
- Undertakes appropriate investigations and interprets results, e.g. urinalysis and fluid diary
- Interprets cystometry, imaging and fluid balance charts in order to reach a diagnosis and develop a management plan

Communication with patients and families

- Discusses the rationale for the plan of care – examination, investigations and treatment in a measured approach
- Demonstrates an ability to give information about urogynaecological examination, investigations and treatment in a manageable amount using patient-friendly language and avoiding jargon
- Demonstrates an understanding of the psychological issues and sensitivities surrounding vault prolapse surgery and incontinence
- Apologises for missing notes

Communication with colleagues

- Describes the differential diagnoses of urinary symptoms and formulate management plans
- Clearly communicates the requirements and the situation with the staffs, assistants and anaesthetists
- Involves specialist in the management of the symptoms

Patient safety

- Has an understanding of the principles of safe surgery, including WHO safe surgery checklist
- Has an understanding of safe prescription in relation to urogynaecological problems, such as detrusor overactivity and urodynamic stress incontinence
- Has an understanding of the contraindications and interactions of urogynaecological drugs and common medical co-morbidities
- Ascertains any allergies and safe prescription

Applied clinical knowledge

- Knowledgeable of the complications of the surgical management options of urogynaecological disorders, including pelvic organ prolapse (in this case, sacrocolpopexy), acute voiding disorders, overactive bladder and stress urinary incontinence
- Ability to critically appraise the literature/evidence in relation to vault prolapse treatment options
- Familiarity with the NICE guideline on urinary incontinence and ROCG Green-top Guideline on vault prolapse

Reference: Urinary incontinence and pelvic organ prolapse in women: management. NICE guideline [NG123] 02 April 2019. Last updated 24 June 2019

Task 10: Complete Molar Pregnancy. Module 12 – Early Pregnancy Care

Candidates Instructions

This is a simulated patient task assessing:

- Information gathering
- Communication patients and families
- Communication with colleagues
- Patient safety
- Applied clinical knowledge

You are an ST5 who is about to see a 33-year-old Mrs Peta Smith in the gynaecology clinic for a follow-up. The conclusion of her histology report is given below.

Conclusion of histology report: Complete hydatidiform mole
Histology report on products of conception
Name: Peta Smith Age: 33 years old

You have 10 minutes within which to:

- Obtained a relevant history
- Explain the diagnosis to the patient
- Explain the management and follow-up
- Explain the prognosis of the diagnosis to the patient

Simulated Patient's Information

You are Mrs Peta Smith, a 33-year-old beautician, who came to the hospital 3 weeks ago bleeding. You were about 8 weeks pregnant when you started bleeding. You were admitted and had surgery (suction) to remove whatever was left in your womb as the bleeding was not stopping. You were discharged home the same day (after surgery) and were told to see your GP for a follow-up but to your surprise, you had a phone call saying you should come to the hospital today. You are not sure what to make of this but hope it's nothing to worry about. You and your husband will like to start trying for a baby straight away as you are not getting younger.

You are one of four children to your mother. You have two brothers and one sister, and they are all well. Your parents are all alive and well.

You live with your husband in your own home, and this was your first attempt at having a baby. You do not smoke although he smokes. You drink socially and have no known allergies.

You are fit with a BMI of 26 kg/M^2 and regularly exercise yourself.

If not covered, you should ask the following questions:

1. What causes a molar pregnancy?
2. What will happen to me now?
3. When can we start trying for a baby?
4. What are the chances that this will happen again?
5. How will I prevent myself from getting pregnant?
6. Why is pregnancy to be avoided?

A good candidate will cover the following:

Information gathering

- Reviews records
- Locates the histology report
- Obtains further history of the plan for pregnancy
- Ascertains anxieties and addresses them

Communication with patients and families

- Explains the diagnosis to the patient in layman's language and the need for baseline investigations (hCG and CXR)
- Explains the implications with respect to increased risk of choriocarcinoma or persistent trophoblastic disease
- Explains the need to register and have a follow-up with one of three regional centres (Sheffield, London Charing Cross or Dundee) in the UK or such centres overseas
- Offers patient information leaflets and liaises with support groups
- Explains the follow-up through tests on urine samples sent in the post and blood tests with the GP

Communication with colleagues

- Liaises with specialist centre and gestational trophoblastic disease (GTD) support team
- Informs the GP

Patient safety

- Explains the risks of unprotected intercourse and contraceptive options
- Empowers patient to make the right choices
- Ascertains allergies (if any) and demonstrates safe prescription (contraception etc.)

Applied clinical knowledge

- Discusses the pathogenesis of molar pregnancy
- Discusses the recurrence rate after one molar pregnancy (increased 10% i.e. from 1:600 to 1:60)
- Discusses the need to prevent pregnancy while hCG levels are being monitored (rising or falling)
- Provides information on pregnancy after molar pregnancy
- Explains why follow-up and why hCG – levels plateauing or rising may indicate persistent disease or choriocarcinoma and therefore the need for chemotherapy
- Demonstrates having up-to-date knowledge on contemporary literature, including RCOG Green-top Guideline on gestational trophoblastic disease

Examiner score sheet		
Information gathering		
Standard not met	Standard partly met	Standard met
0	1	2

Communication with patients and families		
Standard not met	Standard partly met	Standard met
0	1	2
Communication with colleagues		
Standard not met	Standard partly met	Standard met
0	1	2
Patient safety		
Standard not met	Standard partly met	Standard met
0	1	2
Applied clinical knowledge		
Standard not met	Standard partly met	Standard met
0	1	2

Examiner Expectations and Basis for Assessment

Information gathering

- Takes comprehensive history about the pregnancy, including family history of molar pregnancy and review histology
- Requests appropriate investigations and interprets results – baseline, CRX and histology
- Knowledgeable of history of future pregnancy plans and contraception (past and future)

Communication with patients and families

- Counsels about the diagnosis and that this will delay trying for another pregnancy
- Discusses sensibly the implications of the diagnosis – the risk of gestational trophoblastic tumour requiring chemotherapy
- Describes clearly the logical approach to different management options (pros and cons, especially of contraception), including complications and rationale for care and follow-up
- Summarises discussions about diagnosis, implications and the need for a follow-up and checks patient's understanding at appropriate intervals

Communication with colleagues

- Liaises with regional gestational trophoblastic disease centres (Sheffield, Charing Cross or Dundee, depending on where the patient lives in the UK and if outside the UK – specialist follow-up) for registration of the patient and follow-up

- Able to communicate with the patient about diagnosis and the need for a follow-up
- Communicates with GP the diagnosis and plans for follow-up, including contraception

Patient safety

- Ascertains allergies
- Safe prescription of appropriate contraception during the period of follow-up
- Discusses the complications that the patient should look out for
- Counsels about when to present for emergency (e.g. unscheduled vaginal bleeding or symptoms of distance metastasis, e.g. haemoptysis)
- Discusses future pregnancies, preparing for these and what to do when pregnancy test is positive

Applied clinical knowledge

- Being up to date with the current literature on gestational trophoblastic disease
- Has an understanding of the recurrent risk as well as the risk of progression to GTD during counselling
- Has an understanding of the current literature, including RCOG Guidelines on trophoblastic disease and the most recent evidence on contraception and follow-up

Reference: The management of gestational trophoblastic disease. The Royal College of Obstetricians and Gynaecologists Green-top Guideline No. 38 4 March 2010

Task 11: Referral Letters. Module 9 – Gynaecological Problems

Candidate's Instructions

This is a structured discussion assessing:

- Information gathering
- Communication with patients and families *(there is very little on this domain here)*
- Communication with colleagues
- Patient safety
- Applied clinical knowledge

You are the ST5 who has been asked by your consultant's secretary to come and undertake some tasks on her behalf. You have five referral letters to review and categorise them as one of the following:

(a) Routine – to be seen within 6–12 weeks
(b) Soon – to be seen within 4–6 weeks
(c) Urgent – to be seen within 2 weeks

In addition, you should mention (1) any additional investigation(s) that should be performed on each of the patients (if appropriate) following their visit to the clinic and (2) the most likely diagnosis/ pathology and (3) most likely treatment option(s)

You have 10 minutes in which you should:

- Read each letter and categorise it as routine, soon or urgent
- Decide which additional information/investigation/precautions (additional steps) is required when the patient comes to the clinic
- Provide a possible working diagnosis based on the information on the letter
- State the most likely diagnosis and the treatment option(s) for each patient

Examiner's Instructions

Familiarise yourself with the instructions to the candidates. You should guide the candidate on the use of their time. Each letter should take approximately 2 minutes. Candidates are at liberty to review the letters in any order.

Referral Letter Number 1

Date

Dear Doctor,

I would be grateful if you could see this 78-year-old retired teacher, who experienced an episode of unprovoked vaginal bleeding 3 days ago. She is diabetic on insulin and is hypertensive. Her blood pressure is well controlled on bendrofluoride and methyldopa. There are no associated urinary symptoms.

When she was examined in the clinic, it was difficult to identify the source of the bleeding, as there was a prolapsed lesion at the introitus close to the anterior vaginal wall. She has a mild cystocele and rectocele. She had a vaginal hysterectomy and pelvic floor repair 3 years ago.

Yours sincerely

Dr Clive Jeswitt

Referral Letter Number 2

Date

Dear Doctor,

Thank you for seeing Mrs Beryl John, a 42-year-old theatre nurse, who presented 1 month ago with abdominal discomfort and erratic vaginal bleeding. She has never been sexually active, and her periods were previously regularly occurring every 30 days and lasting for 5 days. For the past 1 year, however, she observed that bleeding had increased, including mid-cycle spotting. Her abdomen also gets bloated mid-cycle, often associated with significant discomfort. She feels otherwise well within herself and has a normal appetite. Her weight has not changed.

On examination, she is found to have a hard, palpable mass, which appears to arise from the uterus reaching the level of the umbilicus. She was unable to tolerate a vaginal examination. An urgent ultrasound scan was therefore arranged (copy enclosed). She is extremely keen to preserve her fertility and has been on the internet where she has found information about embolisation and magnetic resonance-guided focused ultrasound surgery. She is fit and does not have a significant past surgical or medical history and is not on any medications.

The mass is causing quite a lot of discomfort and urinary symptoms. I would be grateful for an early assessment.

Yours sincerely

Dr Patrician Brown

Ultrasound report – date

The uterus is enlarged containing numerous discrete masses, the largest measures 12 × 15 cm. The size of the uterus is difficult to measure because of the masses. The appearances of the masses are typical of uterine fibroids. The ovaries appear normal in size. The endometrial cavity is irregular in shape.

Referral Letter Number 3

Date

Dear Doctor,

Would you be kind enough to see this 42-year-old woman, Mrs Shantal Breya, who came to see me today with severe anxiety and loss of appetite. She recently lost her husband to cancer and has been suffering from mood swings and loss of concentration. Over the last 12 months, her periods have been completely unpredictable and the last one was 4 months ago and very light. I suspect that she may be perimenopausal, and hence I am referring her for a gynaecological opinion. I have placed her on mild anxiolytics in the meantime.

Her past medical history is as follows:

1. Three elective caesarean sections
2. Previous two abnormal smears; all treated by LLETZ – now back on routine follow-up. Her last smear was 12 months ago and was normal
3. Mild hypertension but not on treatment
4. Irritable bowel syndrome treated intermittently with colpermin

Thank you for seeing her.

Yours sincerely

Dr Jaydeep Kaur

Referral Letter Number 4

Dear Doctor,

I would be grateful if you could see Miss Preti Hopkins, a 25-year-old single mother of three, who is requesting for sterilisation. She has had difficulties remembering her oral contraceptive pills and feels that her family is complete and does not, therefore, want any more children. Her present partner is 40 years old and has three children from his previous relationships. They live together with six children.

   She is generally healthy, although has had a persistent vaginal discharge for the past 4 months. I have given her treatment for thrush but this does not seem to have made a significant difference to the discharge.

Yours sincerely

Dr Helma Bounty

Referral Letter Number 5

Date

Dear Doctor,

I would welcome a gynaecological assessment of this 18-year-old student (Susan Jones), virgo intacta, who came to see me very concerned that she has not started menstruating. She is the second of her mother's two children. She has some vague lower abdominal pain, which is intermittent, but there was nothing abnormal found on examination. Her secondary sexual characteristics are well developed (breast, axillary and pubic hair). Many thanks for seeing her.

Yours sincerely

Dr Josephine Plumb

A good candidate will cover the following:

Case Number	Category	Additional information/investigations/precautions/steps to take when admitted	Most likely diagnosis/ differential diagnoses	Treatment option(s)
1	Soon	Pelvic examination including speculum Using any topical HRT? Urinalysis Urea and electrolytes FBC	Urethral prolapse Atrophic vaginitis	Excision Topic oestrogen cream

2	Soon	Any associated urinary symptoms? Abdominal and pelvic examination FBC and urea and electrolytes (renal function) Renal ultrasound scan	Uterine fibroids	Myomectomy Magnetic resonance focus ultrasound (MRgFUS) Uterine artery embolisation Ulipristal acetate GnRH agonist
3	Urgent	Abdominal and pelvic examination CA125 Abdominal and pelvic ultrasound scan Serum FSH and LH	Ovarian cancer Perimenopause	Staging laparotomy Hormone replacement therapy (previously known as HRT)
4	Routine	Contraindications for hormonal contraception Abdominal and pelvic including speculum examination Endocervical/HVS swabs	Unwanted fertility Cervical erosion	Long-acting reversible contraception (LARC) Vasectomy Tubal ligation
5	Routine	Ultrasound scan of pelvis and abdomen	Mullerian abnormality	Referral to paediatric and adolescent gynaecologist Neovagina Excision of rudimentary horn

Examiner score sheet		
Information gathering		
Standard not met	Standard partly met	Standard met
0	1	2
Communication with patients and families		
Standard not met	Standard partly met	Standard met
0	1	2
Communication with colleagues		
Standard not met	Standard partly met	Standard met
0	1	2

Patient safety		
Standard not met	Standard partly met	Standard met
0	1	2
Applied clinical knowledge		
Standard not met	Standard partly met	Standard met
0	1	2

Examiner Expectations and Basis for Assessment

Information gathering

- Identifies additional information/appropriate investigations for each patient
- Discusses appropriate investigations for each of the patients and the information to be obtained from the investigation
- Synthesises the information provided in each letter and then uses it correctly in planning and management

Communication with patients and families

- Able to communicate to each patient the need for further investigations and when to come to the clinic
- Able to explain the rationale for classifying cases as routine, soon or urgent

Communication with colleagues

- Able to prioritise the letters appropriately into urgent, soon (semi-urgent) and routine (non-urgent) cases
- Able to form a logical differential diagnosis for each of the cases
- Provides appropriate amount of detail to ensure management plans are clear and easily understood by colleagues
- Able to identify additional expertise required for each case as its prioritised

Patient safety

- Aware of possible consequences of a delay in seeing a patient on the waiting list
- Has an understanding of the need for additional investigations to ensure correct diagnosis and treatment
- Appreciates the complications of treatment

Applied clinical knowledge

- Knowledgeable of various common gynaecological problems
- Able to critically appraise the information provided in the letters to arrive at a diagnosis
- Able to initiate appropriate investigations to confirm diagnosis and make management plans
- Has a working knowledge of the roles of other members of the multidisciplinary team to ensure best care for patient (in discussing the additional precautions to be taken)
- Knowledgeable at an appropriate level of various NICE/RCOG Guidelines in gynaecology and the governments recommendation for waiting times for oncology cases

---

Task 12: Long-Acting Reversible Contraception. Module 11 – Sexual and Reproductive Health

Candidate's Instructions

This is a simulated patient task assessing:

- Information gathering
- Communication with patients and families
- Communication with colleagues
- Patient safety
- Applied clinical knowledge

You are an ST5 in the gynaecology clinic. The GP has referred a 34-year-old for counselling on contraception. The referral letter is given below.

Winchester Road Surgery
12 Winchester Road
Southend-on-Sea
SO19 7TY

Dear Dr,
Re: Mrs Heather French, Age 34 years
I saw this woman in my surgery requesting contraception. She wanted to go on the combined oral contraceptive pill. Her history is very complicated and I was not comfortable starting her on this. I would be grateful if you could see and offer her the best option. The family planning services are too far from here, and hence I am referring her to the gynaecology clinic.

Yours sincerely

Dr Sanjay Prabhu MBChB, FRCGP

You have 10 minutes in which you should:

- Take focused history
- Initiate any investigations considered appropriate
- Offer contraceptive advice

Simulated Patient's Information

You are Mrs Heather French, a 34-year-old teacher who went to your GP 3 weeks ago for contraceptive advice. He referred you to the hospital because he was unsure which option would best suite you.

You have had two children – the first was an emergency caesarean section 4 years ago, because you had remained at the same stage in labour for 6 hours. Your son weighed 3,400 g. Your second was an elective caesarean section (it was your choice as you did not want to have an emergency CS) 12 months ago. You breast fed exclusively for 6 months and after that your husband started using the condom. You are not very comfortable with this as it can fail. You are not sure you will have more children, hence will like an alternate reliable form on contraception. You have never used any form of contraception before. You discussed this with your husband who himself wanted to go for a vasectomy as he does not want more children but because you are unsure you were against it.

Your periods are regular. The last one was 1 week ago. They occur every 28–30 days, and you bleed for 3–4 days. The first day is always heavy but you do not pass clots and the bleeding never gets through the pad. You do no suffer from any bleeding in between periods.

You had diabetes in the first pregnancy and after that the diabetes did not go away. You are currently taking Glucophage (metformin) which controls your blood sugars very well. Your father and mother also have type II diabetes and are on similar medication. You suffer from high blood pressure and take methyldopa 250 mg three times a day. When you were pregnant, you were given daily injections to thin your blood as you were told your risk of having a blood clot was high. You have never had pelvic infection before and your husband is your third partner.

You neither drink alcohol nor smoke, but your husband Craig, who is 40 years old, is a social drinker but does not smoke.

You are allergic to aspirin. Your last smear test was 3 months ago and was normal. You last weighed yourself in pregnancy and were 93 kg.

If not covered, you may ask the following:

- Why can I not have the combined oral contraceptive pill?
- What are the side effects of the contraception you are recommending for me?
- What will happen if I want to have a baby?
- Does this contraceptive affect my diabetes and high blood pressure?

A good candidate should cover the following:

Information gathering

- Focused history
  - Menstrual cycles – duration and regularity; heavy or not?
  - Sexual health history – no previous history of STIs

- Obstetric history – two previous CS and complicated by GDM, given anticoagulants during pregnancy (not sure why)
  - Medical disorders – type II diabetes and hypertensive
  - Smear history and allergy
  - Contraception history – previous use and whether vasectomy was considered as an option
- Examination
  - Check weight and blood pressure – measure and then abdomen and pelvis examination
- Investigations
  - Thrombophilia screen – this may be necessary
- Reviews obstetrics records/notes to understand rationale for thromboprophylaxis, and if not clear, investigates for thrombophilia
- Performs pregnancy test to rule out pregnancy

Communication with patients and families

- Discusses the various options and outlines the rationale for why other forms are contraindicated, especially the combined contraception (UK Medical Eligibility Criteria – UKMEC)
- Able to identify a chosen method for patient – copper intrauterine device – best option followed by the levonorgestrel intrauterine system
- Discusses the pros and cons of the recommended method of contraception – (frequency of application, side effects, duration of action and reversibility)
- Explains why depot and Nexplanon are not preferred options
- Obtains consent to insert copper IUD/levonorgestrel IUD (Mirena)

Communication with colleagues

- Knows limits of one's own abilities and may consider referral to family planning services if needed
- Feedback to the GP

Patient safety

- Confirms patients details at the start of the task
- Establishes drug allergy
- Safe prescription, with respect to contraception
- Uses the UKMEC to discuss the reasons why other methods of contraception cannot be used
- Able to determine when to insert the IUD and make sure the patient is not pregnant
- Offers appropriate advice after inserting the IUD, depending on the day in the cycle
- Education on when to seek for help – indications for this(strings not felt, missed period, irregular periods, abnormal discharge and suspected pregnancy)

Applied clinical knowledge

- Most suitable option – LARC and why?
- Contraindications to combined hormonal contraception (weight, diabetes, hypertensive and high risk for venous thromboembolism)
- Timing of insertion and counselling and advice for post insertion care
- Demonstrates knowledge of NICE LARC, FSRH and RCOG Guidelines on contraception

Examiner score sheet		
Information gathering		
Standard not met	Standard partly met	Standard met
0	1	2
Communication with patients and families		
Standard not met	Standard partly met	Standard met
0	1	2
Communication with colleagues		
Standard not met	Standard partly met	Standard met
0	1	2
Patient safety		
Standard not met	Standard partly met	Standard met
0	1	2
Applied clinical knowledge		
Standard not met	Standard partly met	Standard met
0	1	2

Examiner Expectations and Basis for Assessment

Information gathering

- Takes comprehensive sexual health history as well as relevant history
- Requests for and reviews obstetrics notes
- Requests for appropriate investigations, including general examination, BP check, abdominal and pelvic examination

Communication with colleagues

- Able to document in detail and prioritise chosen method in communication/feedback to GP
- May consider referral to family planning centre if unable to provide chosen method or insert the IUD

Communication with patients and families

- Outlines clearly the chosen methods of contraception (pros and cons)
- Explains the rationale for contraindications for other methods especially the combined hormonal contraception
- Summarises discussions succinctly and checks understanding by the patient at appropriate intervals, encouraging questions and answering all of them

Patient safety

- Confirms patients identify at the start of the task
- Contraindications to combined hormonal contraception
- Screens for thrombophilia
- Establishes drug allergy
- Safe prescription

Applied clinical knowledge

- Knowledgeable of the various forms of contraception
- Demonstrates an understanding of the UKMEC
- Familiar with NICE guidelines on long-acting reversible contraception (LARC), RCOG and FSRH Guidelines on the provision of contraception

Reference: Long-acting reversible contraception. NICE Clinical guideline [CG30] 26 October 2005. Last updated 02 July 2019

Task 13: Secondary Haemorrhage Presenting after Hysterectomy. Module 3 – Post-Operative Care

Candidate's Instructions

This is a structured discussion task assessing:

- Communication with colleagues
- Communication with patients and families
- Patient safety
- Applied clinical knowledge

You are the ST5 in the unit and have been called to see a patient who had a hysterectomy (laparoscopic) 24 hours ago. This was straightforward, and the patient is supposed to go home today. The sister has called you, concerned about her vital signs. Her vital signs chart for the last 11 hours is given below.

Time	2000	2100	2200	2300	2400	0100	0200	0300	0400	0500	0600
Pulse/min	88	92	78	60	84	88	90	94	98	100	110
RR/min	16	20	22	18	20	18	20	22	22	20	20
Systolic BP (mmHg)	120	125	135	130	132	128	125	120	120	122	118
Diastolic BP (mmHg)	70	75	70	78	73	70	68	70	65	65	64
Temperature (°C)	36.5	36.7	36.4	37.1	36.8	36.4	36.9	37.0	36.6	36.4	36.6

She has not passed any urine in the past 6 hours.

You have 10 minutes in which you will discuss the management of the patient with the examiner who has four questions to guide the discussion.

Examiner's Instructions

Familiarise yourself with the candidate's instructions.

Use the following four questions to guide the discussion you will have with the candidate. Provide some guidance on how much time the candidate spends on each question.

1. What would be your initial response to this patient?
2. What are the possible reasons for her vital signs?
3. What would be your management for this patient?
4. How will you deal with governance issues around her management?

A good candidate should cover the following:

What would be your initial response to this patient?

- Review her notes (operation notes, looking for any difficulties at surgery, estimated blood loss, risk factors for bleeding (e.g. difficulties securing haemostasis), vital signs etc.)
- Enquire after symptoms that may suggest the cause of deterioration in signs (e.g. increasing pains in the abdomen)
- Perform an examination – general, abdomen and vaginal
- Insert two large-size cannulae (16 FG)
- Blood for group and cross-match four units of blood
- Inform consultant
- Inform theatre
- Counsel patient and inform ward staff
- Obtain consent for exploratory laparotomy

What are the possible reasons for her vital signs?

- Pain post surgery
- Internal haemorrhage (most likely)
- Ureteric injuries
- Infection leading to septic shock

What would be your management for this patient?

- Obtain consent for exploration (surgery)
- Arrange exploratory laparotomy with consultant
- Resuscitate (IV fluids – plasma expanders)
- FBC, urea and electrolytes and cross-match blood
- Exploratory laparotomy
- Identify bleeders and stop them
- Drain in abdomen
- Antibiotics
- Thromboprophylaxis
- Discharge with communication to GP and follow-up in the clinic to see consultant

How will you deal with governance issues around her management?

- Complete incident form (Datix form)
- Inform risk manager and team
- Debrief patient as soon as possible, reinforcing the message and ensuring that all questions are answered
- Undertake root cause analysis and communicate report findings with patient, welcoming questions and being honest (duty of candour)
- Institute steps to address any deficiencies identified by the root cause analysis
- Arrange a follow-up to complete debrief

Examiner score sheet		
Information gathering		
Standard not met	Standard partly met	Standard met
0	1	2
Communication with patients and families		
Standard not met	Standard partly met	Standard met
0	1	2
Communication with colleagues		
Standard not met	Standard partly met	Standard met
0	1	2
Patient safety		
Standard not met	Standard partly met	Standard met
0	1	2
Applied clinical knowledge		
Standard not met	Standard partly met	Standard met
0	1	2

Examiner Expectations and Basis for Assessment

Communication with patients and families

- Communicates with the patient about the complication
- Debriefs after surgery
- Shares risk management report with the patient (duty of candour)

Communication with colleagues

- Communicates with the nursing staff
- Informs consultant, anaesthetist, theatres and blood bank
- Completes incident form
- Informs GP with a detailed follow-up plan as well and short-term and long-term management plan

---

Applied clinical knowledge

- Knowledgeable on how to diagnose post-operative complications, especially haemorrhage
- Aware of the differential diagnoses of possible deteriorating post-operative patient
- Knows when to re-operate
- Demonstrates knowledge of current literature on management of major complications of surgery

---

Patient safety

- Fluid resuscitation
- Quick exploration and arrest of bleeding
- Antibiotics
- Thromboprophylaxis
- Checks allergy and safe prescription

Task 14: Ovarian Cancer. Module 13 – Gynaecological Cancer

Candidate's Instructions

This is a structured discussion assessing:

- Information gathering
- Communication with patients and families
- Communication with colleagues
- Patient safety
- Applied clinical knowledge

You are an ST5 and have been asked to see a patient referred by her GP because of dyspeptic symptoms and bloating. The letter from the GP is given below. The examiner has a set of questions to ask you about the patient.

Summerway Bank Surgery
Wellington
Somerset
TA12H44

Dear Dr,
Re: Mrs Blanche Stricker Age 57 years
Will you be kind enough to see this patient urgently? She is a 56-year-old saleswoman, with a high-street store. She saw me today complaining that she has been feeling bloated and also suffering from indigestion. Her tummy is getting bigger. She has never been diagnosed to be suffering with irritable bowel syndrome. I feel that in light of the NICE guideline on ovarian cancer screening, we need to screen her. I could feel a mass in the lower abdomen on palpation. I have requested for a CA125, and the result should be with you by the time she sees you.

Yours sincerely

Dr Tunde Fagbomi MBBS, MRCP, DCH, DRCOG

You have 10 minutes in which you should study the referral letter and then discuss the management of the patient with the examiner, who has four questions to use. The examiner will guide your time management.

Additional Patient Information

Mrs Blanche Stricker is a 57-year-old saleswoman with a high-street store. She has two children, aged 30 and 32. She had been healthy until now. Her husband is a 65-year-old retired storekeeper.

Mrs Stricker has been struggling to fit into her dresses lately, and in fact, feels that her tummy has got bigger. At first, she did not bother about this but is now worried as she is suffering from severe indigestion to the extent that she dreads eating. She has not lost weight.

Her mother died from cancer of the breast and her father who is alive has a heart problem.

She is up to date with her smears, and apart from two caesarean sections for her children, she has not had any surgery. She does not smoke but drinks occasionally.

Examiner's instructions

Familiarise yourself with the information above, and use the four questions below to discuss the management of the patient with the candidate. You should direct the candidate as to the use of their time, ensuring that the candidate attempts the four questions.

1. The CA125 has come back as 450 iu/L. Justify the investigations you will undertake on the patient?
2. Having completed the investigations, what will be the next step in the management of this patient? Why is this important?
3. What would be the approach to managing this patient? Describe the treatment that she will be offered?
4. How will she be managed after this treatment (if the candidate does not mention surgery, ask the question as what will the treatment be after surgery)?

A good candidate should cover the following:

Information gathering

- Justifying the investigations: Her RMI is >250, and therefore the working diagnosis is ovarian cancer. Investigations would be two-fold – confirmation and enabling planning and treatment
  - Liver and renal function tests, FBC, group and safe (will require surgery)
  - Ultrasound scan of the pelvis and abdomen – to define the type of tumour
  - MRI/CT of the abdomen and liver to define the presence of secondaries in the abdomen
  - CXR – for secondaries in the chest

Communication with patients and families

- Explains the rationale for the investigations being ordered
- Discusses the differential diagnosis (with ovarian cancer being the most likely diagnosis on the basis of symptoms) sensitively and in a language that the patient will understand
- Briefly outlines management of ovarian cancer as this the most likely diagnosis here
- Explains referral to gynaecological oncologist
- Provides information in a step-wise approach and pauses to confirm understanding and also take questions

Communication with colleagues

- Most important step after completing investigations is referral to MDT, including a gynaecological oncologist, pathologist, radiologist, radiotherapy, oncologist, cancer nurse and GP (if possible)
- Cancer support team to be involved

Patient safety

- Confirms patients details at the start of the task
- Empowering patient to make informed choices
- Safety of prescribing therapy

Applied clinical knowledge

- Most likely diagnosis – ovarian cancer; management will be for ovarian cancer
  - Staging laparotomy – mid-line, TAH, BSO, infracolic omentectomy, peritoneal washing and omental biopsies – for staging and also debulking (best result of surgery is if residual disease is <1 cm)
    - Subject specimen to histology for confirmation of cancer and type
- Adjuvant chemotherapy for 6 months
- Follow-up with clinical and radiological with CA125; clinical examination not very reliable to identify recurrence
- Use of guidelines to inform clinical discussions and management

Examiner score sheet		
Information gathering		
Standard not met	Standard partly met	Standard met
0	1	2
Communication with patients and families		
Standard not met	Standard partly met	Standard met
0	1	2
Communication with colleagues		
Standard not met	Standard partly met	Standard met
0	1	2
Patient safety		
Standard not met	Standard partly met	Standard met
0	1	2
Applied clinical knowledge		
Standard not met	Standard partly met	Standard met
0	1	2

Rationale for Scoring under Each of the Domains – Expectations from Candidates

Information gathering

- Takes comprehensive history of the insidious onset of symptoms suggestive of malignancy
- Requests appropriate investigations (abdominal and pelvic examination), chest X-ray, tumour markers, full blood count and liver and renal function tests and biopsies
- Uses given CA125 to calculate RMI
- Imaging – ultrasound followed by MRI/CT scan of the pelvis and abdomen

Communication with patients and families

- Counsels about the diagnosis and how these relate to symptoms
- Describes clearly the logical approach to different management options (pros and cons), including complications and rationale for care and follow-up – investigations, referral to gynaecological oncologist and most likely treatment

Communication with colleagues

- Ability to refer an oncology centre
- Has an understanding of the role of MDT in the management of ovarian cancer
- Has an understanding of the role of support groups in the management of the patient

Patient safety

- Confirms patients details at the start of the task
- Safe prescription – adjuvant chemotherapy for managing ovarian cancer – asking about allergies and medical disorders that could be considered contraindications to the medications
- Principles of safe surgery – WHO safe surgery checklist

Applied clinical knowledge

- Good knowledge of implications of ovarian cancer as evidence from explaining diagnosis and management options
- Has an understanding of the contents of NICE/RCOG Guidelines on ovarian cysts/cancer, with regard to management, follow-up and implications for fertility
- Refers to patient educational materials on endometriosis (e.g. from the RCOG)

Reference: Ovarian cancer: recognition and initial management. NICE Clinical guideline [CG122] 27 April 2011

14
Paper III

Task 1: Perineal Repair. Module 1 – Teaching

Candidate's Instructions

This is a simulated trainee task assessing:

1. Information gathering
2. Communication with patients and families
3. Communication with colleagues
4. Patient safety
5. Applied clinical knowledge

You are the ST5 who is required to teach a Specialist Trainee in her first year to perform a repair of a perineal tear.

You have 10 minutes in which you should:

- Outline to the trainee the principles of perineal repair
- Teach in a step-wise manner how to undertake a repair
- Educate on the follow-up after a repair

A competent candidate will cover the following in the session *(the information contained in the narrative below is too detailed to be covered in 10 minutes but it provides the platform for better understanding of the basis for this type of assessment):*

a. **Introduction and establishment of knowledge level and experience**
   - Introduce yourself and the purpose of the task
   - Ask if they have observed, done or read about a perineal repair
b. **State clearly the objectives of the session and the goals to be achieved at the end.**
   At the end of the session, you should be able to:
   - Understand the principles involved in repairing an episiotomy and a second-degree perineal tear
   - Repair an episiotomy or a second-degree perineal tear
   - Assess the patient to ensure that the procedure has been completed safely
c. **Explain and obtain consent from the patient and prepare for procedure**
   - Explain to the patient what is to be done and why
   - Offer inhalational analgesia such as Entonox and local infiltration, or if already has an epidural, no need for further analgesia if appropriately topped up

- Ensure good lighting is available
- Position the patient so that she is comfortable and that the genital structures can be seen clearly

d. **Systematic assessment of genital or perineal trauma should include:**
- An initial examination, if none was done immediately following birth, to define the degree of perineal trauma (vaginal and anal) – a per vaginal (PV) and per rectal (PR) examination should be performed in the presence of any degree of genital trauma, including vaginal or perineal trauma
- A confirmation by the patient that tested effective local or regional analgesia is in place
- A visual assessment of the extent of perineal trauma. Commence the examination anteriorly; examine the periurethral area and descent laterally to include the labia, vaginal vault, lateral vaginal walls, anterior and posterior vaginal walls, the perineal body and the anal sphincter
- The apex of the injury should be clearly identified and assessment of bleeding noted
- A per anal (PA) and per rectal (PR) examination to assess whether there has been any damage to the external or internal anal sphincter if there is any degree of genital trauma, including vaginal or perineal trauma

e. **Classification of perineal trauma – explain the classification of perineal trauma to the trainee**

Degree	Trauma (description)
First degree	Superficial lacerations to the vaginal and perineal skin only
Second degree	Injury to the posterior vaginal wall, subcutaneous fat, perineal skin and superficial muscle (bulbocavernosus and superficial transverse perinei) and deep muscle. But not involving the anal sphincter, includes damage resulting from an episiotomy
Third degree	Injury to the perineum involving the anal sphincter muscles
3a	Less than 50% of external anal sphincter thickness torn
3b	More than 50% of external anal sphincter thickness torn
3c	Internal sphincter torn
Fourth degree	Complete disruption of the external and internal anal sphincter complex and the anal epithelium

f. **Preparation for procedure – what is required (this will depend on the type of analgesia needed) – assuming that the patient does not have an epidural**
- Sterile suture/delivery pack
- Suture instrument set
- 20 ml syringe
- Green needle
- Obstetric cream
- Clean tap water
- Lidocaine 1%, 20 ml
- Sterile gloves
- Vicryl rapide 0 or 2/0 (1–2 packets)

g. **Performing the procedure**
- This is a sterile procedure and referral should be made to the 'Standard Infection Prevention' guideline
- Count swabs and sutures prior to the procedure with a second person
- Swab perineum with gauze soaked in clean tap water (one swipe only)
- Carefully visualise tear/episiotomy to ensure the extent of the tear is recognised prior to the commencement of suturing and to identify landmarks (i.e. hymen ring) that will facilitate correct tissue realignment
- Infiltrate perineal tear with 1% lidocaine 20 ml (as per standing orders)
- Infiltrate through the wound. Take care to infiltrate symmetrically to prevent distortion of the wound and subsequent repair
- Allow time for lidocaine to work. Alternatively, if patient has an epidural in, ensure it is topped up prior to suturing

h. **Procedure: Principles – vagina, perineal muscle and skin**
- Identify the apex of the tear/episiotomy. Insert first suture about 1 cm above the apex of the tear and tie a knot. Avoid placing first stitch too deep – remember close proximity to the rectum
- Close posterior vaginal wall using continuous non-locking sutures, using vicryl rapide 2/0, on a tapercut needle 0.5 cm from the edge of the wound, 1 cm apart and 1 cm deep
- Continue suturing until the introitus is reached using the hymenal remnants as a landmark. Bring the needle through the tissue underneath the hymenal ring into the muscle layer
- Define the depth of the wound, close the perineal body (muscle layer) and close with continuous non-locking sutures
- Finally repair the perineal skin using continuous subcuticular or interrupted transcutaneous sutures. Continuous subcuticular are less painful

i. **On completion**
- Check vagina. Ensure it easily admits two fingers and for any further high vaginal wall lacerations
- Perform a rectal examination to check for any sutures that have penetrated the rectal mucosa (if they have, undo and repeat procedure)
- Consider voltarol® 100 mg per rectum for analgesia if there are no contraindications
- Swab the perineum and place a sterile pad in situ
- With a second person, count the needles, swabs and instruments, recording the findings on the clinical data collection system

Communication with colleagues

- State the objectives of teaching and what the outcome of the exercise will be
- Ascertain if the trainee has seen a repair before and their experience with repairs
- Elaborate/explain the principles involved in perineal repair
- Describe different types of tears and what the requirements for undertaking a repair are
- Take the trainee in a step-wise manner through how perineal repairs are done
- Discuss the indications for referral to seniors for repair

Communication with patients and families
- Explain what the patient should be told
  - Obtain consent

- Adequate analgesia
- Duration of repair and course of the recovery

Patient safety

- Ensure the trainee understands the risk of improperly repaired perineal tears
- Confirm patients details before embarking on the procedure
- Minimise complications from anaesthesia and provide the right dosage of local anaesthetic to be administered
- Take steps to identify and deal with complications of the repair
- Teaching should show that steps have been taken to minimise the long-term consequences of repair, especially as relates to subsequent pregnancies

Applied clinical knowledge

- Explain the principles of perineal repair
- Teach on the different types of perineal tears
- Justify the use of instruments, place of repair and lighting
- Justify the checking procedure after a successful repair
- Demonstrate awareness of current literature, including RCOG Green-top Guidelines

Examiner score sheet		
Information gathering		
Standard not met	Standard partly met	Standard met
0	1	2
Communication with patients and families		
Standard not met	Standard partly met	Standard met
0	1	2
Communication with colleagues		
Standard not met	Standard partly met	Standard met
0	1	2
Patient safety		
Standard not met	Standard partly met	Standard met
0	1	2
Applied clinical knowledge		
Standard not met	Standard partly met	Standard met
0	1	2

Examiner Expectations and Basis for Assessment

Information gathering

- Has an understanding of the need to first determine the skills of the tutee – what are they
- The expectations of the tutee – state clearly the expectations at the end of the teaching

Communication with patients and families

- Appropriate introduction to the patient and partner
- Explain the role of the tutee and nature of the interaction to the patient
- Informed consent is obtained for teaching from the patient

Communication with colleagues

- Introduces self and role
- Has an understanding of the principles of adult learning and giving feedback
- Takes appropriate steps in increasing the clinical and technical skills of the learner (tutee), with respect to a perineal tear repair
- Ability to use appropriate verbal and non-verbal communication to encourage learning
- Invites questions and encourages dialogue
- Shows a logical approach to building the pre-existing skills of the learner

Patient safety

- Confirms patient identity prior to commencement of suturing
- Patient safety is maintained when teaching a practical skill, showing an understanding of when to continue teaching and when to intervene to halt the teaching session
- Appropriate checks are undertaken to ensure procedure has been appropriately undertaken
- Safe prescription, especially with respect to the administration of local anaesthetics
- Ensures there is a pelvic examination to eliminate the risk of injury from the repair
- Maintains patient dignity during teaching

Applied clinical knowledge

Demonstrates:

- An understanding of the steps in the tasks being undertaken (teaching task)
- An understanding of the learning objectives and outcomes in relation to the tasks being taught
- An ability to conduct and give feedback on using a work-based assessment tool in this task
- Current knowledge of the literature on perineal repair, especially RCOG Green-top Guidelines

---

Reference: The management of third- and fourth-degree perineal tears. The Royal College of Obstetricians and Gynaecologists Green-top Guideline No. 29 June 2016

Task 2: Macrosomia. Module 6 – Management of Labour

Candidates Instructions

This is a four-part structured discussion assessing:

- Information gathering
- Communication with patients and families
- Communication with colleagues
- Patient safety
- Applied clinical knowledge

You are an ST5 in the clinic and have been asked to see a patient who has just returned from an ultrasound scan. This is a 29-year-old primigravida, who is now 34 weeks pregnant. She booked for antenatal care at 11 weeks of gestation. This was an unplanned pregnancy. Her BMI at booking was 34 kg/M². All the investigations performed at boking came back as normal. She is blood group O Rhesus D positive. She had a combined biochemical and NT screening at 13 weeks, and this was low risk. At 26 weeks, she had an oral glucose tolerance test which was normal (fasting 4.8 mmol/l and 2 hours 6.0 mmol/L). At 20 weeks, she had a detailed ultrasound scan which was normal. Her care so far has been with the midwife. When she saw the midwife last week, the fundal height measured 38 cm. The midwife, therefore, referred her to the hospital for an ultrasound scan and a follow-up in the clinic. The baby's movements are normal.

She had her ultrasound scan today, and the baby's abdominal circumference is >95th centile, and there is polyhydramnios (with the single deepest vertical pool of 12 cm and an AFI of 25 cm). The fetus is in cephalic presentation and the placenta is fundal.

You have 10 minutes to discuss the diagnosis and management of the problems this patient presents with. The examiner has four questions around which to structure the discussion. You will be guided as to how your time is distributed to each of the questions.

Examiner's Instructions

You have four questions around which to structure your discussion with the candidate. The discussion should be completed in 10 minutes. At each stage, you should tell the candidate any additional information and then begin the discussion by covering the following points:

1. What investigations will you like to order for her and why?
2. These investigations come back as normal, what would be the plan for the rest of the pregnancy including counselling?
3. She presents in labour at 38 weeks' gestation with intact membranes, what would be your management of the patient?
4. She progresses to full dilatation but there is a delay in crowning of the head. After an initial delay, she delivers the head but the shoulders are stuck. Outline how you will manage this patient from now until she leaves the hospital.

A good candidate will cover the following:

1. Reviews the scan report to check if structural abnormalities associated with polyhydramnios have been excluded (such as duodenal atresia, diaphragmatic hernia, gastro-oesophageal atresia and cranial); if these were not mentioned in the report, request for a scan to exclude them
   Screens for diabetes – although the OGTT was normal, a screening test should be repeated – an OGTT is not reliable at this stage, and so a blood sugar series is best (fasting and post prandial)
2. Counsels the patient about the diagnosis and implications (increased risk of prelabour rupture of fetal membranes and cord prolapse and abdominal pain). Arranges for a serial ultrasound scan – for the estimation of the fetal weight and liquor volume quantification, including presentation
3. Continues the rest of the antenatal care in a consultant-led clinic
4. Manages the anticipation of complications: IV line, group and safe and watch out for cord prolapse with rupture of membranes, especially if head if not engaged; placental abruption and anticipate shoulder dystocia and postpartum haemorrhage
5. Calls for help – experience midwife, anaesthetist, neonatologist, consultant obstetrician or ST6/7. Asks a staff member to document and time duration of manoeuvres. Documents and start manoeuvres (each lasting not more than 30 seconds) – start by placing patient in McRobert's position, follow by applying pressure on the anterior shoulder and traction, and if unsuccessful, internal manoeuvres
6. Nasogastric tube to be passed before the baby is fed. Completes delivery and placenta and explores genital tract for trauma and repair. Completes incident form and debriefs patient

Examiner score sheet		
Information gathering		
Standard not met	Standard partly met	Standard met
0	1	2

Communication with patients and families		
Standard not met	Standard partly met	Standard met
0	1	2
Communication with colleagues		
Standard not met	Standard partly met	Standard met
0	1	2
Patient safety		
Standard not met	Standard partly met	Standard met
0	1	2
Applied clinical knowledge		
Standard not met	Standard partly met	Standard met
0	1	2

Examiner Expectations and Basis for Assessment

Information gathering

- Able to to interpret ultrasound findings
- Requests for additional investigations, for example, to exclude GDM and fetal abnormalities
- Investigates in labour in the anticipation of complications (FBC and IV line)

Communication with patients and families

- Introduces self and role
- Discusses investigations, follow-up and plan for antenatal care with the patient
- Able to bring out the concerns of the patient and address them sensitively and appropriately, encouraging questions
- Communicates the plan of management for the rest of the pregnancy and during labour, including complications that may arise
- Informs parents of neonatal management after delivery, prior to feeding – passage of nasogastric tube

---

Communication with colleagues

- Liaises with imaging for serial ultrasound scan and/or exclusion of structural causes of polyhydramnios, if not already done
- Able to communicate with colleagues in primary care and other specialties, e.g. obstetric anaesthetists and neonatologists

---

Patient safety

- Awareness of complication of cord prolapse and shoulder dystocia and takes appropriate precautions for this during labour
- Has an understanding of clinical governance and risk management for women declining usual antenatal care
- Active management of second stage of labour
- Being prepared for management of recurrent postpartum haemorrhage (IV line, group and safe and syntocinon in 500 ml Ringer's lactate/normal saline)

Applied clinical knowledge:

- Knowledgeable of antenatal care of women with polyhydramnios and macrosomia, including gestational diabetes
- Has an understanding of management of shoulder dystocia
- Knowledgeable of the recent guidelines on shoulder dystocia and literature on macrosomia and polyhydramnios, RCOG Green to guidelines and current literature

---

1. *Reference:* Intrapartum care for healthy women and babies. NICE Clinical guideline [CG190] 03 December 2014. Last updated 21 February 2017
2. *Reference:* Management of shoulder dystocia. The Royal College of Obstetricians and Gynaecologists Green-top Guideline No. 42 23 March 2012. Last updated February 2017

Task 3: Epilepsy in Pregnancy. Module 5 – Maternal Medicine

Candidate's Instructions

This is a simulated patient task assessing:

- Information gathering
- Communication with patients and families

- Communication with colleagues
- Patient safety
- Applied clinical knowledge

You are the ST5 working with your consultant Dr Jones. He is away, and you have been asked to see Lauren Fay in his absence. The referral letter from her General Practitioner is given below.

Hamilton Road Surgery
Queensferry
Burton
QS1 4SR

Dear Obstetrician,
Re: Mrs Lauren Fay
I would like you to see this 30-year-old who is an epileptic on treatment since the age of 5 years.
She was diagnosed with grand mal epilepsy at the age of 5 years and has been on treatment since then. She is currently on sodium valproate (Epilum), which controls her fits very well. I tried to switch her to something else but this was not as effective as Epilum, and she wanted to continue with it. Her last fit was 12 months ago.
She is married and would like to become pregnant.
She has never been pregnant and her periods are regular. She has been married for 2 years and it was always their plan to start trying for a baby 2 years after marriage. She does not smoke but drinks alcohol socially.
She does not suffer from any other medical disorders. She had a laparoscopy 3 years ago as an emergency for acute lower abdominal pain and was found to have a ruptured ovarian cyst that bleed. This was treated by simply cauterising the bleeding vessels.
Her BMI is 24 kg/M².
She is allergic to penicillin (this is a severe allergy with breathing difficulties and severe rashes; she had it once and had to be given intravenous steroids – she carries an Epipen).

Yours sincerely

James Blamforth MBBS, FRCP, DRCOG

You have 10 minutes in which you should:

- Take a focused history
- Discuss the antenatal management of this patient
- Explain the impact of pregnancy on her condition and pregnancy on her condition and how to minimise these

Simulated Patient's Information

You are Mrs Lauren Fay, a 30-year-old teacher who was diagnosed with epilepsy from the age of 5 years. You have had several investigations (your mother tells you), and the exact cause was not found. You have been on medication since then, and in the last 1 year, you have had fits once. You were told that it is grand mal epilepsy, and you take Epilum (sodium valproate) every day.

When you mentioned to your doctor last year that you wanted to start trying for a baby, he tried to switch you to one of the newer preparations (Lamotrigine) but you took it for a few days and was afraid that your fits will return. You, therefore, went back to him to change you back to Epilum.

You have been married for 2 years and want to start trying for a baby now. This was always your plan, and up to now, you have been very cautious about becoming pregnant, although you do not use any form of contraception.

Your periods are regular, and the last one was 1 week ago. You are fit and exercise regularly. You are not overweight (BMI 24 kg/M^2) and do not smoke but take alcohol occasionally.

You had laparoscopy for a ruptured ovarian cyst three years ago and are allergic to penicillin. You had this antibiotic when you had an infection in your throat and had a terrible rash and could not breathe. You had to have a steroid into your vein to help. You currently carry a card saying you are allergic and an Epipen.

You mother had three children – all were delivered normally but she had diabetes in pregnancy. She is otherwise well and so is your father.

If not covered, you should ask the candidate the following questions:

- *Will the epilepsy affect my baby? Are the tablets I am taking dangerous for the baby?*
- *Will my epilepsy get worse in pregnancy?*
- *How will I be delivered?*
- *Will my baby have epilepsy?*

A good candidate will cover the following:

Information gathering

- History of epilepsy diagnosis, investigations and treatment; how long ago was the last fit
- Menstrual cycles and gynaecological history
- Contraception
- Other medical and surgical history including medications and allergies
- Social history/husband's health

Communication with patients and families

- Introduces self and role
- Recommends coming off Epilum – not advisable in pregnancy because of teratogenicity and potential effect on fertility
- Contraception while stabilising on new anti-epileptic
- Folic acid – 5 mg
- Referral to neurologist
- Discusses the impact of epilepsy on pregnancy and vice versa
- Management of pregnancy – referral to an obstetrician with an interest in epilepsy in pregnancy or a Medical Disorders in Pregnancy Clinic
- Involvement of fetal medicine team for screening for congenital malformations
- Delivery and postnatal follow-up, including the risk of epilepsy on the baby

Communication with colleagues

- Consultation with neurologist
- Provision of information leaflet

- Multidisciplinary team when pregnant – primary care (GP), specialist midwife, obstetrician with an interest in medical disorders in pregnancy, fetal medicine, neurologist and anaesthetist

Patient safety

- Confirms patients details at the start of the task
- Safe prescription
- Ascertains drug allergy
- Provision of patient leaflets on planning pregnancy

Applied clinical knowledge

- Demonstrates good knowledge of managing epilepsy in pregnancy and being up to date with the current medical literature, especially RCOG Green-top Guideline on women with epilepsy in pregnancy

Examiner score sheet		
Information gathering		
Standard not met	Standard partly met	Standard met
0	1	2
Communication with patients and families		
Standard not met	Standard partly met	Standard met
0	1	2
Communication with colleagues		
Standard not met	Standard partly met	Standard ct
0	1	2
Patient safety		
Standard not met	Standard partly met	Standard met
0	1	2
Applied clinical knowledge		
Standard not met	Standard partly met	Standard met
0	1	2

Examiner Expectations and Basis for Assessment

Information gathering

- Able to take concise and relevant medical history on a patient with epilepsy planning pregnancy
- Skilled in signposting and guiding the consultation

- Able to ensure that the patient understands and encourages questions
- Able to describe to the patient with epilepsy a clear pre-pregnancy care plan and the rationale for a follow-up based on discussion

Communication with patients and families

- Introduces self and role to the patient
- Able to tackle the sensitivity of teratogenicity and delaying pregnancy until the timing is best for the fetus and the mother
- Able to give information to the patient with epilepsy of both its impact of the pregnancy on her condition and her condition on the pregnancy and the fetus

Communication with colleagues

- Able to communicate with or refer to colleagues in primary care and within the multidisciplinary team, including specialist midwife, physicians and fetal medicine

Patient safety

- Ensures patient's details are confirmed at start of task
- Awareness of safety of investigations and therapeutics pre-conception, during pregnancy and in the postnatal period, including safe prescription for the patient with epilepsy
- Has an understanding of both the impact of pregnancy on epilepsy conditions and the impact of epilepsy on the pregnancy and the fetus
- Drug allergy history and safe prescription

Applied clinical knowledge

Demonstrates he/she:

- hasappropriate knowledge of pre-conception, antenatal and postnatal care, including the risks of maternal morbidity and mortality related to epilepsy in pregnancy
- has appropriate knowledge of RCOG Green-top Guidelines on the management of women with epilepsy in pregnancy

Reference: Epilepsy in pregnancy. The Royal College of Obstetricians and Gynaecologists Green-top Guideline No. 68 June 2016

Task 4: Sickle Cell Anaemia. Module 4 – Antepartum Care

Candidate's Instructions

This is a simulated patient task assessing:

- Information gathering
- Communication with patients and families
- Communication with colleagues
- Patient safety
- Applied clinical knowledge

You are the ST5 working with a consultant with an interest in high-risk obstetrics in a district general hospital. You are in the antenatal clinic and are about to see Mrs Jennifer Dawood, who has been sent to the antenatal clinic for booking on account of her medical history.

You have 10 minutes in which you should:

- Obtain relevant history
- Discuss prenatal diagnosis and why
- Explain the effect of her medical condition on her pregnancy
- Explain the impact of pregnancy on her medical condition
- Outline and justify your management of her pregnancy and labour

Simulated Patient's Information

You are Mrs Jennifer Dawood, a 26-year-old lawyer originally from Nigeria, who is attending your fist visit to the hospital in what is your first pregnancy. You are about 10 weeks, and this was a planned pregnancy. You have been married for 3 years, and prior to conceiving, were on folic acid 400 µg per day, which you are still taking.

You have always known that you have sickle cell anaemia since you were old enough to understand why you kept going to the hospital. You have had several admissions, including blood transfusions. You recall suffering from severe pain in your bones and abdomen at various times in the past years. You are happy to say that it's been quite good for the last 3 years, with little pain and hardly any admission into the hospital, but you have had a blood transfusion in the last 1 year.

You have had several admissions for various problems, including chest infections and infections in the bones of your legs and your kidneys. When you were 6 years old, you suffered from very yellow eyes (jaundice). You have a haematologist but she does not know that you are pregnant. You last saw her 3.5 months ago.

You have no other medical or surgical problems but take paracetamol from time to time for pain. You are allergic to powder.

You have two siblings – one has the same problem but the other is normal. You are told that both your parents are sickle cell carriers. Your husband is also of Nigerian descent but does not have any family history of sickle cell disease. He is an engineer.

You neither smoke nor drink alcohol. Your BMI is 21 kg/M² and you are in general fit.

If not covered by the candidate, you should ask the following questions:

- How will you make sure that my baby is not affected by sickle cell anaemia?
- Is my baby normal and what may happen to the baby?

- What problems may I have in this pregnancy?
- What steps will you take to make sure that I am safe during the pregnancy?
- When and how will I be delivered?
- Is there a risk that I may die in this pregnancy?

A good candidate will cover the following:

Information gathering

- Takes a good history – past medical history including previous treatments, family history and social history – partner (origin/ethnicity) – and current medication
- Information on investigations already done by GP or haematologist
- Reviews recent investigations – especially renal function test and full blood count

Communication with the patients and families

- Introduces self and roles
- Explains implications of sickle cell anaemia in pregnancy – increased complications – maternal and fetal. Discusses some of the maternal complications to watch out for
- Explains the details of antenatal care and how to avoid complications
- Explains the management and monitoring, including regular scans, blood tests and need for transfusion etc.
- Time of delivery – to be determined by obstetric reasons – place and mode of delivery
- Involvement of haematologist – multidisciplinary care team

Patient safety

- Confirms patients details at the start of the task
- Prophylaxis – folic acid (higher dose) and avoiding iron unless iron deficiency anaemia
- General health measures – hydration avoidance of risk of DVT
- Avoidance of precipitating factors of crises (e.g. extremes of temperatures, dehydration, infections and overexertion)
- Administers influenza vaccine if not given in the previous year
- Ascertains drug allergy and demonstrates safe prescription

Applied clinical knowledge

- Hb genotyping of husband
- Prenatal diagnosis by NIPD – if husband is a carrier
- Treatment of complications – infections, acute chest syndrome and haemolysis
- Knowledgeable of current literature, including RCOG Green-top Guidelines on sickle cell disease and thalassaemia

Alternate questions (task discussion). This particular problem lends itself to a discussion with the examiner where specific questions could be asked:

1. What will you do after booking this woman?
2. She presents with chest pain; how will you manage her assuming she has acute chest syndrome?
3. What complication may the baby have and how will you manage these?
4. She is admitted into labour. How will you manage her labour and puerperium?

Examiner score sheet		
Information gathering		
Standard not met	Standard partly met	Standard met
0	1	2
Communication with patients and families		
Standard not met	Standard partly met	Standard met
0	1	2
Communication with colleagues		
Standard not met	Standard partly met	Standard met
0	1	2
Patient safety		
Standard not met	Standard partly met	Standard met
0	1	2
Applied clinical knowledge		
Standard not met	Standard partly met	Standard met
0	1	2

Examiner Expectations and Basis for Assessment

Information gathering

- Able to take concise and relevant antenatal history
- Skills in signposting and guiding the antenatal consultation
- Able to ensure that the patient understands and encourages questions
- Able to describe to the antenatal patient with sickle cell anaemia a clear action plan and the rationale for a follow-up based on the discussion

Communication with patients and families

- Introduces self and role
- Able to discuss investigations, follow-up and plan for antenatal care, including prenatal diagnosis by NIPD
- Able to sensitively discuss the complications of sickle cell anaemia in pregnancy and how to minimise them
- Able to succinctly summarise discussions with antenatal patients

---

Communication with colleagues

- Appropriate involvement of other disciplinarians in the care of pregnant women with sickle cell anaemia (haematologist, obstetrician with an interest in haematological disorders, specialist midwife, GP and fetal medicine)
- Ability to know when to interact with other specialties, e.g. obstetric anaesthetics antenatally

---

Patient safety

- Confirms patients details at the start of the task
- Ability to triage patient to different patterns of antenatal care according to risk factors
- Awareness of safety of investigations and therapeutics during pregnancy, including safe prescription, e.g. with regard to iron supplementation (contraindicated), immunisation etc.
- Has an understanding of the clinical governance and the risk management for women declining antenatal testing/prenatal diagnosis

---

Applied clinical knowledge

- Knowledgeable of antenatal care and of women with haematological disorders, especially sickle cell anaemia
- Ability to interpret clinical examination findings and results of investigations in the context of sickle cell anaemia
- Awareness of the risks and benefits of various different management options balancing the needs of the mother and the fetus
- Knowledgeable of the current literature, including RCOG Green-top Guidelines on haematological disorders in pregnancy (specifically sickle cell disease)

Reference: Management of sickle cell disease in pregnancy. The Royal College of Obstetricians and Gynaecologists Green-top Guideline No. 61 July 2011

Task 5: Vaginal Birth after CS. Module 7 – Management of Delivery

Candidate's Instructions

This is a simulated patient task assessing:

- Information gathering
- Communication with patients and families

- Communication with colleagues
- Patient safety
- Applied clinical knowledge

You are Dr Patchett's ST5 working in a unit that delivers 4,500 babies per year. You are in the antenatal clinic and have been called by the midwife to see a patient who has been referred by her GP for counselling at 34 weeks of gestation. The referral letter is given below.

Featherstone Surgery
Stockdale
Yorkshire
YK2 4TT

Dear Dr Patchett,
I will be grateful if you would be kind enough to see Mrs Modiwe Sikuwjabe, a 30-year-old teacher in her second pregnancy, for counselling about the mode of delivery. Her first pregnancy ended in an emergency caesarean section when she was 8 cm dilated. She would like to review her options for this pregnancy.

Yours sincerely

Dr Suhbit Arora MBChB, MRCP, DFFP, DRCOG

You have 10 minutes in which you should:

- Take focused history
- Discuss the management of the patient
- Answer any questions she may have

Simulated Patient's Information

You are Mrs Modiwe Sikuwjabe, a 30-year-old teacher, who is now 34 weeks into your second pregnancy. You live in a rented (you have just moved into the area) detached house at the outskirts of the city with your husband Desmond Sikuwjabe, who is 36 years old and works in the bank. This pregnancy has been uneventful so far, and the midwife who has been looking after you feels you could go for a vaginal delivery. The GP therefore referred you to the hospital.

Your first pregnancy was uncomplicated, and you went into labour 2 days after your due date. You were admitted and told you were in early labour and had to wait for a while. You waited for 6 hours and then they broke the baby's waters. Your contractions became very strong and you asked for and had an epidural for pain relief. You dilated to 8 cm, and after 4 hours, the doctor examined you and said you had not changed, and therefore started you on a drip with oxytocin. Shortly after, the baby's heart rate dropped and was not coming back up even though they switch off the drip. They therefore rushed you to theatre where your son was delivered by CS. He weighed 3,450 g and cried at birth. He stayed with your husband while they finished the CS. You remained in the hospital for 3 days and went home with your baby.

In this pregnancy, you have discussed options with the midwife, and she is uncertain what you should be going for. You are worried about going into labour and ending up having another emergency CS. You had an ultrasound scan today, and the baby is estimated to weigh 2,800 g.

You have no medical or surgical problems in the past and are not on any drugs other than iron tablets as your Hb was low at 28 weeks (it was 100 g/l). You are not aware of any allergies. You drink alcohol occasionally and do not smoke.

If not covered, you could ask the candidate the following questions:

- What are my chances of having a normal vaginal delivery?
- What are the risks of trying to deliver vaginally?
- If I go past my due dates, what will happen?
- Is there a way you can predict whether I will have a successful delivery or not?
- If I want to have a CS, when will it be done?

A good candidate should cover the following:

Information gathering

- Obtains relevant history that will highlight the course of the last CS
- Reviews notes from the previous hospital, if available, or request for them and reviews
- Ascertains the fears and worries of the woman
- Confirms that this pregnancy is progressing without any issues or anxieties

Communication with patients and families

- Introduces self and role
- Discusses the pros and cons of an elective versus a trial of labour after caesarean section (TOLAC)
- Offers to review again at 37 weeks to confirm decision on mode of delivery with an ultrasound scan
- If chosen, elective repeat caesarean section (ERCS) should be performed at 39^{+0} weeks
- Discusses the risk of uterine rupture (approximately 1:200 or 0.5%)
- Discusses intrapartum monitoring of progress of labour and fetal health (wellbeing) and the need for continuous electronic fetal monitoring
- Risk of uterine rupture increased two- to three-fold with induction of labour and 1.5 fold increased CS rate (urgent) compared with vaginal birth after caesarean section (VBAC)
- Repeats CS associated with increased risk of placenta creta/praevia in subsequent pregnancies and pelvic adhesions
- Slightly increased risk of respiratory distress with CS, especially if before 39 weeks
- Provides information at a pace that allows comprehension and encourages questions

Communication with colleagues

- Referral to VBAC clinic, if there is one, or to a team with expertise in managing patients who have had one previous CS and are considering trial of vaginal delivery
- Anaesthetist consultation if considered appropriate

Patient safety

- Confirms patients details at the start of the task
- Informed choice – ultimately the patient
- Delivery should be in a consultant unit with facilities for immediate CS
- Recommends epidural analgesia
- Cautions about the use of oxytocin if needed
- Discusses the pros and cons of induction of labour if goes past due dates

Applied clinical knowledge

- Demonstrates knowledge of the RCOG Green-top Guidelines on VBAC

Examiner score sheet		
Information gathering		
Standard not met	Standard partly met	Standard met
0	1	2
Communication with patients and families		
Standard not met	Standard partly met	Standard met
0	1	2
Communication with colleagues		
Standard not met	Standard partly met	Standard met
0	1	2
Patient safety		
Standard not met	Standard partly met	Standard met
0	1	2
Applied clinical knowledge		
Standard not met	Standard partly met	Standard met
0	1	2

Examiner Expectations and Basis for Assessment

Information gathering

- Obtains information from patients and clinical notes about previous pregnancy and birth
- Obtains information about current pregnancy, explores wishes and concerns of the patient and partner and seeks more information upon which to base the decision on options
- Reviews current notes (investigations and especially placental localisation)

Communication with patients and families

- Introduces self and role
- Able to communicate to the woman and her partner the plans and the rationale for the recommendation
- Able to explain the risks and benefits of vaginal birth for both the mother and the fetus

---

Communication with colleagues

- Signposts the patient to see a consultant
- Involvement of anaesthesia antenatally

Patient safety

- Confirms patients details at the start of the task
- Has an understanding of the risks from interventions such as regional analgesia during labour in VBAC
- Accurate prescription in labour, including the management of intravenous infusions
- Has an understanding of the risk management and the clinical governance processes in relation to intrapartum care
- Discusses continuous monitoring in labour and rationale for it

---

Applied clinical knowledge:

- Knowledgeable of intrapartum care, including the induction of labour, management of normal and abnormal labour, obstetric interventions and the interpretation of CTG
- Ability to critically appraise the literature, including guidelines (RCOG Green-top Guidelines on VBAC and NICE guidelines on intrapartum care and caesarean section)

Reference: Birth after a previous caesarean section. The Royal College of Obstetricians and Gynaecologists Green-top Guideline No. 45 October 2015

Task 6: Postpartum Dyspareunia. Module 8 – Postpartum Problems (The Puerperium)

Candidate's Instructions

This is a simulated patient task covering:

- Information gathering
- Communication with patients and families
- Communication with colleagues
- Patient safety
- Applied clinical knowledge

You are the ST5 who has been asked to see Mrs Nkumasi Alice, a 25-year-old technician working in the hospital laboratory who delivered 6 weeks ago. The GP has written to your consultant asking for a review. The letter from the GP is given below.

Gleeson Surgery
Scarthope Hill
Grimsby
GM2 6GD

Dear Mr Swan,
Re: Mrs Alice Nkumasi
I would like you to arrange to see Mrs Nkumasi Alice, who is a staff in your hospital. She delivered 6 weeks ago and came to see me today complaining of painful sexual intercourse. I did not examine her as I felt it would be better to have a proper assessment in the hospital – she was having real anxieties when I broached the subject of examination.

Yours sincerely

Dr Gladys Stern MBBS, MRCGP, DCH

You have 10 minutes in which to cover the following:

- Obtain focused history
- Discuss possible causes
- Outline the plan of management
- Answer any questions she may have

Simulated Patient's Information

You are Mrs Alice Nkumasi, a 25-year-old technician working in the blood bank of the hospital. You live with your husband, who is a nurse in the hospital, and your son in a rented semi-detached house. Neither of you smokes nor drink alcohol. You do not have anyone living with you, and you are worried about going back to work without making provisions for the care of your son.

You had your son 6 weeks ago. The pregnancy was complicated by pre-eclampsia, and you had to be induced at 37 weeks. You laboured for 14 hours and had a ventouse delivery because he was in distress. You were very frightened by the experience as he did not cry when he was born. The doctors had to give him oxygen, and he was admitted into the neonatal unit for 3 days. A scan of his head was done, and this was said to be normal. You had a terrible tear inside the vagina and also on the outside and had to be taken to the theatre for this to be repaired. It was initially very painful, but with time, it got better, and you are now pain free. You are, however, very scared of allowing anything into your vagina as you are worried that it will tear again. Your husband has been very understanding, and you have just started having sexual intercourse but it's very painful. When he attempts to go inside you during sexual intercourse, you just seem to freeze and become very tight. He has used lubricants, which have made it easier. You feel guilty for pushing him away but it's because of the fear of pain. You are breastfeeding exclusively.

You did not have any abnormal vaginal discharge after the delivery, and the midwife who saw you at home examined your bottom and was happy with the healing.

You do not have any urinary symptoms, and your bowel habits are normal.

In the past, you have had an ovarian cyst removed by keyhole surgery but do not have any other medical problems. You have no known allergies.

If not covered, you should ask the following questions:

- Why am I experiencing so much pain during sexual intercourse? It was not like this before I had my baby.
- What will you do to help me?
- Will my next delivery be the same or could I go for a caesarean section?

A good candidate will cover the following:

Information gathering

- Reviews details of the pregnancy and of the operative delivery
- Ascertains the psychological impact of the traumatic experience
- Explores the potential impact of this on her fear of penetrative sexual intercourse
- Indicates that the notes of her delivery will be/have been reviewed to have a better understanding of what happened, including the details of the repair
- Justifies the need for examining her
- Identifies the fact that they have no support at home and she is about to go back to work

Communication with patients and families

- Introduces self and role
- Explains the need for examination and the details of the expected examination
- Explains the possible causes of the painful sexual intercourse
  - Fear of damaging the vagina
  - Trauma from bad birthing experience
  - Scarred/narrow introitus and vagina
- Attempts to counsel and provides reassurance that this is not unusual and will be addressed
- Encourages involving husband at the next visit

Communication with colleagues

- Referral to psychosexual counselling
- Involvement of perineal trauma team in counselling and management

Patient safety

- Confirms patients details at the start of the task
- Empowers the patient to make informed choices
- Appreciates and takes into consideration her fears
- Discusses any potential safety of any medications to be used on breastfeeding
- Allays fears of involving social workers – to support rather that judge her fitness to be a mother
- Addresses the fear of another vaginal tear
- Ascertains drug allergy

Applied clinical knowledge

- Explains that scarring is likely a contributing factor
- Assures that the healing is complete and the risk of tear with penetrative intercourse is minimal
- Offers the use of lubricants and even dilators
- If the scar is considered the major problem, offers refashioning – e.g. Fenton's repair (this may be delayed and conservative approaches such as massaging with almond and tea tree oil to soften it, considered that surgery is regarded as a last option)
- Refers to clinical/psychosexual counsellor
- Knowledge of current literature on perineal trauma

Examiner score sheet		
Information gathering		
Standard not met	Standard partly met	Standard met
0	1	2
Communication with patients and families		
Standard not met	Standard partly met	Standard met
0	1	2
Communication with colleagues		
Standard not met	Standard partly met	Standard met
0	1	2
Patient safety		
Standard not met	Standard partly met	Standard met
0	1	2
Applied clinical knowledge		
Standard not met	Standard partly met	Standard met
0	1	2

Examiner Expectations and Basis for Assessment

Information gathering

- Able to take concise and relevant intrapartum and postnatal history
- Skilled in signposting and building the postnatal consultation
- Ensures the patient understands and encourages questions
- Able to succinctly summarise discussions with the postnatal patient

---

Communication with patients and families

- Introduces self and role
- Able to tackle the difficulty of painful sexual intercourse post delivery
- Able to describe to the postnatal patient a clear action plan and the rationale for a follow-up based on the discussion
- Explains the treatment option clearly and sensitively, encouraging and answering questions

---

Communication with colleagues

- Ability to communicate with colleagues in primary care and other specialties, e.g. urogynaecologists and perineal trauma team physiotherapists
- Referral to psychosexual counselling or clinical psychologist

---

Patient safety

- Confirms the patients details at the start of the task
- Awareness of safety investigations and treatment for postpartum dyspareunia

---

Applied clinical knowledge

- Knowledgeable of postnatal care, including the risks of maternal morbidity, especially dyspareunia, mortality and psychiatric disorders related to the postnatal period
- Knowledgeable of NICE and RCOG Green-top Guideline

Task 7: Secondary Postpartum Haemorrhage. Module 8 – Postpartum Problems (The Puerperium)

Candidate's Instructions

This is a simulated patient task assessing:

- Information gathering
- Communication with patients and families

- Communication with colleagues
- Patient safety
- Applied clinical knowledge

You are the ST5 who has been asked to see a 28-year-old woman, Ms Aisha Bhandwarna, in the emergency unit. She has been referred by the GP. The letter from the GP is given below.

Blaiby Surgery
Margate
Kent
KT3 7VX

Dear Dr,
Re: Ms Aisha Bhandwarna
I would be grateful if you could see this 28-year-old who delivered 10 days ago and now presents with heavy bleeding which is bright red and associated mild lower abdominal pain. She is breastfeeding.

Yours sincerely

Dr Mamta Gurmind, MBBS, MRCP

You have 10 minutes in which you should:

- Take focused history
- Discuss the management of the patient
- Answer any questions she may have

Simulated Patient's Information

You are Ms Aisha Bhadwarna, a 28-year-old apprentice, who delivered 10 days ago. You live with your partner of 6 years in your own detached home. You smoke about 10 cigarettes per day and also drink alcohol but cut down on both when it was confirmed you were having your daughter (after you had a positive pregnancy test).

This was your second pregnancy. The pregnancy was not complicated, and you were induced because you had gone past your due date. You had two pessaries and then the baby's waters were broken after which you were started on a drip. You laboured for 10 hours and then delivered by yourself. The placenta took a bit of time to come out but was eventually delivered by pulling by the midwife. You were discharged home 12 hours after delivery because of no beds. You remained well at home and was visited by the midwife a few days after delivery. You are breastfeeding exclusively, and your daughter is eating well and putting on weight.

Two days ago, you started experiencing a brownish discharge. At first you wondered whether this was a period but was surprised as with your first child you went for months without a period, who you also breastfed exclusively. This was associated with mild tummy ache. The bleeding became red today and more than a period. You are experiencing cramps and had to take paracetamol. You have been feeling very hot and sometimes sweaty. You do not have any other symptoms. You have not resumed sexual intercourse with your partner yet.

Your first baby was a vaginal delivery on your due date. You had gone into labour on your own and, the labour lasted for about 7 hours from when you were admitted into the hospital. Your daughter weighted 2,900 g and breastfed for 6 months. She is alive and well.

You do not have any other medical problems and you have no known allergies.

If not covered, you should ask the following questions:

- Why am I bleeding?
- What tests will you undertake to help find the cause of this bleeding?
- How will you treat me?
- Will the treatment affect breastfeeding as I am doing it exclusively?

A good candidate should cover the following:

Information gathering

- Obtains details of the pregnancy and delivery
- Establishes the symptoms of bleeding, abdominal pain and possible pyrexia (feeling very hot)
- Establishes exclusive breastfeeding
- Establishes the history of previous pregnancy
- Examines patient – temperature, pulse rate, respiratory rate, BP, abdomen and pelvis
- Indicates that case notes will be reviewed for additional information – for example, were placenta and membranes complete?
- Initiates investigations – CBC, ultrasound scan of the pelvis and swabs if vaginal discharge (very rarely βhCG may be quantified to exclude a trophoblastic disease)

Communication with patients and families

- Introduces self and role
- Explains of possible causes – retained products of conception, such as membranes with or without infections
- Management – may require admission into hospital
  - Antibiotics
  - Evacuation of products
  - Antipyretics/analgesics
- Explains the complications of surgery

Communication with colleagues

- Discusses imaging - specifically regarding ultrasound scan
- Involvement of microbiology and other disciplines

Patient safety

- Confirms patients details at the start of the task
- Empowers the patient to make informed choices
- Safety of treatment, with respect to breastfeeding baby – inhibition and effects of drugs on the baby
- Establishes drug allergy and demonstrates safe prescription for a lactating woman

Applied clinical knowledge

- Presentation is with secondary postpartum haemorrhage
- Causes of secondary postpartum haemorrhage
- Treatment options and associated complications
- Knowledgeable of NICE guidelines on intrapartum care and current literature on secondary postpartum haemorrhage

Examiner score sheet		
Information gathering		
Standard not met	Standard partly met	Standard met
0	1	2
Communication with patients and families		
Standard not met	Standard partly met	Standard met
0	1	2
Communication with colleagues		
Standard not met	Standard partly met	Standard met
0	1	2
Patient safety		
Standard not met	Standard partly met	Standard met
0	1	2
Applied clinical knowledge		
Standard not met	Standard partly met	Standard met
0	1	2

Examiner Expectations and Basis for Assessment

Information gathering

- Able to take concise and relevant postnatal history to identify possible causes of secondary PPH
- Skilled in signposting and building the postnatal consultation
- Ensures patient understanding and encourages questions
- Instigates appropriate investigations to aid the diagnosis of causes of secondary PPH
- Able to interpret investigations' results to help with the management

Communication with patients and families

- Introduces self and role
- Ability to describe to the patient a clear action plan of management of secondary postpartum haemorrhage and the rationale for a follow-up based on the discussion
- Discuss the possible causes and investigations, including explaining the need for examination

Communication with colleagues

- Able to communicate with colleagues in imaging and microbiology the need for specific investigations to aid the diagnosis and the plan management
- Liaises with different specialties for management depending on the cause – e.g. microbiology for antibiotics
- Knows when to call senior colleagues – for example, a consultant if the patient requires evacuation

Patient safety

- Confirms patients details at start of task
- Awareness of safety investigations and treatment for secondary PPH
- Has an understanding of psychological co-morbidities, including increased risk of VTE If infection
- Safe prescription, with respect to breastfeeding and the baby

Applied clinical knowledge

- Knowledgeable of the causes and the management of secondary PPH
- Knowledgeable of NICE and RCOG Guidelines on the management of secondary PPH

Reference: Prevention and management of postpartum haemorrhage. The Royal College of Obstetricians and Gynaecologists Green-top Guideline No. 52 16 December 2016

Task 8: Results for Interpretation. Module 4 – Antenatal Care

Candidate's Instructions

This is a structured discussion task assessing:

- Information gathering
- Communication with patients and families
- Communication with colleagues
- Patient safety
- Applied clinical knowledge

You are an ST5 working with Miss Sriven Tobin, one of five consultants in the hospital. Below are summaries of pregnant patients booked under your team, who have either been to the hospital and undergone investigations or have had some investigations at their current visit.

You have 10 minutes in which you should:

- Read the patient summary and results
- Identify what is abnormal with the result and the implication if any
- Discuss your immediate action with the examiner
- Where appropriate, discuss any additional information you may require to help manage the patient properly

Patient Summary and Results

1. A 30-year-old primigravida was seen in the clinic in the delivery suite with loin pain and frequency of micturition. A urinalysis showed nitrites ++, leucocytes ++ and protein ++. She was sent home on analgesics and an MSU sent. This has now been reported as *Pseudomonas species* sensitive to tetracycline, gentamycin and amoxicillin.

2. A primigravida books for antennal clinic at 11 weeks' gestation. The booking ultrasound scan shows a single viable fetus of appropriate gestation. The nuchal translucency measures 4 mm.

3. A 29-year-old primigravida attends for her routine detailed ultrasound scan at 20 weeks' gestation. This demonstrates bilateral choroid plexus cyst with no other anomalies.

4. A 34-year-old gravida 3 para2 booked for antenatal care and was screened for hepatitis. Her report has come back as hepatitis B surface antigen positive.

5. A primigravida attends for a booking ultrasound scan at 12 weeks' gestation and is found to have a unilateral simple ovarian cyst measuring 10×13 cm. The fetus is viable and of appropriate gestation.

6. Mrs B is in her second pregnancy, the first was complicated by placental abruption. She is Rhesus (D) positive. At 28 weeks' gestation, an antibody screen is reported as 8 iu of anti-c in maternal blood.

A good candidate should cover the following:

Case No	Abnormal result and implication if any	Immediate action	Additional information required that may help
1	UTI with *Pseudomonas spp* Untreated is associated with increased risk of preterm labour and pyelonephritis	Contact patient to have antibiotics and GP to prescribe amoxicillin for 5 days	Renal ultrasound scan to rule out renal calculi or congenital malformations
2	Raised NT Associated with increased risk of aneuploidy, and if normal, congenital structural abnormalities, especially of the heart	Counsel and offer karyotyping by CVS. Consider NIPT if declines CVS and wishes non-invasive testing. This is not diagnostic and only excludes major trisomies	Age of patient to allow for the calculation of risk of aneuploidy
3	Bilateral choroid plexus cyst	Reassurance if the only finding	None
4	Hepatitis B surface antigen positive Carrier of hepatitis B and increased risk of vertical transmission to the fetus	Inform the women and alert neonatal team at birth Newborn to receive hepatitis vaccine and hepatitis B immune globulin (HBIG) within 12 hours of birth	Check for hepatitis S antibodies Offer screening for other blood born infections – hepatitis C and HIV (if not already done)
5	Unilateral ovarian cyst Risk of accident in pregnancy – torsion or haemorrhage or rupture	Offer cystectomy at 14–18 weeks	Any associated symptoms
6	Rhesus isoimmunised with small c antibodies. Increased risk of haemolytic disease of the fetus and newborn	Serial measurement of anti-c antibodies Refer to fetal medicine for monitoring with Middle Cerebral Doppler PSV	Any blood transfusions Was the previous pregnancy affected – was the baby affected with jaundice

Examiner score sheet		
Information gathering		
Standard not met	Standard partly met	Standard met
0	1	2
Communication with patients and families		
Standard not met	Standard partly met	Standard met
0	1	2
Communication with colleagues		
Standard not met	Standard partly met	Standard met
0	1	2

Patient safety		
Standard not met	Standard partly met	Standard met
0	1	2
Applied clinical knowledge		
Standard not met	Standard partly met	Standard met
0	1	2

Examiner Expectations and Basis for Assessment

Information gathering

- Able to interpret information from investigations appropriately
- Is able to initiate additional investigations to help make a diagnosis and plan management
- Has an understanding of additional information that may be required to help arrive at a diagnosis and plan care

Communication with patients and families

- Gives information sensitively and in manageable amounts regarding results of investigations in pregnancy and management
- Communicates implications of an abnormal result for the patient and the fetus, including future pregnancies
- Describes a clear, logical action and rationale for a follow-up

Communication with colleagues

- Ability to prioritise cases appropriately and refer them for timely investigations in pregnancy, recognising the importance of time, especially in relation to prenatal diagnosis
- Describe the differential diagnoses and formulate an appropriate management plan
- Refers appropriately to other specialties, e.g. fetal medicine and haematology

Patient safety

- Has an understanding of their limits of their clinical abilities and demonstrates an understanding of when to refer patients to senior colleagues and other disciplines
- Initiates steps to mitigate risks
- Articulates clearly the risk of inaction

Applied clinical knowledge

- Knowledgeable of the routine antenatal care investigations and actions to be taken when these are abnormal
- Has an understanding of the role of imaging in the investigation/management of pregnancy
- Ability to present management options and their risks and benefits using non-directional counselling
- Knowledgeable of antenatal care pathways and investigations and management as detailed in the current literature and guidelines (NICE and RCOG)

Reference: Intrapartum care for healthy women and babies. NICE Clinical guideline [CG190] 03 December 2014. Last updated 21 February 2017

Task 9: Hirsutism. Module 9 – Gynaecological Problems

Candidate's Instructions

This is a simulated patient task assessing:

- Information gathering
- Communication with patients and families
- Communication with colleagues
- Patient safety
- Applied clinical knowledge

You are the ST5 in the gynaecology clinic today with your ST1, a GP trainee. The consultant is away and all his referrals will have to see you. One of them was referred because of excessive hair growth. The letter is given below.

> *Bradgate Hill Surgery*
> *Thornfield Farm Estate*
> *Richmond*
> *Surrey SR23 8UG*

Dear Mr Grundstaff,
Could you please see Ms Jess Brindle, a 26-year-old city council staff, who is complaining of having excessive hair on her face. She is single and does not have any other medical problems. Thank you for seeing her.

Yours sincerely

Dr JM Smith MBBS, MRCGP, DRCOG

You have 10 minutes in which you should:

- Take relevant history
- Explain the most likely causes of her hirsutism
- Discuss possible investigations that will help confirm the diagnosis
- Discuss/explain treatment options and course of treatment
- Answer any questions

Simulated Patient's Information

You are Jess Brindle, a 26-year-old city council staff, who is single and living on your own. You have had a steady boyfriend for 3 years. You would like to have a family but only after you get married.

You smoke about 5–10 cigarettes per day and drink alcohol over the weekends when you go out with the girls.

You have noticed since you had your periods that you have more hair on your face than other girls. You have been shaving for the past 1 year as what started like fine hair is more obvious and is getting longer and darker. You were getting too self-conscious and shaving was the only option you had to avoid being embarrassed. You also noticed that there is more hair on your tummy extending right up to your belly button as well as some hair around your nipples. The hair on your legs extends to your thighs and you again have to shave almost every week. You suffer from acne and are concerned about how thick the back of your neck feels.

Your weight has been difficult to control – you now weigh 80 kg and last year you were 72 kg.

You have not taken tablets in the past and are not aware of anything that could have caused the excessive hair growth. You do not have any unusual headaches and there's no milky discharge from your breasts.

You started having your periods when you were 13 years old. Your periods are irregular but they have always been like that since you had the first one. The longest you have gone without a period is 2 months. Often when you go for a long time without a period and then when they come, they tend to be heavy. You usually menstruate for 4–6 days, with the passage of occasional clots when the periods are long.

You have regular sexual intercourse with your boyfriend and do not use any contraception but have not been pregnant yet. Sexual intercourse is not painful.

Your last menstrual period was 1 week ago and you are up to date with your smears.

You are not taking any medicines at the moment and have no known allergies.

Your mother says that she had a lot of hair as well but that it was always thought to be normal for her family. You have one brother who is 30 years old. He is married and has two children.

If not covered, you should ask the following questions:

- What is wrong with me?
- What tests will you do on me?
- What treatment will you give me?
- Will this ever go away and will it affect my chances of having a baby?

A good candidate will cover the following:

Information gathering

- Detailed history of the hirsutism
- Associated symptoms – acne, weight gain, acanthosis nigricans and irregular periods

- Family history
- Exclusive factors – drugs or other medical problems
- Investigations – biochemistry (follicular phase) and ultrasound scan of the ovaries and adrenals
- Explains need for examination, including quantification of hirsutism – Ferriman–Gallwey score

Communication with patients and families

- Introduces self and role
- Explains of the possible diagnosis – PCOS but differentials include iatrogenic, familiar and adrenal tumours
- Discusses investigations – biochemistry (e.g. FSH, LH, testosterone, sex hormone binding globulin and prolactin) and ultrasound scan (of the pelvic – ovaries and abdomen – adrenals)
- Explains the treatment options (mechanical – e.g. shaving, creams, laser and electrolysis; hormonal – combined hormonal contraception and anti-androgen, e.g. cyproterone acetate or others)
- Implications for periods, fertility and long-term health – showing sensitivity in discussing these

Communication with colleagues

- Liaises with endocrinologist
- Referral to reproductive medicine
- Involvement of clinical psychologist – poor self-esteem, especially with weight
- Links with sleep team to discuss sleep apnoea
- Connects the patient to patient support groups

Patient safety

- Confirms patients details at the start of the task
- Empowers the patient to make informed choices
- Safe prescription bearing in mind the weight
- Counsels about long-term medical implications of pathology
- Ensures allergy is ascertained
- Counsels on medication and pregnancy, including risks of medication

Applied clinical knowledge

- Demonstrates being up to date with current literature on hirsutism as evidenced from
  - Discussion of diagnosis of PCOS and differentials
  - Treatment options – focus on hirsutism – mechanical (bleaching, shaving, depilatory, waxing, laser and drugs – hormones – combined hormonal contraception and anti-androgens)
  - Discussion on weight control and lifestyle modification
  - Implications for fertility and periods
- Familiarity with current guidelines, e.g. ESHRE and International Consensus Guidelines on diagnosis and management of PCOS

Examiner score sheet		
Information gathering		
Standard not met	Standard partly met	Standard met
0	1	2
Communication with patients and families		
Standard not met	Standard partly met	Standard met
0	1	2
Communication with colleagues		
Standard not met	Standard partly met	Standard met
0	1	2
Patient safety		
Standard not met	Standard partly met	Standard met
0	1	2
Applied clinical knowledge		
Standard not met	Standard partly met	Standard met
0	1	2

Examiner Expectations and Basis for Assessment

Information gathering

- Able to obtain a detailed history about the presenting symptom of hirsutism
- Logical approach to clearly reasoned style of questioning
- Able to initiate appropriate investigations and interpret results in order to develop a clear management plan and rationale for a follow-up

Communication with patients and families

- Introduces self and role
- Gives information in a sensitive manner and in manageable amounts regarding investigations and management of primary hirsutism
- Describes a clear and logical action and rationale for a follow-up
- Able to summarise discussions succinctly and checks patient's understanding at appropriate intervals

Communication with colleagues

- Ability to involve other specialties (endocrinologist, clinical psychologist and support groups)
- Describe the differential diagnoses and formulates an appropriate management plan

Patient safety

- Confirms patients details at the start of task
- Has an understanding of safe prescription in this woman with hirsutism, including recognising drug interactions, allergies and special circumstances, e.g. renal and liver impairment

Applied clinical knowledge

- Knowledgeable of the treatment of gynaecological disorders, specifically hirsutism
- Ability to critically appraise medical literature in relation to treatment of hirsutism
- Has an understanding of the role of imaging in the investigation/management of hirsutism
- Has an understanding of referral pathways – endocrinology
- Ability to present management options and their risks and benefits using non-directional counselling
- Knowledgeable of contemporary literature on hirsutism, including RCOG and ESHRE Guidelines

Task 10: Male Infertility. Module 10 – Subfertility

Candidate's Instructions

This is a stimulated patient task assessing:

- Information gathering
- Communication with patients and families
- Communication with colleagues
- Patient safety
- Applied clinical knowledge

You are an ST5 who is about to see Mr John Pearson, a 32-year-old engineer, who is attending the gynaecology clinic to discuss the results of investigations of his and his partner who have been trying for a baby for 2 years. His partner Andrea Pearson is 30 years old and is a teacher. She has unfortunately travelled with the school to France for 4 days. This is John's first marriage but his partner has a 6-year-old son from a previous relationship although she was never married. They had been to the gynaecology clinic 6 weeks ago, and a series of investigations were performed.

You have been told that the case notes of Andrea cannot be located for this clinic but the team has succeeded in printing the investigations results for the consultation.

You have 10 minutes to:

1. Obtain a brief, targeted clinical and fertility history
2. Explain the likely cause of the couple's subfertility
3. Establish the issues involved in the management of this couple and discuss them sensitively

Summary of Investigations

1. Semen analysis on John Pearson (partner of Andrea Smith) of two occasions, no spermatozoa seen. Normal volume with <10 WCC/HPF
2. 21-day progesterone on Andrea Smith – ovulatory (40 iu/L)
3. Follicular phase hormone profile
   a. FSH – 5.8 iu/L (3.0–9.0 iu/L)
   b. LH – 6.1 iu/L (2.5–9.0 iu/L)
   c. Prolactin – 520 miu/L (normal <400 miu/L)
   d. Testosterone – 0.4 iu/L (0.2–2.5 iu/L)
   e. Sex hormone binding globulin – 48 nmol/L (40–120 nmol/L)
4. HSG – normal uterine cavity and fallopian tubes with bilateral spillage into the peritoneum/pelvis

Simulated Patient's Information

Mr John Pearson. Age 32 years
3 Forest Street
Stretton ST2 4RG

You are Mr John Pearson, a 32-year-old engineer. You live with your wife for 4 years, Andrea, a teacher.

Andrea has a 6-year-old son, Jason, from her previous relationship. You have never fathered a pregnancy to the best of your knowledge. You had two long-term relationships before but pregnancy was never an issue, and you are not sure any of the women used a form of contraception. You never tried for a baby and were very sure that they were not trying either. You broke up with your last steady girlfriend because she was promiscuous. Six months after you broke up she sent you a text saying get yourself tested for chlamydia. You went for a test and it was positive. You received antibiotics. This was before you met Andrea.

You have sexual intercourse two to three times a week and are aware of your wife's fertile periods. You try as much as possible to have intercourse during this time.

Your stepson was conceived spontaneously and the pregnancy was uncomplicated. Andrea went into spontaneous labour but had to have an emergency caesarean section because the baby was in distress. She says she was discharged home 2 days after surgery and did not have any problems after. She breastfed for 6 months.

You are not aware of anything of relevance in her medical history, and you yourself are well. You live in your own four bedroom detached house in the village with Andrea and her son. Neither of you smokes but you drink alcohol at least three times per week – usually with your evening meals and sometimes with friends when you go out over the weekends. Neither of you is overweight although you do not know Andrea's weight but your BMI is 25 kg/M^2.

Andrea's mother and your father suffer from high blood pressure and are on treatment. You have no siblings but Andrea has two – one brother and one sister. Both have two children each.

Acting requirements

You understand what is being told to you and you are very unhappy and disappointed with the results.

You are angry and feel you have let down your wife. You blame the chlamydia infection for the problem.

If not covered by the candidate, you could ask the following questions:

1. Why do you think my sperm count is zero or so poor?
2. What are our options?
3. What is the next test that you can do to find out why this is the case?
4. Can we have IVF on the NHS?

A good candidate will cover the following:

Information gathering

- Obtains appropriate fertility-focused history
- Obtains specific information relevant to azoospermia, e.g. previous mumps orchitis, trauma, endocrine pathology and radiotherapy
- Interprets correctly and explains clearly the investigation results and their implications
- Reassures the patient to obtain the case notes and look through to check all the relevant facts about past medical history and previous pregnancy and to record this consultation in detail

Communication with patients and families

- Introduces self and role
- Explains possible reasons for the azoospermia
- Explores the man's fears and concerns
- Expresses empathy for the situation and the patient's bitter disappointment (chlamydia contracted from ex-partner may be the cause of current situation)
- Explains rationale for recommending karyotyping and testicular biopsy
- Conveys suggested management plan and offers hope: recommend ICSI/PESA and ICSI through self-funded IVF (give estimated costs, e.g. £3–4K per cycle as of 2020, less for subsequent cycles if embryos frozen)
- Encourages and welcomes his partner to attend consultation in the future

Communication with colleagues

- Referral to reproductive medicine
- Involvement of urologist in management of azoospermia
- Liaises with clinical psychologist/nurse counsellor
- Gives contact of support groups

Patient safety

- Confirms patients details at the start of the task
- Demonstrates an understanding of the processes and procedures to keep individual patients safe
- Presents the pros and cons of proposed management in a balanced way
- Recognises the limits of their clinical abilities and refers appropriately
- Highlights all governance issues and necessary actions to reduce risks and mishaps in future
- Identifies any allergies and demonstrates safe and accurate prescribing techniques
- Only discusses the results of Andrea if there is evidence of her permission otherwise defer until she is present

Applied clinical knowledge

- Appreciates different causes of azoospermia, e.g. chlamydia trachomatis infection leading to obstruction, mumps, trauma, endocrine pathology and genetic/karyotypic abnormalities
- Demonstrates a sound and comprehensive evidence-based clinical knowledge
- Interprets and explains the clinical findings accurately
- Justifies investigations, management options (ICSI and IVF) and demonstrates a rationale for each
- Synthesises a comprehensive and well-organised management plan based on the history and investigations and takes into consideration the various factors
- Demonstrates knowledge of current literature on management of the infertile couple, especially of NICE guidelines

Examiner score sheet		
Information gathering		
Standard not met	Standard partly met	Standard met
0	1	2
Communication with patients and families		
Standard not met	Standard partly met	Standard met
0	1	2
Communication with colleagues		
Standard not met	Standard partly met	Standard met
0	1	2
Patient safety		
Standard not met	Standard partly met	Standard met
0	1	2
Applied clinical knowledge		
Standard not met	Standard partly met	Standard met
0	1	2

Examiner Expectations and Basis for Assessment

Information gathering

- Takes a comprehensive and focused history from both partners of an infertile couple
- Requests appropriate investigations and interprets results from both female and male partners and operative findings in order to develop a clear and rationale management plan

Communication with patients and families

- Introduces self and role
- An ability to give information about infertility, investigations and treatment options sensitively and in manageable amounts, using patient-friendly language and avoiding jargon
- Honest around benefits, side effects, complications and outcomes of fertility treatments
- Has an understating of the psychological needs of the partner as well as the infertile woman
- Has an understanding of the psychological issues and sensitivities surrounding infertility
- Has an understanding of consent in discussing investigation results of couples in their absence
- Summarises discussions succinctly and checks that the patient understands at appropriate intervals

Communication with colleagues

- Ability to describe the differential diagnosis and formulate an appropriate management plan
- Ability to know when to refer and who to refer to for further management

Patient safety

- Confirms patient's details at the start of task
- Has an understanding of the risk management and the clinical governance and regulatory processes in relation to infertility, including issues of confidentiality
- Acknowledges the need to consider the welfare of the child in providing fertility treatment
- Informs the risks of multiple pregnancies associated with fertility treatment
- Issues of missing records and consequences on safety and management

Applied clinical knowledge

- Knowledgeable of the treatment of infertility, including surgical management of tubal disease, endometriosis and male infertility
- Sound evidence-based clinical knowledge of ovulation induction, assisted conception and gamete donation, including the risks and limitations of these treatments
- An ability to critically appraise medical literature in relation to infertility treatment
- Understands and demonstrates the role of HEFA and the NHS funding restrictions and rationing of assisted conceptions
- Understands the role of counselling for the infertile couple
- Understands culture issues and issues relating to same-sex partners and single parents
- Knowledgeable about current ESHRE and HFEA Guidelines on assisted reproduction techniques

Reference: Fertility problems: assessment and treatment. NICE Clinical guideline [CG156] 20 February 2013. Last updated 06 September 2017

Task 11: Urgency Incontinence. Module 14 – Urogynaecology and Pelvic Floor Problems

Candidate's Instructions

This is a simulated patient task assessing:

- Information gathering
- Communication with patients and families
- Communication with colleagues
- Patient safety
- Applied clinical knowledge

You are an ST5 in the clinic and are about to see your next patient who has been referred from the GP with urinary incontinence. The letter from the GP is given below.

The Maiden Surgery
Maidenhead
MD4 9py

Dear Mr Coswell,
Thank you for seeing Mrs Sasha Gurdip, a 40-year-old teacher complaining of a variety of urinary symptoms. She is struggling to cope with her symptoms and work. I have not examined her but feel that she will benefit from an assessment by your team.

Yours sincerely

James Standtrip MBBS, MRCGP

You have 10 minutes in which you should:

- Take focused history
- Discuss appropriate investigations
- Management of this patient's symptoms
- Answer any questions she may have

Simulated Patient's Information

You are Mrs Sasha Gurdip, a 40-year-old secondary school teacher, who has been having issues with your waterworks for the past 9 months. The problems started after you had a cold that was associated with severe, and sometimes violent, coughing. You leaked a lot of wee then but when the coughing stopped you realised that every time you had to go, you had to rush otherwise an accident will happen. As time went by, this got worse, and you were struggling to teach and dash out to the toilet. The students started talking and making fun of you, and you found it very embarrassing.

You also go more frequently than you used to, and furthermore, have to wake up several times (two to three) at night to stop yourself from wetting the bed. You do not experience any burning sensation when you are voiding and there is no feeling of incompletely emptying the bladder. When you cough, you also wet yourself.

You drink five to six cups of coffee every day and also like coke. You drink alcohol socially and smoke 10–15 cigarettes per day.

Your weight at the last check was 87 kg.

You have three children. All were vaginal deliveries. The first was 15 years ago. She was born at 42 weeks and weighed 3,400 g. You laboured for 14 hours and pushed for 2 hours before they used a suction to deliver her head. The second was born 12 years ago at 40 weeks. He came on time and you laboured for 10 hours. He weighed 3,500 g. Your last is 8 years old. He was born at 41 weeks and weighed 3,600 g. You had a forceps delivery because he was distressed. For all of them, you had an episiotomy that was repaired. You have not had any problems with your back passage and sexual intercourse is not a problem although it's very infrequent.

You do not have any dragging sensation down below and are not constipated. You are diabetic on Glucophage (metformin). Most members of your family have diabetes as well.

You do not suffer from any other medical problem apart from the fact that you are allergic to plaster. You have not had any surgery in the past.

If not covered, you should ask the candidate the following questions:

- What is the problem with my waterworks?
- What test will you recommend I do at this stage?
- What are the treatment options for me?
- I do not like taking tablets and will rather have surgery – is this possible?
- What are the side effects of the drugs you have given me and how long will it take for me to know that they are working or not?

A good candidate should cover the following:

Information gathering

- Obtains good history which demonstrates an understanding of the clinical problem
- Initiates appropriate investigations to help make a diagnosis
  - Fluid diary
  - Urinalysis

- Blood glucose
- Urodynamics

Communication with patients and families

- Introduces self and role
- Explains the need for carrying out an examination of the genital tract
- Explains the diagnosis of overactive bladder with a differential of mixed urinary incontinence
- Explains the need for investigations
- Discusses the treatment options including physiotherapy and drugs
- Explains that drugs may take up to 4–6 months before the effects are noticed
- Explains the follow-up process

Communication with colleagues

- Referral to urogynaecology
- Liaises with and involvement of physiotherapist and incontinence nurse
- Counsellor – incontinence

Patient safety

- Confirms the patients details at the start of the task
- Empowers the patient to make informed choices
- Discusses the safety of drugs prescribed for control of symptoms
- Establishes drug allergy and demonstrates safe prescription

Applied clinical knowledge

- Explains the pathophysiology of stress incontinence
- Discusses the basis of treatment – physiotherapy, drugs and surgery
- Discusses the rationale behind urodynamics and that this will most certainly exclude a mixed urinary incontinence
- Benefits of physiotherapy
- Lifestyle modification – fluid intake (avoidance of caffeine containing fluids, e.g. coffee and coke, quit smoking and weight loss)
- Bladder training
- Explains the type of follow-up and for how long
- Demonstrates knowledge of contemporary literature on urinary incontinence, including NICE guidelines

Examiner score sheet		
Information gathering		
Standard not met	Standard partly met	Standard met
0	1	2
Communication with patients and families		
Standard not met	Standard partly met	Standard met
0	1	2

Communication with colleagues		
Standard not met	Standard partly met	Standard met
0	1	2
Patient safety		
Standard not met	Standard partly met	Standard met
0	1	2
Applied clinical knowledge		
Standard not met	Standard partly met	Standard met
0	1	2

Examiner Expectations and Basis for Assessment

Information gathering

- Takes comprehensive history of urinary incontinence and excluding prolapse
- Interprets urodynamic investigations and microbiological and urine microscopy results
- Interprets fluid balance charts in order to reach a diagnosis and develop a management plan

Communication with patients and families

- Introduces self and role
- Demonstrates an ability to give information about urogynaecological examination, investigations and treatment in a manageable amount, using patient-friendly language and avoiding jargon
- Discusses honestly the pros and cons of treatment options, including clinical uncertainty about long-term outcomes of stress urinary incontinence treatment options
- Demonstrates an understanding of the psychological issues and sensitivities surrounding urinary incontinence

Communication with colleagues

- Describes the differential diagnoses and formulates management plans to colleagues
- Communicates clearly the requirements and the situation with theatre staff, assistants and anaesthetists
- Determines when and who to refer to (urogynaecologist, urodynamics, physiotherapy etc.)

Patient safety

- Confirms patients details at the start of the task
- Understands the principles of safe surgery, including WHO safe surgery checklist
- Understands safe prescription in relation to urinary incontinence
- Understands the contraindications and interactions of urinary incontinence drugs and common medical co-morbidities
- Ascertains drug allergy and demonstrates safe prescription

Applied clinical knowledge

- Knowledgeable of the surgical, non-surgical and medical management options of urinary incontinence
- Able to critically appraise the literature/evidence in relation to urinary incontinence treatment options
- Knowledgeable of NICE and RCOG Guidelines on urinary incontinence and pelvic floor prolapse

---

Reference: *Urinary incontinence and pelvic organ prolapse in women: management. NICE guideline [NG123] 02 April 2019. Last updated 24 June 2019*

Task 12: Cervical Cancer. Module 13 – Gynaecological Oncology

Candidate's Instructions

This is a structured discussion assessing:

- Information gathering
- Communication with patients and families
- Communication with colleagues
- Patient safety
- Applied clinical knowledge

You are an ST5 and have been asked to see a patient referred by her GP because of coital and post-coital bleeding and an irregular vaginal discharge. The letter from the GP is given below.

> *Coventry Road Surgery*
> *West Midlands*
> *BM12 5TS*

Dear Dr,
Re: Mrs Deborah Styme Age: 43 years
I would be grateful if you would see this woman urgently. She came to see me today complaining of bleeding during and after sexual intercourse. She also has a brownish and sometimes foul smelling

discharge. Her last smear was 5 years ago. She has a child who was delivered 10 years ago. When I examined her, I thought the cervix looked very suspicious. I have informed her that she may well have cervical cancer.

Yours sincerely

Dr Prathi Suwas MBBS, MRCP, DFFP, DRCOG, DCH

You have 10 minutes in which you should:

Read the information provided and

- Discuss this case with the examiner
- Answer the questions asked by the examiner

The examiner has five questions to ask that will help inform the discussion. If there is need for further information, the examiner will provide it.

Examiner's Instructions

Familiarise yourself with the candidate's instructions. Use the following five questions to form the basis of a discussion with the candidate about the diagnosis and management of the patient. Provide additional information prior to the third question. You should guide the candidate as to the use of time.

1. What will you find on examining the patient that will make you suspect cervical cancer?
2. What investigations will you undertake?
3. What would be the next step in her management?
   Read this out before posing question 3: 'She has an EUA and is found to have a lesion that is limited to the cervix and upper third of the vagina but not the parametrium. An ultrasound scan does not show renal involvement. An MRI and chest X-ray show no secondaries in nodes or in the chest'.
4. What surgical treatment will you recommend for her and what are the complications that she may have as a result of the surgery?
5. The surgical specimen shows no involvement of lymph nodes What will determine whether she will have further treatment or not?

A good candidate will cover the following points:

Information gathering

- General examination – looking for cachexia, anaemia and features of renal failure
- Vaginal examination – discharge, lesions on the vagina – exophytic or friable lesion of the cervix on inspection/abnormal looking cervix bleeding easily on contact; parametrial wall thickness
- Investigations
  - Ultrasound scan of the pelvis, kidneys and bladder
  - Biopsy for histology
  - Examination under anaesthesia to stage cancer
  - Checks kidney, liver function and full blood count
  - Chest X-ray and MRI of the pelvis

229

Communication with colleagues

- Liaises with MDT (oncologist, gynaecology oncologist, radiologist and cancer nurse/ McMillan nurse)
- Liaises with support team
- Liaises with GP and community nurse

Patient safety

- Confirms patients details at the start of the task
- Empowers the patient to make the right choice of treatment option
- WHO safety surgical patient checklist
- MDT within 2 weeks

Applied clinical knowledge

- Staging of cervical cancer
- Justifies the investigations
- Discusses treatment options – radiotherapy versus surgery
- Complications – immediate and long term
- Prognostic factors – presence of lymph node disease and need for adjuvant therapy
- Demonstrates knowledge of the current literature on management of cervical cancer

Examiner score sheet		
Information gathering		
Standard not met	Standard partly met	Standard met
0	1	2
Communication with patients and families		
Standard not met	Standard partly met	Standard met
0	1	2
Communication with colleagues		
Standard not met	Standard partly met	Standard met
0	1	2
Patient safety		
Standard not met	Standard partly met	Standard met
0	1	2
Applied clinical knowledge		
Standard not met	Standard partly met	Standard met
0	1	2

Examiner Expectations and Basis for Assessment

Information gathering

- Describes clinical features of cervical cancer
- Requests appropriate and timely investigations; interprets results and operative findings in order to develop a clear management plan and rationale for a follow-up

---

Communication with patients and families

- Gives information in a sensitive way and in manageable amounts to the patient and family regarding investigations, diagnosis and management of cervical cancer
- Describes a clear and logical action plan

Communication with colleagues

- Involves different specialties in the investigation and care of patient with cervical cancer (e.g. radiology)
- Discusses gynaecological oncological cases with different specialties, including oncology nurses, oncologists (gynaecology and internists), counsellors (nurses and psychologists), radiotherapists and support groups
- Able to recognise limits of their clinical abilities and demonstrates an understanding of when to call for help and involve senior colleagues and other disciplines like radiotherapy and chemical oncology

---

Patient safety

- Confirms patients details at the start of the task
- An ability to apply referral pathways and targets for investigations in the treatment of cervical cancer
- Has an understanding of safe prescription in gynaecological oncology, including recognition of drug interaction, allergies and special circumstances, e.g. renal and liver impairment
- Has an understanding of the principles of surgery including WHO safe surgery checklist

---

Applied clinical knowledge

- Understands the roles and responsibilities of the members of the multidisciplinary team
- Able to critically appraise the literature/evidence in relation to cervical cancer
- Understands the role of screening and imaging in cervical cancer
- Understands referral pathways in cervical cancer
- Able to present management options and their risks and benefits using non-directional counselling
- Knowledgeable of the epidemiology, presentation, investigation and treatment of cervical cancer, including palliation
- Familiar with contemporary literature on cervical cancer

Reference: *Urinary incontinence and pelvic organ prolapse in women: management. NICE guideline [NG123] 02 April 2019. Last updated 24 June 2019*

Task 13: Vaginal Hysterectomy. Module 2 – Core Surgical Skills

Candidate's Instructions

This task is a structured discussion assessing:

- Information gathering
- Communication with colleagues
- Patient safety
- Applied clinical knowledge

You are the ST5 working with Mr Kemp, your consultant, and you are preparing to assist him today in the theatre. The next case is a vaginal hysterectomy. The details of the patient are as follows:

'A 49-year-old sexually active mother of two was seen in the clinic with irregular vaginal bleeding of 6 months duration. She has had two normal vaginal deliveries; the last was 12 years ago. She was investigated by an ultrasound scan, a hysteroscopy and an endometrial biopsy and a diagnosis of simple endometrial hyperplasia was made. She was placed on cyclical progestogens which failed to control the irregular bleeding. She was being seen in the clinic, and following counselling, opted for a hysterectomy. She is on the list for a hysterectomy? Vaginal today'.

You have 10 minutes to explain to the examiner how this surgery will be performed. The examiner will direct the discussion using four questions and timings for each question.

Examiner's Instructions

Familiarise yourself with the candidate's instructions. Use the four questions to structure the discussion with the candidate. Direct the candidate to the use of time.

1. What initial steps will you take after the patient has been anaesthetised in preparation for the surgery, assuming the hysterectomy will be vaginal?
2. What will you be looking for when you examine the patient?

3. Describe the various steps you will take in performing a vaginal hysterectomy in this patient. You should identify the instruments you will be using.
4. What will be your post-operative instructions?

A good candidate will cover the following under each of the questions:

1. *What initial steps will you take after the patient has been anaesthetised in preparation for the surgery, assuming the hysterectomy will be vaginal?*
    *   WHO checklist with team
    *   Position patient – lithotomy position
    *   Clean and drape
    *   Empty bladder
    *   Perform a pelvic examination
2. *What will you be looking for when you examine the patient?*
    *   Laxity of the vagina
    *   Size and position of the uterus (anteverted or retroverted) – hysterectomy easier with retroverted uterus
    *   Descent of the uterus/cervix
    *   Presence or absence of an adnexal mass – if adnexal mass – hysterectomy preferably abdominal or laparoscopically assisted
    *   Associated vaginal wall prolapse – cystocele, rectocele or enterocele or a combination
3. *Describe the various steps you will take in performing a vaginal hysterectomy in this patient. You should identify the instruments you will be using. (**The following narrative is one approach – principles are same but approaches can vary. Be familiar with one and be able to describe and defend it.**)*
    *   Apply vulsellum to anterior and posterior lips of cervix
    *   Infiltrate with xylocaine 1:1,000 with adrenaline (inform the anaesthetist)
    *   Make circumferential incision, or one you are familiar with, around the internal cervical os
    *   Push the bladder up anteriorly to expose the uterovesical peritoneum and the rectum posteriorly to expose the posterior peritoneum; incise the peritoneum and feel for the adnexa (to ensure there are no masses and there are no adhesions)
    *   Apply clamps to the transverse cervical ligaments (Mackenrodt's ligaments), making sure that the bladder is pushed away to avoid the ureters
    *   Divide ligaments close to the uterus and transfix with the end of the stich anchored to clamp
    *   Retrovert the uterus to expose the U-V peritoneum and then divide it
    *   Apply clamps to the infundibulo-pelvic fold containing round ligament and fallopian tube, and divide and transfix
    *   Identify peritoneum and anchor it with small forceps; close peritoneum with continuous suture (this step may be omitted and the peritoneum not closed)
    *   Identify the angle of vagina and tie transverse ligaments to it. Close vagina with interrupted sutures
    *   Insert Foley's catheter in bladder
    *   Pack the vagina (again this may be omitted if there is no bleeding and there has been no repair)

4. *What will be your post-operative instructions?*
- Leave pack for 24 hours – remove the following day and document it
- Remove catheter either a few hours after pack comes out or after 48 hours
- Advice the patient that she should expect to have some mild bleeding, which should not be bright but will be brownish for a few days
- May also expel some of the suture material after about a week
- Avoid sexual intercourse or douching or tampons for at least 4 weeks
- Inform when to call the GP or come back to hospital

Examiner score sheet		
Information gathering		
Standard not met	Standard partly met	Standard met
0	1	2
Communication with colleagues		
Standard not met	Standard partly met	Standard met
0	1	2
Patient safety		
Standard not met	Standard partly met	Standard met
0	1	2
Applied clinical knowledge		
Standard not met	Standard partly met	Standard met
0	1	2

Examiner expectations and basis for assessment

Information gathering

- Has an understanding of essential pre-operative investigations and relevant clinical assessment
- Ability to interpret clinical findings and investigations when making decisions about surgical technique and approach
- Ability to describe clear action plan, including ongoing management plan after surgical procedure

Communication with colleagues

- Able to communicate legibly and with an ordered approach (date, time, etc.), e.g. clinical and operation notes
- Demonstrates when and who to call when complications arise
- Able to recognise one's own ability and limitations and when to call for help or refer to another specialty

Patient safety

- Understands the principles of safe surgery, including WHO safe surgery checklist
- Understands moving, preparing and positioning the unconscious for vaginal hysterectomy
- Recognition of limitations of abilities and demonstrates an understanding of when to call for help and involve senior colleagues and other disciplines
- Knows the principles of safe surgery, including use of prophylactic antibiotics, bladder catheters and vaginal packs
- Ensures drug allergy is excluded for safe prescription

Applied clinical knowledge

Demonstrates:

- Appropriate knowledge in relation to gynaecological surgery, including techniques and the risks and benefits of various procedures
- An ability to critically appraise medical literature in relation to surgical procedures

Task 14: Consent for Hysterectomy. Module 2 – Core Surgical Skills

Candidate's Instructions

This is a stimulated patient task assessing:

- Information gathering
- Communication with patients and families
- Communication with colleagues
- Patient safety
- Applied clinical knowledge

You are an ST5 who has been asked by your consultant, Mrs Smith, to obtain consent from a 46-year-old mother of two and also place her on the waiting list for an abdominal hysterectomy. This was the fifth visit of the patient to the clinic. She has a very busy clinic and has acceded to the woman's request for a hysterectomy. She does not perform surgery laparoscopically but there are other consultants in the hospital who offer laparoscopic hysterectomy.

You have 10 minutes in which you should:

- Take focused history
- Counsel appropriately
- Obtain consent for surgery and add her onto the waiting list
- Answer any questions the patient may have

Simulated Patient's Information

You are Mrs Serine Falvoir, a 45-year-old mother of two. You have been suffering from heavy periods for the past 3 years. Your periods initially lasted for 3–4 days, but in the last 3 years, they have been lasting for 5–8 days. You use super pads and often have to change them so many times per day. When you first attended Mrs Smith's clinic a year ago, you were told your womb is enlarged. You had an ultrasound scan which showed multiple fibroids and something called adenomyosis. Your periods are not only heavy but very painful. The pain which starts a few days before your periods last for 7–10 days after. You had to be transfused on one occasion as you had become very anaemic. You have had various medical treatment options that include tranexamic acid, norethisterone and the contraceptive pill but none has been effective. You are fed up and want a hysterectomy. You have completed your family, and both you and your husband are happy not to have more children. The bleeding is affecting your job (you are a manager with the city council) and you are fearful of losing it, as you have had to take time off work on several occasions.

You are not allergic to anything. Your last smear test was 6 months ago and was normal. You live with your husband, who is a banker, and your two sons, who are aged 10 and 8 years. They were normal deliveries, following uncomplicated pregnancies. You are currently taking iron tablets, and each time you bleed, you take tranexamic acid which slows down the bleeding. You do not use any form of contraception as your husband uses the condom.

You do not suffer from any medical illness and have not had any surgery in the past. Your mother is hypertensive and diabetic. Your father is alive and well.

You saw Mrs Smith today, and following discussions, she agreed to your request for a hysterectomy.

Your last menstrual period was 2 weeks ago.

If not covered, you may ask the following questions:

1. How long will I stay in the hospital after the surgery?
2. Why can I not have the hysterectomy through keyhole surgery?
3. How soon will I be able to get back to work?
4. Who will be doing my surgery?

Clinical Examiner's Instructions

Familiarise yourself with the candidate's and simulated patient's information and instructions and use the standard marking sheet to score them on the five domains. Discuss with the lay examiner and agree a common approach to assessment.

Lay Examiner's Instructions

Familiarise yourself with the candidate's instructions as well as the simulated patients' instructions. Score the candidate's performance in the two domains of information gathering and communication with patients and families. Discuss with the clinical examiner and agree on how to approach the assessment.

A good candidate should cover the following:

Information gathering

- Reviews notes to familiarise self with history, investigations (including imaging and definition of the size of the uterus and any adnexal masses) and treatment so far
- Confirms information in notes – main symptom, duration, impact on patient (life and otherwise), investigations and treatment
- Explores other options not offered so far – Mirena and endometrial ablation, progesterone receptor modulators, MRI guided focused ultrasound scan (MRgFUS)
- Excludes pregnancy and advice to take appropriate contraception prior to surgery
- Initiate appropriate investigations to ensure suitability for surgery – FBC, urea and electrolytes if necessary (for example if fibroids are huge and could potentially be compressing the ureters)
- Any contraindications to laparoscopic surgery?

Communication with patients and families

- Confirms that the patient wants the procedure
- Explains the procedure in layman's language (including the fact that the tubes will be removed but ovaries will be preserved), including the course of recovery – immediate and long term
- Ascertains if alternatives such as endometrial ablation and the levonorgestrel intrauterine system (Mirena) have been explored and if not, discusses them including pros and cons
- Informs the patient of the options to surgery (in this case, endometrial ablation, the levonorgestrel intrauterine system, ulipristal acetate (demonstrating that they are familiar with current Regulatory recommendations on the use of this in patients – currently not recommended for use pending further safety reviews) and magnetic resonance focused ultrasound) – pros and cons
- Discusses alternate approaches to hysterectomy – laparoscopic/vaginal, depending on the size of uterus and associated pathology
- Explains the intended benefits of hysterectomy
- Discusses significant, unavoidable or frequently occurring risks (haemorrhage, infections and injury to viscera – bowel, bladder and ureters, vault prolapse, urinary incontinence or symptoms and early menopause)
- Informs patient that she may require blood transfusion
- Discusses what would happen if surgery is not performed
- Documents the procedure and complications on the form, ensuring that the procedure is in layman's language with no abbreviations
- Documents procedure that may become necessary during the procedure like oophorectomy
- Discusses blood transfusion and documents that the patient will be happy to be transfused (if not, discusses options as in the case of Jehovah Witness)
- Discusses anaesthesia

- Explains that consent is only valid if it's not withdrawn and that she can withdraw the consent even on the day of surgery
- Provides information in a step-wise approach, ensuring a good understanding at each stage, encouraging questions and answering them
- Offers information leaflet on hysterectomy and post-surgery recovery

Communication with colleagues

- Communicates with waiting list team
- Arranges anaesthetic review
- Provides feedback to GP on date for surgery (if consultant's letter does not mention date)

Patient safety

- Confirms patients details at the start of the task
- Ascertains that there are no allergies
- Ensures that the patient understands and signs and dates consent form
- Gives copy of consent form to patient
- Ensures that the patient is fit for surgery
- Counsels about pregnancy – advice to use effective contraception leading up to surgery and indicates that there'll be a pregnancy test on the day of surgery

Applied clinical knowledge

- Demonstrates knowledge of what constitutes valid consent (patient has the capacity to consent, understands the operation being offered, the alternatives and what are the consequences of not having surgery)
- Familiar with contemporary approach to hysterectomy (including the current thinking that the tubes should be removed because of the risk of epithelial ovarian cancers, which are now thought to arise from the fimbrial ends of the fallopian tubes)
- Familiar with the different approaches to hysterectomy and why

Examiner score sheet		
Information gathering		
Standard not met	Standard partly met	Standard met
0	1	2
Communication with patients and families		
Standard not met	Standard partly met	Standard met
0	1	2
Communication with colleagues		
Standard not met	Standard partly met	Standard met
0	1	2

Patient safety		
Standard not met	Standard partly met	Standard met
0	1	2
Applied clinical knowledge		
Standard not met	Standard partly met	Standard met
0	1	2

Examiner Expectations and Basis for Assessment

Information gathering

- Offers to review notes
- Confirms symptoms and request for hysterectomy
- Establishes an understanding of what the procedure entails
- Enquires after tried treatment options
- Initiates appropriate investigations or checks that results are available
- Establishes the capacity to consent for surgery through questioning

Communication with patients and families

- Introduces self to patient
- Discusses the details of the procedure, including complications and post-operative course
- Explores routes of surgery – if uterus is not above 16 weeks (laparoscopic and vaginal)
- Discusses anaesthesia and options
- Explains options – endometrial ablation, Mirena and others
- Follows the procedure for obtaining consent

Communication with colleagues

- Confirms date of surgery with consultant
- Refers patient to pre-surgery anaesthetic review
- Informs waiting list to the team/manager
- Considers referral to laparoscopic team if uterus is less than 16 weeks

Patient safety

- Confirms details of the patient at the start of the task
- Ensures there are no contraindications to surgery (makes sure patient is fit for surgery)
- Ascertains no allergies that could affect safe prescription, including the use of anaesthetic drugs
- Confirms that transfusion will be accepted, and if not, as in the case of Jehovah Witness – makes appropriate arrangements
- Consent form signed and dated and copy given to patient

Applied clinical knowledge

- Discusses the details of the procedure and the indication
- Aware of the alternatives to management
- Aware of the principles of consenting in medicine (various domains that must be covered)
- Familiar with the NHS consent form and the procedure and able to use information leaflets from RCOG

15
Paper IV

Task 1: Previous Postpartum Haemorrhage. Module 4 – Antepartum Care

Candidate's Instructions

This is a simulated patient task assessing:

- Information gathering
- Communication with the patients and families
- Communication with colleagues
- Patient safety
- Applied clinical knowledge

You are an ST5 working with a consultant in the general obstetrics clinic of your hospital. You have been called by the midwife to see a patient, who has been referred by her GP for counselling at 28 weeks of gestation. The referral letter is given below.

Backstrougton Surgery
Peckham
East London
EC1 5DR

Dear Dr Abimbola,
I will be grateful if you would be kind enough to see Ms Alice Glumster, a 34-year-old home care assistant in her second pregnancy at 28 weeks for counselling about the mode of delivery. Her first pregnancy was complicated by gestational diabetes, which was managed by diet only. She went into spontaneous labour at 40 weeks. Labour was complicated by severe postpartum haemor-rhage, for which she was transfused four units of blood. The baby who weighed 3,500 g is healthy. She will like to review her options for this pregnancy.

Yours sincerely

Dr Kate Adcock MBChB, MRCGP, DRCOG

You have 10 minutes in which you should:

- Take focused history
- Initiate appropriate investigations
- Counsel the patient about her management
- Answer any questions she may have

Simulated Patient's Information

You are Ms Alice Glumster a 34-year-old home care assistant in your second pregnancy. You live with your partner John Partridge, who is 30 years old, and your daughter who is 4 years old. You are healthy and neither smoke nor drink. You are allergic to penicillin (you had it once and developed a severe rash). This is a planned pregnancy, and your partner is the father of your daughter. You live in your own house – a three bedroom semi-detached house.

Your first pregnancy was at another hospital in South East London. The pregnancy had so many problems. You were first admitted with excessive vomiting around 8 weeks and had to stay in the hospital for 3 days. You then had some bleeding around 32 weeks and again had to be admitted into the hospital. You were told that the placenta was low and in front. However, a few days after the admission, the bleeding settled, and you were discharged home. You had another scan at 36 weeks and the placenta was said to have moved. You were very happy as you did not want a caesarean section.

At 41 weeks, you went into labour and came into the hospital. Everything was going very well, and you had a normal delivery 6 hours after coming into the hospital. What followed was a nightmare. As soon as your daughter was born (she weighed 3,500 g), you started bleeding. The placenta had not come out. You just bled and bled. The midwives pushed the alarm bell and everyone rushed in. You had drips and a tube in your bladder, and it was very frightening. The doctor tried to explain to you but you could not take it in. John remembers being told that your womb was not contracting very well. You were eventually taken to the theatre where a balloon was put inside your womb. The bleeding then slowed down and finally stopped after about 12 hours. This balloon stayed in for 24 hours. You breastfed exclusively for 6 months during which time you had no periods. You saw the consultant 6 weeks after your delivery, and he explained everything to you. You are very scared of it happening again.

Your periods returned as soon as you stopped breastfeeding and were regular. You have no medical problems and have not had any surgery in the past.

If not covered, you may wish to ask the candidate the following questions:

- What are the chances of this happening again?
- What steps will be taken to reduce the risk of this happening again?
- If it did happen, will it be possible to avoid the commotion that ensued last time, as that really frightened John and I?
- What if I have a caesarean section?
- Can this happen in CS?

A good candidate should cover the following:

Information gathering

- Obtains a detailed history of the previous experience
- Requests for and reviews notes from previous hospital
- Ascertains concerns – fear of recurrence and traumatic experience
- Reviews ultrasound to confirm the position of the placenta

Communication with the patient

- Introduces self and role
- Affirms concerns of patient and addresses them

- Discusses the recurrence and the plans to minimise recurrence
- Explains the possible reasons for PPH and precautions to be taken
- Explains the risks versus benefits of vaginal versus CS

Patient safety

- Confirms patients details at the start of the task
- Ensures emotional support for patient – seemed to have had a traumatic experience – any evidence that psychological support was offered?
- Empowers patient to make an informed choice
- Option of CS available but does not avoid PPH
- Will have to have blood grouped and saved in labour and also to have an IV line
- Ascertains allergy and safe prescription

Applied clinical knowledge

- Discusses the causes of PPH – tone, tissues, trauma and thrombin (4Ts)
- Explores the haematological issues if any
- Demonstrates sound knowledge of current literature, including RCOG Green-top (postpartum haemorrhage) and NICE guidelines (intrapartum care)

Examiner score sheet		
Information gathering		
Standard not met	Standard partly met	Standard met
0	1	2
Communication with patients and families		
Standard not met	Standard partly met	Standard met
0	1	2
Communication with colleagues		
Standard not met	Standard partly met	Standard met
0	1	2
Patient safety		
Standard not met	Standard partly met	Standard met
0	1	2
Applied clinical knowledge		
Standard not met	Standard partly met	Standard met
0	1	2

Examiner Expectations and Basis for Assessment

Information gathering

- Obtains information from patients about current and past pregnancies, including complications
- Reviews obstetrics notes of previous pregnancy
- Reviews current obstetrics notes, including placental location on ultrasound scan and any maternal or fetal complications
- Establishes concerns of the patient and her fears, including counselling offered with plans for subsequent pregnancies

---

Communication with patients and family

- Introduces self and role
- Reviews with the woman the reasons for the PPH in the previous pregnancy and the plans for subsequent pregnancies and delivery
- Outlines that there are no risk factors antenatally for PPH but that this does not guarantee that this will not reoccur
- Explains the risks and benefits of vaginal versus caesarean delivery (emphasising that PPH can also occur with CS)
- Discusses the plan for delivery in detail – providing incremental information and encouraging questions and ensuring understanding

---

Communication with colleagues

- Knows when (offers to) to refer to consultant for further counselling (if required) and confirmation of outline plan of the management
- Liaises with midwife to reinforce counselling and plan of care

---

Patient safety

- Confirms patients details at the start of the task
- Understands risks from interventions, such as intravenous uterotonics regional analgesia, and other therapeutics in labour to prevent PPH
- Accurate prescription in labour, including management of intravenous infusions

- Has an understanding of risk management and clinical governance processes in relation to intrapartum care
- Takes appropriate steps to reduce the risk of recurrence of PPH – IV line, group and safe, active management of the third stage of labour, minimising prolong labour, use of uterotonics with delivery of the anterior shoulder etc.

Applied clinical knowledge

- Knowledgeable of intrapartum care, including induction of labour, management of normal and abnormal labour and timely interventions to reduce the risk of PPH, and even when it occurs to arrest it
- Has a working knowledge of the roles of other members of the multidisciplinary team in the management of PPH
- Ability to critically appraise the recent literature, including RCOG Green-top Guidelines on the management of PPH guidelines, protocols and scientific papers

Reference: *Antenatal care for uncomplicated pregnancies. NICE Clinical guideline [CG62] 26 March 2008. Last updated 04 February 2019*

Task 2: Teaching Breech Delivery. Module 1 – Teaching

Candidate's Instructions

This is a simulated trainee task assessing:

1. Information gathering
2. Communication with patients and families
3. Communication with colleagues
4. Patient safety
5. Applied clinical knowledge

You are an ST5 who is required to teach a Specialist Trainee in her first year to conduct a vaginal breech delivery.

You have 10 minutes in which you should:

- Outline to the trainee the principles of vaginal breech delivery
- Teach in a step-wise manner how to undertake a vaginal breech delivery

A good candidate should cover the following:

a. **Introduction and establishment of the knowledge and experience level**
   - Introduce yourself and the purpose of the task; inform the patient and obtain consent for teaching
   - Ask if they have seen a breech deliver or read about the conduct of a vaginal breech delivery

b. **State the aims of the teaching**

By the end of this session, you should be able to:

- Understand the conditions that have to be fulfilled before you can conduct a breech delivery
- Conduct an assisted breech delivery
- Understand the various techniques available for delivering the upper limbs and the head in an assisted breech delivery

c. **Patient selection**

- The fetal neck is not hyperextended on ultrasound scan (i.e. it is flexed)
- The estimated weight is between 1,500 and 3,800 g
- The type of breech – its either frank or complete (a footling breech is considered a contraindication for a vaginal breech delivery unless this is an emergency or the second twin)

d. **Conditions that need to be fulfilled before conducting a breech delivery**

- Appropriate analgesia has been offered and skilled assistance is available (always inform consultant) or someone senior enough to supervise
- No contraindication for a vaginal delivery – inadequate pelvis, a compromised fetus and footling breech
- Neonatologist is available
- Hospital setting with facilities for emergency CS

e. **Preparing for breech delivery**

- For patients seen prior to labour and those presenting in labour, where time and circumstances permit, the position of the fetal neck and legs and the fetal weight should be estimated using ultrasound
- Discuss the pros and cons of vaginal breech delivery (including risks, especially with difficulties in the delivery of the after-coming head); perinatal mortality and the consensus in terms of delivery of breech – elective CS in most cases

f. **Conduct of breech delivery** – Assisted breech delivery (means being passive until well into the second stage)

- Always empty the bladder as you may have to use a forceps to assist the delivery of the after-coming head
- Position the patient – best in the semi-recumbent or dorsal position, with the buttocks right at the end of the bed
- Adequate descent of the breech in the passive second stage is a prerequisite for encouragement of the active second stage. While involuntary pushing may occur earlier, encouragement of maternal effort should not start until the breech is visible
- Assistance, without traction, is required if there is delay or evidence of poor fetal condition
- Once the buttocks have passed the perineum, significant cord compression is common, watch out for this – a loop of cord may be pulled down to minimise this
  i. Traction should also be avoided; a 'hands-off' approach is required, but with appropriate and timely intervention, if progress is not made once the umbilicus has delivered or there is poor tone, extended arms or an extended neck
  ii. Avoid tactile stimulation of the fetus as it may result in reflex extension of the arms or head, making delivery difficult
- Care must be taken in all manoeuvres to avoid fetal trauma: the fetus should be grasped around the pelvic girdle (not soft tissues) and the neck should never be hyperextended

- Selective rather than routine episiotomy is recommended
- Signs that delivery should be assisted include lack of tone or colour, or delay, commonly due to extended arms or an extended neck
  i. In general, intervention to expedite breech birth is required if there is evidence of:
     1. A poor fetal condition
     2. If there is a delay of more than 5 minutes from delivery of the buttocks to the head
     3. More than 3 minutes from the umbilicus to the head
- If the back starts to rotate posteriorly, gentle rotation without traction should be used to ensure that it remains anterior
- Once the scapula is visible, the arms can be hooked down by inserting a finger in the elbow and flexing the arms across the chest
- If arms are nuchal, Lövset's manoeuvre is advised (with fetal back to the left, introduce hand along the anterior arm and flex the forearm at the elbow over the chest, and once delivered, rotate the fetus so the posterior shoulder is anterior and repeat the procedure)
- Delivery of the after-coming head:
  i. Is achieved either with the Mauriceau–Smellie–Veit manoeuvre, or
  ii. With forceps
  iii. Suprapubic pressure will aid flexion if there is delay due to an extended neck. Delivery using the Burns–Marshall technique (rarely used nowadays)

g. **Deliver the head**
- *Mauriceau–Smellie–Veit manoeuvre*
  i. Lay the baby face down with the length of its body over your hand and arm
  ii. Place the first and third fingers of this hand on the baby's cheekbones and place the second finger beneath the chin, ease the cheeks down and flex the head
  iii. Use the other hand to grasp the baby's shoulders
  iv. With two fingers of this hand, gently flex the baby's head towards the chest, while applying downward pressure on the cheeks to bring the baby's head down until the hairline is visible
  v. Pull gently to deliver the head
- *Forceps*
  i. Catheterise the bladder
  ii. Have an assistant hold the baby up towards the mother's abdomen
  iii. Apply forceps
  iv. Use the forceps to flex the baby's head and deliver the head
  v. If unable to use forceps, apply firm pressure above the mother's pubic bone to flex the baby's head and push it through the pelvis

h. **Clamp and cut the cord early and continue with active management of the third stage**

Examiner score sheet		
Information gathering		
Standard not met	Standard partly met	Standard met
0	1	2

Communication with patients and families		
Standard not met	Standard partly met	Standard met
0	1	2
Communication with colleagues		
Standard not met	Standard partly met	Standard met
0	1	2
Patient safety		
Standard not met	Standard partly met	Standard met
0	1	2
Applied clinical knowledge		
Standard not met	Standard partly met	Standard met
0	1	2

Examiner Expectations and Basis for Assessment

Information gathering

- Understands the need to first determine the skills of the tutee
- Outlines the expectations of the tutee
- Understands timings during a breech delivery (from delivery up to the buttocks and up to the cord to the delivery of the head – 5 and 3 minutes, respectively)

Communication with patients and families

- Appropriate introduction of the self and tutee and the task to the patient and partner
- Explains the roles of trainer and the tutee and nature of the interaction to the patient
- Obtains informed consent for the procedure (teaching and vaginal breech delivery) from the patient

Communication with colleagues

- Understands the principles of adult learning and giving feedback with regard to vaginal breech delivery
- Takes appropriate steps in increasing clinical and technical skills of the learner (tutee)
- Ability to use appropriate language and non-verbal language to encourage learning
- Invites questions and encourages dialogue
- Shows logical approach in building the pre-existing skills of the learner

Patient safety

- Patient safety is maintained when teaching conduction of a breech delivery, showing an understanding of when to continue teaching and when to intervene to halt the teaching session
- Appropriate safety checks are in place and knows when to sought assistance when conducting a vaginal breech delivery
- Appropriate checks are in place to ensure that the procedure has been appropriately undertaken

Applied clinical knowledge

- Understands the steps in the tasks being undertaken (teaching task)
- Has an understanding of the learning objectives and outcomes in relation to the tasks being taught
- Ability to conduct and give feedback on using a work-based assessment tool in this task
- Knowledgeable of the principles of twin delivery as detailed in standard Operative Obstetrics and RCOG Green-top Guidelines on the management of breech presentation and operative vaginal deliveries

Conduct of Breech Delivery – Teaching (Details to Provide to the Trainee)

Encourage pushing with contractions until full dilatation is confirmed and the buttocks have entered the vagina. Maternal expulsion delivers the frank breech from the lower birth canal, while the contractile forces of the uterus maintain flexion of the fetal head.

Inappropriate traction on the breech at this point may lead to extension of the fetal head, or entrapment of an arm behind the head (nuchal arm). Let the buttocks deliver until the lower back and inferior angle of the scapula are seen.

Gently hold the buttocks in one hand, but do not pull. If the legs do not deliver spontaneously, deliver one leg at a time: do this by splinting the thigh whilst flexing and abducting the hip. Note the lateral rotation of the thighs on the hips to deliver the legs. Avoid the instinctive manoeuvre of hooking the thigh down, thus bending the knee in the wrong direction.

At this point, the breech should hang downwards, while maternal efforts expel the infant until the lower border of the scapula is visible below the pubic arch.

Wrap the baby in a towel and hold the baby by the hips. Do not hold the baby by the flanks or abdomen as this may cause kidney or liver damage. Ensure that the back does not rotate posteriorly. For delivery of the shoulders and arms, the clinician's thumbs overlie the sacrum with the fingers around the iliac crests, so that the hands cradle the fetal pelvis. Allow the arms to disengage spontaneously one by one. Only assist if necessary. If the fetal arms have not become extended, the clinician passes the index and middle fingers over the shoulder and sweeps the left arm medially across the chest, thus delivering it. Repeat for the right arm

If the fetal arms have extended, the clinician applies Lövset's manoeuvre. The clinician rotates the body with the back uppermost, 180 degrees. The posterior shoulder has been rotated anteriorly and lies beneath the symphysis. The clinician hooks the arm downwards and then rotates the body back 180 degrees to deliver the other arm in the same manner. Gentle elevation of the fetal trunk allows the clinician access to the fetal airway. You must avoid over-extension, because of the risk of fetal cervical injury and hyperextension of the fetal head.

Reference: Management of breech presentation. The Royal College of Obstetricians and Gynaecologists Green-top Guideline No. 20b March 2017

Task 3: Crohn's Disease. Module 5 – Maternal Medicine

Candidate's Instructions

This is a simulated patient task assessing:

- Information gathering
- Communication with patients and families
- Communication with colleagues
- Patient safety
- Applied clinical knowledge

You are an ST5 in the antenatal clinic with your team, including the consultant. This is a combined booking and follow-up clinic. Your consultant has an interest in gastrointestinal disorders associated with pregnancy. You are about to see a patient who is booking for antenatal care having been triaged by the Community Midwife to the consultant clinic because of her medical history. The summary of the information on the patient from the GP is provided below.

Treefield Surgery
Assumcion Road
Crowley CR2 5RT

Dear Mr Alfonse Dean, FRCOG,
Re: Ms Gail Timothy
I would be grateful if you can book this woman into your medical disorders antenatal clinic.
Ms Gail Timothy is 32 years old and suffers from Crohn's disease for which she is taking infliximab and prednisolone. She has been symptom free for the past 6 months and finds herself pregnant.
This is her second pregnancy, and she is about 8 weeks. The first was 3 years ago and was complicated by growth restriction. She was delivered by a caesarean section at 36 weeks of gestation. This pregnancy has so far been problem free, and she is on folic acid 400 µg.
Her current medications are infliximab-abda, folic acid, prednisolone and vitamin D.

Yours sincerely

Dr Grace Mbonzi MBBS, MRCGP

You have 10 minutes in which you should:

- Take focused history
- Discuss the management of the pregnancy including complications
- Answer any questions that the patient may have

Simulated Patient's Information

You are a 32-year-old married nurse, who works full-time. You find yourself pregnant, and though very pleased, you are worried as your last pregnancy was very difficult. Your periods were regular, and the last one was 8 weeks ago.

You have been suffering from Crohn's disease for the past 8 years and have been on infliximab-abda (you do not know the dose) given through your vein every 8 weeks and prednisolone 5 mg three times a day for the past 2 years. It seems to control your symptoms well, although there are the occasional flares of bouts of diarrhoea and colicky abdominal pain.

You had an elective caesarean section 3 years ago for your son who is healthy and doing very well. The pregnancy was very troublesome. He was very small, and you had several ultrasound scans during pregnancy and had a planned caesarean section at 36 weeks because he had stopped growing. When he was born, he weighed 1,800 g and was admitted into the neonatal intensive care unit for 1 week. The surgery was described as difficult because of adhesions. You spent 4 days in the hospital before going home as your tummy had swollen up shortly after surgery and you could not eat or drink for 2 days.

You have been very well since you went on your present medication which you take with regular pain killers. You do not have any allergies and neither smoke nor drink alcohol. Your weight is 65 kg, and you are generally fit.

You are very worried about the pregnancy, and equally important, you are worried about the effect of the drugs on the pregnancy.

If not covered, you should ask the following questions:

- Will the Crohn's disease get worse with pregnancy or will it get better?
- Is the baby safe or will he be affected by Crohn's disease or the drug?
- I understand that this drug is not licensed in pregnancy. Should I stop it?
- As my last baby was very small, what are the chances of this one being small and how will the baby be monitored?
- How will I be delivered? Will it be CS again, and if so, I am really worried, as last time they said there were lots of adhesions.
- Is Crohn's disease inherited – in other words will I pass it onto my children?

A good candidate will cover the following:

Information gathering

- Able to obtain concise and relevant history – when diagnosis was made, medication (infliximab and prednisolone) and duration of medication, disease active or not (i.e. any symptoms) and physician managing Crohn's disease
- Medication prior to pregnancy and during pregnancy – any folic acid and dose
- Past obstetrics history – complications antenatally, mode of delivery – if vaginal – any associated perineal/vaginal scarring?
- Offers to review medical record and investigations including any antibodies

Communication with patients and families

- Introduces self and role
- Signposts antenatal care and timing of investigations at various stage
- Communicates information at a reasonable pace, ensuring that the patient understands, and encourages questions and provides answers
- Discusses the impact of pregnancy on Crohn's disease (in up to 75% of those with active disease at the beginning of pregnancy, disease becomes quiescent; remission more likely in the puerperium)
- Discusses impact of Crohn's disease on pregnancy – inactive disease has minimal impact on pregnancy, including delivery; active disease may be associated with a slightly increased risk for miscarriage, preterm delivery, small for gestational age and increased CS rate
- Discusses importance to continue with medication throughout the pregnancy – folic acid (5 mg until 12 weeks)
- Discusses prenatal screening, monitoring of the fetus and the timing and the mode of delivery (depends on the mode of delivery of previous baby and state of perineum and vagina – if no scarring, then vaginal delivery anticipated)

Communication with colleagues

- Referral to or involvement of gastroenterologist
- Referral to fetal medicine for fetal assessment (steroids and mildly increased risk of malformations)
- Anaesthetic assessment at 34/36 weeks
- Feedback to GP and community midwife on care pathway

Patient safety

- Confirms patients details at the start of the task
- Ascertains drug allergy
- Discusses safety of anti-TNα medication (infliximab) in pregnancy and the need to continue with medication – need to continue with medication in pregnancy to avoid flares
- Safety of corticosteroids in pregnancy – teratogenicity – and impact on screening for diabetes
- Prednisolone and stress – Iv hydrocortisone in labour

Applied clinical knowledge

- Demonstrates knowledge of current literature on the management of inflammatory bowel diseases as evidence from
- Explains the implications of Crohn's disease on pregnancy and pregnancy on Crohn's disease
- Discusses on medications and their impact on pregnancy
- Discusses on the delivery

Examiner score sheet		
Information gathering		
Standard not met	Standard partly met	Standard met
0	1	2

Communication with patients and families		
Standard not met	Standard partly met	Standard met
0	1	2
Communication with colleagues		
Standard not met	Standard partly met	Standard met
0	1	2
Patient safety		
Standard not met	Standard partly met	Standard met
0	1	2
Applied clinical knowledge		
Standard not met	Standard partly met	Standard met
0	1	2

Examiner Expectations and Basis for Assessment

Information gathering

- Ability to take concise and relevant medical history about Crohn's disease (timing, symptoms and diagnostic tests) and medications – details to include on when it was started and doses
- Skilled in signposting and guiding the consultation
- Ability to obtain information about the past management, including investigations for complications, especially renal
- Offers examination – general and specific
- Ability to ensure that the patient understands and encourages questions – provides information in a step-wise manner in appropriate quantities, checking to ensure understanding

Communication with patients and families

- Introduces self and role
- Ability to tackle difficult or sensitive topics, including the risk of miscarriage, complications during pregnancy and flare up after delivery
- Ability to give information to the patient about Crohn's disease in terms of both the impact of pregnancy on Crohn's disease and Crohn's disease on the pregnancy and the fetus
- Ability to signpost management of Crohn's disease in pregnancy and screening both the fetus and the mother

Communication with colleagues

- Clear and logical approach to the management plan for patients with Crohn's disease, including the need to exclude renal involvement by rheumatologist or internist
- Clear plan of involvement of MDT – internist, rheumatologist, fetal medicine, specialist midwife, anaesthetist and neonatologist and their role
- Ability to communicate with colleagues in primary care and within the multidisciplinary team

Patient safety

- Confirms patients details at the start of the task
- Demonstrates an understanding of both the impact of pregnancy on Crohn's disease and the impact of Crohn's disease on the pregnancy and the fetus
- Safe prescription and implications of, especially, infliximab-abd and corticosteroids in pregnancy
- Safety with regard to allergy

Applied clinical knowledge

Demonstrates:

- Knowledgeable of pre-conception, antenatal and postnatal care, including the risks of maternal morbidity and mortality related to Crohn's disease
- Aware of contemporary literature on Crohn's disease in pregnancy and the puerperium

Task 4: Morbid Obesity. Module 4 – Antepartum Care

Candidate's Instructions

This is a simulated patient task assessing:

- Information gathering
- Communication with patients and families
- Communication with colleagues
- Patient safety
- Applied clinical knowledge

You are an ST5 running a routine antenatal clinic with your consultant. You have been asked to see the next patient whose details are provided below in the referral letter from the GP. This is her first visit.

Hope Hill Surgery
25 London Road
Birmingham
BR2 6TS

Dear Obstetrician,
Re: Nuala Hip
Would you be kind enough to book this 38-year-old woman for antenatal care in your high-risk obstetrics antenatal clinic? She is a mother of two, and just recently found out that she is pregnant. We are not able to triage her to the midwifery clinic because she does not fit the criteria for that clinic. She has a very high BMI.

Yours sincerely

Elaine Butterworth MBBS, FRCGP, DRCOG, DFFP

You have 10 minutes in which you should:

- Obtain detailed and relevant history
- Offer and justify a management plan
- Answer any questions the patient may have

Simulated Patient's Information

You are Nuala Hip, a 38-year-old unemployed mother of two. This is your fourth pregnancy. The first was an uncomplicated pregnancy that ended in a normal vaginal delivery of a 3.4 kg male infant. He is well. The second was a miscarriage at 10 weeks. You had stopped feeling pregnant and an internal ultrasound scan in the hospital showed that the baby had stopped growing at 8 weeks. You were given some pessaries and everything came out. The third was last year. You went into labour 2 weeks before your due date and delivered normally. She weighed 4.6 kg. You wanted an injection in your back for pain relief in labour but the doctor tried twice and failed, and you refused further attempts and used only gas and air.

The father of this pregnancy is different from that of the other two. You have been going out for 6 months. He wants the pregnancy, although you had not been planning for a baby when it happened. Your periods have always been very irregular, and it was only 2 weeks ago that you went to the doctors because you were feeling very sick and your breast were swelling up and becoming very tender. The doctor did a pregnancy test which came out positive. Your last period was about 9 weeks ago, and you are up to date with your smears.

You have always been on the big side and so are your brother, sister, mother and father. You do not know your weight but the GP told you that your BMI is 55 kg/M^2. You smoke about 10–15 cigarettes per day and drink alcohol. The most you take is two pints of lager a day, but since finding out about the pregnancy, you have cut down and only drink over the weekends. If all goes well, you will like to have a home birth as you are worried about your two kids.

You have no major medical problems although you have mild asthma (not taking anything for it at the moment) and have not had any surgery. You are currently on multivitamins and are not aware of any allergies.

You live with your two kids in a council estate with your partner who is also unemployed and smokes 10–20 cigarettes per day and also drinks alcohol almost every day. At times he gets so drunk that you are fearful of him hitting you.

If not covered by the candidate, you should ask the following questions:

1. Why am I not having my care with the midwife as most other women in my estate?
2. Will my baby be very big? The last one was 2 weeks early and was quite big.
3. I will like to deliver at home since my last two deliveries were straightforward.
4. I would like to know whether my baby had Down syndrome as I am an older mother.

A good candidate should cover the following points:

Information gathering

Takes focused history that identifies the following:

- High BMI and family history of obesity
- Irregular periods
- Previous failed epidural
- Lack of appropriate prophylaxis for spina bifida
- Patient's desire to have a home birth – primarily because of fear for her children (domestic violence)
- Asking after domestic violence and potential child safety issues

Communication with patients and families

- Introduces self and role
- Explains the plans at this visit
- Books ultrasound scan to date pregnancy, confirms viability and determines the number of fetuses
- Need for basic bloods – FBC, blood group and antibodies, HIV and others
- Screens for aneuploidy and the limitations
- Implications of high BMI for screening; monitoring of BP and FH and anomaly scan
- Plan of care including regular visit
- Sensitivity about smoking and alcohol
- Screens for gestational diabetes – fasting blood glucose and then OGTT if normal
- Discusses about delivery and where this will occur (preferably in the hospital)
- Acknowledges the issue of alcohol and smoking (for the patient and her husband)

Communication with colleagues

- Referral to dietician
- Referral to anaesthetist to assess back, neck and airway
- Referral to staff about equipment for lifting etc.
- Safeguarding children and the patient – domestic violence

Patient safety

- Confirms patients identity at the start of the task
- Empowers the patient to make an informed decision on the management
- Safe prescription
- Takes into consideration any allergies

Applied clinical knowledge

- Supplementation with vitamin D and increase folic acid to 5 mg daily
- Multidisciplinary care
- Assessment of risk of VTE
- Thromboprophylaxis antenatally and postpartum
- Demonstrates an understanding of the issues of safeguarding children
- Demonstrates the use of guidelines to inform decision on treatment – NICE and RCOG Green-top Guidelines

Examiner score sheet		
Information gathering		
Standard not met	Standard partly met	Standard met
0	1	2
Communication with patients and families		
Standard not met	Standard partly met	Standard met
0	1	2
Communication with colleagues		
Standard not met	Standard partly met	Standard met
0	1	2
Patient safety		
Standard not met	Standard partly met	Standard met
0	1	2
Applied clinical knowledge		
Standard not met	Standard partly met	Standard met
0	1	2

Examiner Expectations and Basis for Assessment

Information gathering

- Able to take concise and relevant antenatal history
- Skilled in signposting and guiding the antenatal consultation
- Able to ensure that the patient understands and encourages questions
- Able to describe to the antenatal patient a clear action plan and the rationale for follow-up based on the discussion of implications of morbid obesity

Communication with patients and families

- Introduces self and role
- Able to discuss investigations, follow-up and plan for antenatal care
- Ability to succinctly summarise discussions with antenatal patients
- Discusses on plan of care and place of delivery (pros and cons of home versus hospital delivery and which hospital delivery is recommended)

Communication with colleagues

- Referral to dietician
- Reviews by anaesthetist at 34 weeks
- MDT – in planning for possible surgery (labour ward theatre staff and anaesthetist) and midwifery colleagues, including specialist midwives and neonatologists

Patient safety

- Confirms patients details at the start of the task
- Ability to triage patient to different patterns of antenatal care according to the risk factors
- Aware of the safety of investigations and therapeutics during pregnancy, including safe prescription
- Aware of issues of drug and alcohol abuse, domestic violence and safeguarding
- Has an understanding of clinical governance and risk management for women declining usual antenatal care
- Discusses and offers thromboprophylaxis

Applied clinical knowledge

- Knowledgeable of antenatal care, including screening for medical complications in morbid obesity
- Ability to interpret clinical examination findings and results of investigations in the context of the clinical scenario
- Aware of the risks and benefits of various different management options, balancing the needs of the mother and the fetus
- Demonstrates being up to date with current medical literature on obesity in pregnancy, especially RCOG Guidelines

Reference: *Antenatal care for uncomplicated pregnancies. NICE Clinical guideline [CG62] 26 March 2008. Last updated 04 February 2019*

Task 5: Prenatal Diagnosis. Module 4 – Antenatal Care

Candidate's Instructions

This is a simulated patient task assessing:

- Information gathering
- Communication with patients and families
- Communication with colleagues
- Patient safety
- Applied clinical knowledge

You are an ST5 working with Mr Sandeep Gupta in a district general hospital. You have been called to see a patient of Mr Gupta who has just had an ultrasound scan at 12 weeks of gestation. The sonographer told her that there is a problem but did not give details other than that the doctor will explain everything to her. Mr Gupta is away. The essential findings on the ultrasound scan report are given below.

Scan report for Joyce Schwanger

Single active live fetus CRL – 75 mm compatible with 12⁺⁶ weeks gestation
There is a complex septate cystic mass around the neck of the fetus, extending down to the upper abdomen. This cystic structure extends to the anterior part of the neck
The fetal stomach is seen below the diaphragm. The kidneys and bladder were also seen.
There are four limbs but the details could not be assessed because of the age of the pregnancy
There is a normal amount of fluid around the baby and the placenta is fundal
There are no adnexal masses
Impression: A large cystic hygroma
Clinic informed and patient to go and see Mr Gupta's ST5

Signed
Hazel Knott
Senior Sonographer

You have 10 minutes in which you should:

- Explain the ultrasound findings and implications
- Discuss management options including complications
- Management of the pregnancy
- Answer any questions the patient may have

Simulated Patient's Information

You are Ms Joyce Schwanger, a 28-year-old trainee accountant with the city council. This is your first pregnancy and is unplanned. You are not married but have had a steady boyfriend of 3 years. He is not sure about the pregnancy though.

You are healthy and have not suffered from any infections or illness that you know of. You neither smoke nor drink alcohol. You are an only child, and there is no family history of any illness like diabetes or hypertension. You are taking pregnancy multivitamins and are allergic to cats.

Your periods were very regular – in fact you describe them as clockwork. You were always very careful about the time of sexual intercourse but you are sure this happened when you celebrated your boyfriend's birthday and he forgot to use the condom.

You and your partner live in a semi-detached house, which you are renting. He is a salesman with a high street store.

You have seen children with disability and do not want to have one if possible.

Although you have not been told a lot, you suspect that there is something wrong as the sonographer who had been talking jokingly suddenly stopped talking, and when you asked her what was wrong, she said your doctor will tell you.

If not covered by the candidate, you should ask the following questions:

1. Will my baby die inside me?
2. Can any test be done that will tell me for sure that the baby is abnormal or not?
3. This swelling on the baby's neck, can it not be removed after the baby is born?
4. Will my baby be handicapped?
5. How will I deliver the baby?
6. I just want to terminate the pregnancy – I do not feel confident to carry on with the pregnancy knowing that there is something wrong with the baby.
7. What kind of a blood test will be done to check chromosomes? Ask this if offered chorionic villus sampling and risks discussed.

A good candidate should cover the following:

Information gathering

- Obtains good history that highlights the lack of pre-pregnancy optimisation
- The fear of having an abnormal baby
- Desires to have a prenatal test
- Reviews ultrasound report and reveals findings

Communication with patients and families

- Introduces self and role
- Goes through the process of breaking bad new
- Explains the ultrasound report with the help of diagrams (this ought to come first before asking for any additional information). It is incorrect to start by telling the woman 'I will like to ask you information about your pregnancy' when she knows that there is something wrong with her baby. This will create a feeling of fear and apprehension, and the patient may lash out
- Explains the options – prenatal testing – chorionic villus sampling at this stage with the risk of miscarriage
- Introduces and discusses NIPT – pros and cons (as an alternative to invasive testing) if CVS is declined
- Discusses the options available if result is normal or abnormal (continuing the pregnancy or termination)

Communication with colleagues

- Involves fetal medicine or referral to centre with fetal medicine expert
- Involvement of geneticist
- Counsellor may be required
- Referral to fetal cardiologist for echo at 22–24 weeks
- Involvement of paediatric surgeon and clinical geneticist – counselling and planning postnatal care if appropriate (i.e. if karyotype if normal and pregnancy is continuing)

Patient safety

- Confirms patients details at the start of the task
- Respects the patient's wishes
- Understands the clauses for termination of pregnancy
- Offers to call partner, relative or friend – this is very important as she may not be able to drive home or take in most of what she is given

Applied clinical knowledge

- Associated risk of aneuploidy, especially 45XO
- Screening for other structural abnormalities – especially cardiovascular
- Surgery for unexplained – prognosis – guarded as baby may be syndromic
- Displays knowledge of the recent literature on prenatal diagnostic testing (invasive and non-invasive) and RCOG Green-top Guidelines on amniocentesis and chorionic villus sampling

Examiner score sheet		
Information gathering		
Standard not met	Standard partly met	Standard met
0	1	2
Communication with patients and families		
Standard not met	Standard partly met	Standard met
0	1	2
Communication with colleagues		
Standard not met	Standard partly met	Standard met
0	1	2
Patient safety		
Standard not met	Standard partly met	Standard met
0	1	2
Applied clinical knowledge		
Standard not met	Standard partly met	Standard met
0	1	2

Examiner Expectations and Basis for Assessment

Information gathering

- Able to take concise and relevant antenatal history
- Skilled in signposting and guiding the antenatal consultation
- Able to ensure that the patient understands and encourages questions
- Able to describe to the antenatal patient a clear action plan and the rationale for follow-up, based on the discussion of implications of a cystic hygroma

---

Communication with patients and families

- Introduces self and role
- Able to discuss investigations, follow-up and plan for antenatal care
- Discusses abnormality (cystic hygroma) and implications
- Discusses investigations, complications and options for management after termination or continuation, depending on results
- Ability to succinctly summarise discussions with antenatal patients
- Appropriate amount of detail to ensure management plans are clear and easily understood by colleagues

---

Communication with colleagues

- Ability to communicate with colleagues in other specialties, e.g. fetal medicine, genetics, paediatrics surgery and paediatric cardiology

---

Patient safety

- Confirms patients details at the start of the task
- Ability to triage patient to different patterns of antenatal care according to the risk factors
- High risk even if karyotypically normal
- Aware of the safety of investigations (risks of invasive testing and limitations of non-invasive testing)
- Has an understanding of clinical governance and risk management for women declining usual antenatal care and options for termination of pregnancy

---

Applied clinical knowledge

- Knowledgeable of antenatal care and pathways for women booking early
- Ability to interpret clinical information and results of investigations (ultrasound) in the context of the clinical scenario
- Aware of the risks and benefits of various different management options, balancing the needs of the mother and the fetus
- Knowledgeable of current literature and of guidelines – RCOG Green-top Guidelines on amniocentesis and chorionic villus sampling

Task 6: Previous Shoulder Dystocia. Module 7 – Management of Delivery

Candidate's Instructions

This is a simulated patient task assessing:

- Information gathering
- Communication with the patients and families
- Communication with colleagues
- Patient safety
- Applied clinical knowledge

You are an ST5 working with a consultant in the high-risk obstetrics clinic of your hospital. You are in the antenatal clinic and have been called by the midwife to see a patient who has been referred by her GP for counselling at 36 weeks of gestation. The referral letter is given below.

Yew Street Surgery
Harrogate
Yorkshire
HG7 2YTM

Dear Dr Gattree,
Re: Ms Baljit Khoor
I will be grateful if you could see Ms Baljit Khoor, a 28-year-old nursing assistant in her second pregnancy, for counselling about the mode of delivery. Her first pregnancy was complicated by gestational diabetes which was managed by diet only. She went into spontaneous labour at 40 weeks. Labour was complicated by shoulder dystocia, although there is no permanent injury to either the baby or the mother. The baby weighed 4,500 g. She is now 36 weeks and will like to review her options for this pregnancy.

Yours sincerely

Dr Sunmi Singh MBChB, MRCP, DFFP, DRCOG

You have 10 minutes in which you should:

- Take a focused history
- Discuss the concerns of the patient
- Management of the pregnancy
- Answer any questions she may have

Simulated Patient's Information

You are a 28-year-old nursing assistant in your second pregnancy. You had your son 2 years ago, and he is well. You live with your partner who is a businessman in his house. You do not smoke but drink alcohol occasionally. You have no known allergies.

You are currently 36 weeks pregnant. You booked at 10 weeks because you had gestational diabetes in your last pregnancy. Your dates were confirmed, and you had an OGTT which was normal at 12 weeks and then again at 24 weeks. You were so relieved to hear that you do not have gestational diabetes this time. You have had ultrasound scans to assess the growth of the baby, and the last scan which was only done yesterday (you are now 36 weeks) estimated the baby's weight to be 3,400 g. You have been told that this baby is unlikely to be as big as your son.

Your last pregnancy was complicated by gestational diabetes. On a few occasions, the diabetic doctor threatened to put you on insulin but you really worked hard on your blood sugar levels, and he did not.

You went into labour on your own at 40 weeks, and the labour progressed very well and within 6 hours of admission, you were fully. You had an epidural for pain relief. After 2 hours of being fully, you started pushing. You pushed for nearly 1 hour but the baby was yet to be delivered. The doctor was called, and he wanted to perform a ventouse delivery but you were determined to do it yourself. With a lot of efforts, you pushed the head out.

When the baby's head was delivered, it took quite some time for the rest of the baby to be delivered. You were informed that the shoulders were not coming. There was commotion as so many people came after the buzzer went off, and they immediately put you flat on your back and put your legs up. After about 2 minutes, the shoulders were delivered and the baby had to be given oxygen. You were torn very badly, and this was repaired.

Although you have been okay since the birth of your son, the thought of going through this again really frightens you. The midwife told you that you could aim for another vaginal delivery but you are scared.

If not covered, you should ask the candidate the following questions:

- What causes shoulder dystocia (makes it difficult for the shoulders to come out)?
- What are the chances of it happening again?
- Can you predict whether it will happen again, and if so, what will be done to reduce the risk of it happening again?
- Which is better for me – a vaginal delivery or a CS?
- Why have I been offered a vaginal delivery?
- As I do not have diabetes now, does that make my chances of having another complication less likely?
- Can I be induced to deliver early as this will ensure that the baby is not too big?

A good candidate will cover the following:

Information gathering

- Obtains relevant history that will reveal previous GDM and shoulder dystocia
- Obtains information about current pregnancy and relevant investigations
- Reviews medical records (informs the woman that notes will be reviewed)
- Ascertains fears and anxieties about having another shoulder dystocia

Communication with patients and families

- Introduces self and role
- Discusses the pros and cons of a vaginal delivery
- Discusses the risk of recurrent shoulder dystocia – average recurrence is 10%
- Need to deliver in hospital under consultant care
- If going for a vaginal birth, should have a fetal scan to estimate birthweight at 38 weeks
- Encourages questions, answers them and able to deliver information in varied quantities, gauging thorough understanding at each stage

Patient safety

- Confirms patients details at the start of the task
- Empowers the woman to make the choice
- Choosing an elective CS is a recognised approach to managing women with a previous shoulder dystocia
- Induction of labour is an option to reduce recurrent shoulder dystocia (contemporary opinion)
- Plan of care must be documented in notes as agreed with the patient, including adequate pain relief and presence of senior staff to perform manoeuvres

Applied clinical knowledge

- Evidence that induction of labour will reduce the risk of shoulder dystocia, except in diabetics/GDM
- Discusses the recurrence risks and the pros and cons of vaginal versus CS delivery
- Discusses the risk factors and how these cannot predict recurrence
- Elective CS could be considered to prevent recurrence and reduce morbidity
- Demonstrates use of NICE and RCOG Guidelines to inform decision making in the management of patient

Examiner score sheet		
Information gathering		
Standard not met	Standard partly met	Standard met
0	1	2
Communication with patients and families		
Standard not met	Standard partly met	Standard met
0	1	2

Communication with colleagues		
Standard not met	Standard partly met	Standard met
0	1	2
Patient safety		
Standard not met	Standard partly met	Standard met
0	1	2
Applied clinical knowledge		
Standard not met	Standard partly met	Standard met
0	1	2

Examiner Expectations and Basis for Assessment

Information gathering

- Obtains information from patients or clinical notes (including the partogram, CTG and maternal vital signs) and use these to formulate a clear clinical picture of the patient
- History of current pregnancy including investigations review ultrasound reports including estimated fetal weight
- Ability to describe a clear action plan and rationale for decisions made based on discussions with the patient
- Ascertains fears and anxieties about recurrence of shoulder dystocia
- Identifies wishes of patient

Communication with patients and families

- Ability to communicate to the woman and her partner and/or family the interventions for abnormal labour and instrumental or operative delivery
- Discusses options – vaginal delivery versus CS
- Discusses prediction of shoulder dystocia and limitations of various models
- Ability to explain the risks and benefits of interventions for both the mother and the fetus
- Agrees a plan for the pregnancy and delivery

Communication with colleagues

- Has an understanding of the limits of one's own competence and when to call for senior help

- Ability to form a logical plan for intrapartum care and anticipatory management of shoulder dystocia
- Appropriate amount of detail to ensure management plans are clear and easily understood by colleagues
- Involvement of other specialties in the care of the patient – anaesthetists for early epidural in labour

Patient safety

- Confirms patients details at the start of the task
- Aware of patient safety in labour
- Has an understanding of risks from interventions such as regional analgesia
- Has an understanding of risk management and clinical governance processes in relation to intrapartum care
- Undertakes the necessary preparations for vaginal delivery (early epidural, skilled stall and ensures good progress of labour) and timely interventions

Applied clinical knowledge

- Knowledgeable of intrapartum care, including induction of labour, management of normal and abnormal labour, obstetric interventions and the interpretation of CTG
- Ability to critically appraise the literature including guidelines, protocols and scientific papers for shoulder dystocia and macrosomia, including RCOG Green-top Guideline on shoulder dystocia
- Has a working knowledge of the roles of other members of the multidisciplinary team – anaesthetist, neonatologist and midwives

Reference: Shoulder dystocia. The Royal College of Obstetricians and Gynaecologists Green-Top Guideline No. 42 28 March 2012. Last updated February 2017

Task 7: Intrauterine Fetal Death. Module 8 – Postpartum Problems (The Puerperium)

Candidate's Instructions

This is a simulated patient task assessing:

- Information gathering
- Communication with patients and families
- Communication with colleagues

- Patient safety
- Applied clinical knowledge

You are the ST5 who is scheduled to run the postnatal clinic for your team. One of the patients you are about to see had an intrauterine fetal death and has come back for follow-up. A summary of the results of the investigations are shown below.

Summary of investigations post delivery showed the following:

Histology – massive placental abruption with multiple infarcts in the placenta
Haematological – positive for anticardiolipin antibody (ACA)
Protein S – 30 (normal 60–140)
Biochemical – normal
Post-mortem – nothing abnormal found

You have 10 minutes in which you should:

1. Take relevant history
2. Explain the results of the investigations after the delivery
3. Institute further investigations if appropriate and justify these
4. Agree a plan for her going forward

Simulates Patient's Information

You are Ms Cindy Loptim, a 21-year-old who lost your first baby 6 weeks ago. The pregnancy was going well and then you developed sudden abdominal pain, which was very severe at 37 weeks. At first, you thought you were in labour but this pain was so severe you had to call the ambulance. When you were taken to the hospital, you had the monitor put on your tummy and your nightmare began. You were told that the baby's heart had stopped beating. You could not believe it and asked the doctors to do something about it but they said you had bled behind the placenta and that it had been severe enough to kill the baby.

They then put up a drip and within 3 hours you had delivered your son, who looked so pale and was lifeless. He weighed 2.9 kg, and all you could remember was a gush of blood down below. There was panic, and you really cannot remember most of what happened thereafter.

You woke up in the intensive care unit, with a tube down your throat and one in your bladder and blood going in on one hand and a drip on the other. You stayed there for 4 days and then moved to the ward where you stayed for 3 days before going home.

You have made very good recovery according to your GP and community midwife, who have been amazingly supportive. You still do not understand exactly what happened and is frightened to embark on another pregnancy although you and your partner really want to have a baby.

You have not resumed sexual intercourse as you are really scared that something is wrong below. You blame yourself for the loss of Jack, as it was you who had the bleeding. You love your partner Luke but it's been very difficult as you do not talk about Jack. All he does is sit in the corner and look at the ultrasound photos that you have.

You have had one period (2 weeks ago) and have no medical problems. You are allergic to aspirin.

You had stopped smoking during pregnancy but started soon after you were able to following the delivery of Jack. It's a relief for you really. You have started drinking again.

If not covered you should ask the following questions:

1. What exactly caused my baby to die?
2. Was it my fault and how can I prevent it from happening again?
3. What are the chances of it happening again?
4. Is something wrong with me down there as I do not want Luke anywhere near me?
5. When can I start trying again?
6. What will be done to monitor the baby and when will the baby be delivered?

A good candidate should cover the following:

1. *Information gathering*
   a. Reviews her notes to see exactly the sequence of events before seeing the patient
   b. Reviews results of investigations
   c. Asks about general health and menstruation
   d. Ascertains the issues about coping, feelings and plans and currently physiology
   e. Establishes current medication and drug allergies
2. *Communication with patients and families*
   a. Introduces self and role
   b. Explains the course of events and confirms an understanding of these (and enquires if this had been offered prior to discharge from hospital)
   c. Explains the course of events after a loss and reassures the patient that the feelings/reactions between her and Luke about Jack are normal and will get better with time
   d. Explores support from bereavement services, SANDS and clinical psychologists
   e. Explains the need for further investigations – repeat ACA 12–14 weeks after previous test, protein S as tends to fall in pregnancy
   f. Outlines the plan of care in next pregnancy
   g. Deals with concerns about anatomy of genital tract and phobia of sexual intercourse
3. *Communication with colleagues*
   a. Liaises with clinical psychologist
   b. Reaches out to the GP and the social worker for support
   c. Reaches out to the support networks locally and nationally
4. *Patient safety*
   a. Confirms patients details at the start of the task
   b. Ensures appropriate follow-up at home by the GP/social worker
   c. Arranges home visit by the support team (midwife, counsellor etc.)
   d. Offers to see again with partner
5. *Applied clinical knowledge*
   a. Discusses the pathology that lead to the IUD
   b. Explains the reasoning behind the pathology (abruption resulted in IUD)
   c. Explains the implications of the investigations

d. Discusses the recurrence rate – 1:20 and plans to minimise reoccurrence
e. Explains and agrees plans for delivery and timing of delivery
f. Demonstrates knowledge of contemporary literature on antepartum haemorrhage and investigations for intrauterine fetal death – RCOG Green-top Guidelines on intrauterine fetal death and antepartum haemorrhage

Examiner score sheet		
Information gathering		
Standard not met	Standard partly met	Standard met
0	1	2
Communication with patients and families		
Standard not met	Standard partly met	Standard met
0	1	2
Communication with colleagues		
Standard not met	Standard partly met	Standard met
0	1	2
Patient safety		
Standard not met	Standard partly met	Standard met
0	1	2
Applied clinical knowledge		
Standard not met	Standard partly met	Standard met
0	1	2

Examiner Expectations and Basis for Assessment

Information gathering

- Obtains information from notes on management prior to discharge
- Obtains/uses information (history, examination and investigations) to help signpost management plans and follow-up
- Ability to obtain information about plans for subsequent pregnancies – when planning to start trying
- Establishes fears and concerns of relationship issues

Communication with patients and families

- Introduces self and role
- Able to communicate with the woman and her partner the details of the complication
- Able to explain the rationale for further/repeating investigations
- An ability to empower the patient to ask questions and also articulate an understanding of the management plans
- Manages communication incrementally, encouraging questions and checking understanding at regular intervals

Communication with colleagues

- Has an understanding of the limits of one's own competence and when to involve consultant where appropriate
- Communicates appropriate amount of detail to ensure that management plans are clear and easily understood by colleagues where appropriate, especially with respect to interpreting investigations
- Team work to support – involvement of bereavement counsellors, SANDs and local support groups

Patient safety

- Confirms patients details at the start of the task
- Understands the impact of loss on risk of depression and relationship breakdown and takes appropriate steps
- Uses appropriate safe prescription where necessary, having established allergies

Applied clinical knowledge

- Knowledgeable of postpartum care of couples with an intrauterine fetal death
- Ability to critically appraise the literature, including guidelines (Green-top Guideline on intrauterine fetal death and other contemporary literature)
- Has a working knowledge of the roles of other members of the multidisciplinary team

Reference: *Late intrauterine fetal death and stillbirth. The Royal College of Obstetricians and Gynaecologists Green-top Guideline No. 55 October 2010*

Task 8: Results for Interpretation. Module 4 – Antepartum Care

Candidate's Instructions

This is a structured discussion task assessing:

- Information gathering
- Communication with patients and families
- Communication with colleagues
- Patient safety
- Applied clinical knowledge

The following are patients with results of various investigations performed on them when they were seen either in the antenatal or gynaecology clinics of your team. You have been called to review the results. For each patient, describe the abnormality and your immediate management plan.

You have 10 minutes in which you should:

- Read the patient summary and results
- Identify what is abnormal with the result and its implication(s)
- Discuss your immediate action, including communication with the patient or others with the examiner

Patient Summary and Results

1. A 36-year-old teacher attended for an ultrasound scan at 26 weeks for reduced fetal movements. She had been generally unwell for a week. The scan showed echogenic bowel in the fetus. As a result, a blood test was performed for virology, and she has now been reported to have IgM and IgG antibodies against parvovirus B19

2. A 17-year-old attended for termination of pregnancy at 10 weeks' gestation. An endocervical swab was obtained at the termination, and this has been reported as positive for *Chlamydia trachomatis*

3. A primigravida attended at 38 weeks' gestation for suspected fetal growth restriction. Ultrasound biometry was ordered and the results are as follows: BPD = 92 mm (37^{+2} days), HC = 325 mm (38^{+3} weeks), AC = 267 mm (33^{+2} weeks), FL = 76 mm (37^{+0} weeks) and AFI = 4.2 (<5th centile for gestational age)

4. A 40-year-old woman has been attending antenatal care for the past 4 months. She is now at 36 weeks of gestation, and a report has just been received from the rheumatologist that she is anti-Ro positive

5. An oral glucose tolerance test was performed on a primigravida at 28 weeks' gestation. She is obese, BMI = 35 kg/M^2 and her mother is diabetic. The results are as follows: fasting (first in the series) = 6.5 mmol/L and 120 minutes (second in the series) = 11.8 mmol/L

6. A 36-year-old teacher had a serum screening test at 16 weeks' gestation. The result is as follows: AFP = 0.5 MoM, hCG = 3.5 MoM and Down's syndrome risk = 1:150

A good candidate will cover most of the following:

Case No	Abnormality and its implication (s) for the fetus	Action to be taken including communication with patient or colleagues
1	Acute parvovirus maternal infection Risk of fetal hydrops and intrauterine fetal death	Refer to fetal medicine for monitoring by means of middle cerebral artery Doppler 5 weeks from acute infection. Intrauterine transfusion if MCA PSV is >90th centile for gestational age
2	Maternal infection with *Chlamydia trachomatis*. Untreated risk of neonatal conjunctivitis	Treat with azithromycin. Screen for other STIs and refer to GUM for contact tracing and counselling about sexual intercourse during treatment
3	Late onset FGR Increased risk of sudden intrauterine fetal death	Ask for Doppler assessment – umbilical artery, middle cerebral and ductus venosus Perform a CTG and assess cervix. Offer induction of labour
4	Positive for anti-Ro antibodies Increased risk of intrauterine fetal death and fetal heart block	Refer to fetal medicine for monitoring of fetal heart at 24, 28 and 32 weeks and growth
5	Abnormal glucose tolerance test (GTT) diagnostic of gestational diabetes Increased risk of fetal macrosomia, polyhydramnios and unexplained intrauterine fetal death	Refer to dietician and diabetic clinic for diet control advice, initiation of treatment (most likely with metformin and insulin) and serial blood glucose monitoring and serial fetal growth measurements
6	High aneuploidy screen Increased risk of trisomy 21 and other aneuploidies in the fetus	Counsel for invasive and non-invasive testing (NIPT). At this state, CVS and its risks or NIPT which is not diagnostic but has an accuracy of >99% for trisomies 21, 18 and 13 with a risk to the fetus

Examiner score sheet		
Information gathering		
Standard not met	Standard partly met	Standard met
0	1	2
Communication with patients and families		
Standard not met	Standard partly met	Standard met
0	1	2
Communication with colleagues		
Standard not met	Standard partly met	Standard met
0	1	2

Patient safety		
Standard not met	Standard partly met	Standard met
0	1	2
Applied clinical knowledge		
Standard not met	Standard partly met	Standard met
0	1	2

Examiner Expectations and Basis for Assessment

Information gathering

- Able to interpret information from investigations appropriately
- Able to initiate additional investigations to help plan management for each case
- Has an understanding of additional information that may be required to help arrive at a diagnosis and plan care

Communication with patients and families

- Gives information sensitively and in manageable amounts, regarding results of investigations in and management of each pregnancy
- Describes a clear and logical action and rationale for a follow-up

Communication with colleagues

- Ability to prioritise cases appropriately and refer them for timely investigations/ interventions in pregnancy, recognising the importance of time, especially in relation to prenatal diagnosis
- Describes the differential diagnoses and formulates an appropriate management plan
- Refers appropriately to fetal medicine and other disciplines

Patient safety

- Has an understanding of the limits of their clinical abilities and demonstrates an understanding of when to refer patients to senior colleagues and other disciplines
- Discusses the risks of interventions, investigations and procedures and takes necessary precautions against it

---

Applied clinical knowledge

- Knowledgeable of the routine antenatal care investigations and actions to be taken when these are abnormal
- Has an understanding of the role of imaging in the investigation/management of pregnancy
- Ability to present management options and their risks and benefits using non-directional counselling
- Knowledge of antenatal care pathways and investigations and management as detailed in current literature and guidelines (NICE and RCOG)

Task 9: Results for Interpretation. Module 9 – Gynaecological Problems

Candidate's Instructions

This is a structured discussion task assessing:

- Information gathering
- Communication with patient and families
- Communication with colleagues
- Patient safety
- Applied clinical knowledge

Below is a series of investigations undertaken in your consultant's clinic. You are his ST5 and have been asked to review them. For each investigation, briefly describe the abnormality and any steps you will take.

You have 10 minutes in which you should:

- Read the patient summary and results
- Identify what is abnormal with the result
- Discuss your immediate action with the examiner

Patient Summary and Results

1. A 26-year-old with secondary amenorrhoea = Prolactin 1,500 miu/l (50–400) Free T4 = 10 pmol/L(9–25), TSH 2.5 miu/L(0.5–4.5)

2. A 26-year-old renal transplant patient at 12 weeks' gestation with proteinuria had an MSU which yielded *Proteus spp.* resistant to amoxycillin but sensitive only to ciprofloxacin

3. Mrs BB, a 30-year-old epileptic had a Down's test at 16 weeks' gestation. AFP = 60 iu (90th centile <35), βHCG 1.75 MoM

4. A 31-year-old whose mother is diabetic and whose previous baby of 4.5 kg had an OGTT at 28 weeks. The results are: fasting = 5.0 and 2 hours = 8.2 mmol/L

5. Mrs Baby is now at 24 weeks of gestation. She had a severe PPH in her first pregnancy and was transfused. This is her second pregnancy. Antibody screen was positive with an anti-c level of 12 iu

275

6. Mrs ST is 57 years old and had breast cancer 4 years ago. She is on 20 mg of tamoxifen and presented with postmenopausal bleeding. An endometrial biopsy was performed. Histology is reported as widespread presence of chronic inflammatory cells and no evidence of atypia

7. A 30-year-old woman is presented with primary infertility and irregular periods. 21-day progesterone = 1.9nnol/L, FSH = 12 iu/L and Rubella immune. Semen = normal

A good candidate will cover most of the following:

Case No	Abnormality	Action to be taken including communication with patient or colleagues
1	Hyperprolactinaemia	Invite patient for a repeat test, and if raised, refer to endocrinologist and consider MRI/CT of the brain
2	Urinary tract infection with *Proteus spp.*	Ask the GP to prescribe antibiotic but counsel about contraindication in pregnancy. Benefits outweigh risks. Repeat urine culture after completion of treatment
3	Raised AFP	Refer to fetal medicine for a detail USS of the fetus. Exclude history of bleeding in pregnancy
4	Abnormal OGTT – impaired glucose tolerance	Refer to dietician in diabetic clinic. Follow-up with blood glucose monitoring and consider metformin if no control. Serial fetal growth scans
5	Isoimmunisation with raised anti-c antibodies	Refer to fetal medicine. Serial (weekly) middle cerebral artery Doppler
6	Non-specific inflammatory endometrial changes	Invite patient for hysteroscopy and directed biopsy, preferably with a sharp curette
7	Anovulatory progesterone levels	Invite patient for serial serum progesterone levels as cycles are irregular

Examiner score sheet		
Information gathering		
Standard not met	Standard partly met	Standard met
0	1	2
Communication with patients and families		
Standard not met	Standard partly met	Standard met
0	1	2
Communication with colleagues		
Standard not met	Standard partly met	Standard met
0	1	2

Patient safety		
Standard not met	Standard partly met	Standard met
0	1	2
Applied clinical knowledge		
Standard not met	Standard partly met	Standard met
0	1	2

Examiner Expectations and Basis for Assessment

Information gathering

• Able to interpret information from investigations appropriately
• Is able to initiate additional investigations to help make a diagnosis and plan management
• Has an understanding of additional information that may be required to help arrive at a diagnosis and plan care

---

Communication with patients and families

• Gives information sensitively and in manageable amounts, regarding results of investigations in pregnancy and management

---

Communication with colleagues

• Able to prioritise cases and refer for timely investigations, recognising the importance of time, especially in relation to implications of abnormality
• Describes the differential diagnoses and formulates an appropriate management plan

---

Patient safety

• Has an understanding of the limits of their clinical abilities and demonstrates an understanding of when to refer patients to senior colleagues and other disciplines
• Initiates steps to mitigate risks
• Establishes drug allergy and demonstrates safe prescription
• Counsels on the risk and benefits of treatment

Applied clinical knowledge

- Knowledgeable of common gynaecology investigations and actions to be taken when these are abnormal
- Has an understanding of the role of imaging in the investigation/management of gynaecology problems
- Able to present management options and their risks and benefits using non-directional counselling
- Knowledgeable of care pathways and investigations and management of common gynaecology problems as detailed in current literature and guidelines (NICE and RCOG)

Task 10: Ovarian Cyst – Suspected Malignancy. Module 13 – Gynaecological Oncology

Candidates Instructions

This is a simulated patient task assessing:

- Information gathering
- Communication with patients and families
- Communication with colleagues
- Patient safety
- Applied clinical knowledge

You are the ST5 in the clinic today, and the referral letter from the GP for your next patient is given below.

The Belway Surgery
George Womsy Way
Branstaple
BK10 15 DL

Dear Doctor,
Would you be kind enough to see this 45-year-old who has just come to my surgery with abdominal pain and complaining that her tummy is getting bigger. I am referring her straight away as I am not happy having felt a mass in her abdomen.
Thank you.

Yours sincerely

Dr Ghada Yassan MBBS, MRCOG, MRCGP

You have 10 minutes in which you should:

- Obtain relevant history
- Explain your suspected diagnosis and investigations to be undertaken
- Discuss treatment options
- Answer any questions she may have

Simulated Patient's Information

You are Ms Chandraseka Patel, a 45-year-old divorcee living with your two children (aged 16 and 20 years) in your own house. You work as a bank counter staff. You ex is very supportive of the children and sees them whenever he wishes.

You had your first child 20 year ago. He was a full-term normal delivery of an uncomplicated pregnancy, weighing 3,200 g. Your second was 16 years ago and weighed 2,960 g. You had placental praevia, hence had to have a caesarean section.

Four months ago, you started having mild pain on the left side. You really did not pay too much attention to this as you thought it was the usual mid-cycle pain that you have always had. The pain, however, did not go away and you started feeling some heaviness on the left side. A month ago, you observed that your skirts were getting tighter and now you cannot fit into them. It was this that made you see the doctor. The pain has persisted although it's not really getting worse. It's just a dull ache which is there all the time.

There have been no changes in your appetite or weight. Your weight is 71 kg. Your periods have remained regular; the last one was 2 weeks ago. There is no associated vaginal bleeding or discharge.

You do not suffer from any bowel problems although you have been more constipated this time than before. You do not have any problems with your waterworks.

You had your tubes tied with your caesarean section and are sexually active (you have a boyfriend but he does not live with you).

You do not have any other medical or surgical history of importance and have no known allergies. You are up to date with your smears. The last one was 1 year ago and was negative.

You do not have anyone in your family with cancer of the ovary, bowel or breast.

If not covered, you should ask the following questions:

- What is the most likely cause of my symptoms?
- What investigations will you perform?
- What treatment will you offer me?
- What complications may I have if I do not have surgery now?

A good candidate should cover the following:

Information gathering

- Insidious onset of symptoms
- Associated bowel symptoms but no associated urinary symptoms
- No weight loss or change in appetite
- Note no family history of cancers
- Offers to undertake a physical, including abdominal and bimanual pelvic examinations
- Discusses the investigations to be performed (ultrasound scan of the pelvis and abdomen, tumour markers such as CA125, LDH and AFP; electrolytes and urea, FBC and LFT)
- Further imaging such as MRI/CT scan if indicated to define tumour type and spread

Communication with patients and families

- Introduces self and role
- Explains of the clinical findings
- Discusses the investigations and management plan

Communication with colleagues

- Consultation with other specialties – imaging and oncology
- Involvement of multidisciplinary team (MDT) – gynaecology oncologist, oncologist, radio-therapist, radiology, oncology nurse, GP, social worker/clinical psychologist and support groups

Patient safety

- Confirms patients identity at the start of the task
- Empowers the patient to make informed choices
- Safe prescription
- Obtains consent for surgery
- Ascertains allergies and safe prescription

Applied clinical knowledge

- Discusses the ultrasound findings
- Risk of malignancy index (RMI) score based on ultrasound and CA125 value
- Management based on RMI and other investigation findings
- Staging laparotomy and hysterectomy and bilateral salpingoophorectomy and omentectomy (but if RMI is less than 250 but more than 200 for laparoscopic surgery by gynaecologist with interest in gynaecological oncology)
- Demonstrates knowledge of the Green-top (ovarian cyst in pre and postmenopausal women) and NICE Guidelines and contemporary literature

Examiner score sheet		
Information gathering		
Standard not met	Standard partly met	Standard met
0	1	2
Communication with patients and families		
Standard not met	Standard partly met	Standard met
0	1	2
Communication with colleagues		
Standard not met	Standard partly met	Standard met
0	1	2
Patient safety		
Standard not met	Standard partly met	Standard met
0	1	2
Applied clinical knowledge		
Standard not met	Standard partly met	Standard met
0	1	2

Examiner Expectations and Basis for Assessment

Information gathering

- Takes comprehensive history of insidious onset of symptoms and symptoms suggestive of malignancy
- Requests appropriate investigations (abdominal and pelvic examinations), chest X-ray, tumour markers, especially CA125, full blood count and liver and renal function tests and biopsies
- Imaging – MRI/CT scan of the pelvis and abdomen

Communication with patients and families

- Introduces self and role
- Demonstrates empathy with communication and breaking possible bad news
- Counsels about the most likely diagnosis and how these relate to symptoms
- Describes clearly the logical approach to different management options (pros and cons), including complications and rationale for care and follow-up
- Discusses the various steps in management (investigations, treatment and follow-up)

Communication with colleagues

- Refers an oncology centre
- Understands the role of MDT (gynaecology oncologist, radiologist, radiotherapist, oncologist, oncology nurse and clinical psychologist) in the management of ovarian cancer
- Has an understanding of the role of support groups in the management of the patient

---

Patient safety

- Confirms patients identity at the start of the task
- Safe prescription for medical options for managing ovarian cancer – asking about allergies and medical disorders that could be considered contraindications to the medications
- Understands principles of chemotherapy, duration and complications as adjuvant treatment for ovarian cancer
- Knows the principles of safe surgery, if it is the chosen option for the patient

---

Applied clinical knowledge

Demonstrates:

- Good knowledge of implications of ovarian cancer as evidence from explaining diagnosis and management options
- An understanding of the contents of NICE/RCOG Guidelines on ovarian cysts/cancer, with regard to management, follow-up and implications for fertility

---

Reference: Ovarian cancer: recognition and initial management. NICE Clinical guideline [CG122] 27 April 2011

Task 11: Female Infertility. Module 10 – Subfertility

Candidate's Instructions

This is a simulated patient task assessing:

- Information gathering
- Communication with patients and families
- Communication with colleagues
- Patient safety
- Applied clinical knowledge

You are an ST5 who is about to see Ms Samantha Smith, a 29-year-old attending the gynaecology clinic with a 3-year history of failure to conceive with her current partner Peter Tomkins, a 35-year-old engineer. The partner has a 5-year-old child from his previous relationship. Ms Smith was married for 7 years and has a 5-year-old daughter from that marriage. They had been seen and investigated by the GP and another trust who sent the results of the investigations with the referral letter. Peter is not able to attend today as he is away on business.

You have 10 minutes in which you should:

- Obtain a brief, targeted clinical and fertility history
- Explain the likely cause of the couple's subfertility
- Establish the issues involved in the management of this couple and discuss them sensitively

---

Investigations accompanying referral letter

I. Semen analysis on Peter Tomkins – Age 35 years, partner of Samantha Smith
Collected 08:20 am; Delivered and examined 09:10 am
Volume – 3 ml
Total count – 25×106
Motility – 50% progressive
Morphology – 40% normal
White cells – 0–4/HPF

2. Investigations on Samantha Smith
   Hormone profile
   Follicular phase (day 2 of cycle) biochemistry
   FSH = 4.5 IU/L (normal 3–10 iu/L)
   LH = 5.7 iu/L (normal 2–8 iu/L)
   Prolactin = 543 miu/L (normal 0–400 miu/L)
   TSH = 4.3 iu/L (normal 0.1–5.5iu/L)
   Testosterone = 20 ng/dl (normal 15–70 ng/dl)
   Sex hormone binding globulin = 50 nmol/L (40–120 nmol/L)
   Free androgen index (FAI) = 10% (normal 5–25%)
   21-day progesterone – 56 nmol/L (non-ovulatory – <10 nmol/L, presumed ovulatory
   10–30 nmol/L and ovulatory >30 nmol/L)
   Hysterosalpingogram (HSG): Normal cervical and uterine cavity, proximal portions of
   fallopian tubes outlined but no filling of the lateral 4/5th of both tubes and no evidence
   of spillage. There is some extravasation into the uterine vessels. Conclusion: Bilateral
   tubal blockage

Simulated Patient's Information

Ms Samantha Smith. Age 29 years
17 Strange Way
Portishead PT2 6BD

You are Ms Samantha Smith, a 29-year-old nurse. You have been living with your current partner Peter Tomkins, aged 35 years, for the past 4 years.

You were married for 7 years and have a 5-year-old daughter Simone. Shortly after Simone was born, your marriage started falling apart. Initially you thought you could work things through but eventually you had to ask for a divorce when you discovered that your ex had given you gonorrhoea. You only found out when you had a burning sensation passing urine and following investigations was told you have acquired a sexually transmitted infection.

A year after your marriage broke down, you met Peter, who is a complete gentleman. He is an engineer and works away from home 2 days a week. He has a child from a previous relationship but was never married. One year after you moved in together, you both wanted to have a child and have been trying for the past 3 years without success. You have sexual intercourse twice a week. You are aware of your fertile periods and try as much as possible to have intercourse during this time.

You daughter was conceived spontaneously, and the pregnancy was uncomplicated. You went into labour at 41 weeks and had a normal uncomplicated vaginal delivery. You breastfeed for 6 months.

You suffer from asthma and take Ventolin and Becotide, otherwise you are healthy and do not suffer from any allergies.

You live in your own semi-detached house with Peter and your daughter Simone. You drink alcohol occasionally – mostly over the weekends; about 1–2 glasses of wine per day. You do not

smoke. You regularly exercise by walking about 1–2 miles every day. You eat healthy and watch your weight – your BMI is 24 kg/M².
Your mother suffers from diabetes and is on insulin, and your sister has two children.

Acting requirements

You understand what is being told to you, and you are very unhappy and disappointed with the results.

You are angry and feel let down by your ex-husband for infecting you with gonorrhoea that is likely to have caused problems with getting pregnant.

If not covered by the candidate, you could ask the following questions:

1. Why do you think my tubes are blocked?
2. What are our options
3. Can my tubes be unblocked?
4. If I need IVF, can I have it on the NHS trust?

A good candidate will cover the following:

Information gathering

- Obtains appropriate fertility-focused history
- Ensures to obtain specific information relevant to tubal blockage STIs excluding other. Causes such as previous surgery and use of Cu-IUD
- Interprets correctly and explains clearly the investigation results and their implications
- Reassures the patient that case notes will also be obtained and looked through to check all the relevant facts about the past medical history and previous pregnancy and to record in this consultation in detail

Communication with patients and families

- Introduces self and role
- Explains possible reasons for tubal blockage (STI salpingitis)
- Explores the women's fears and concerns
- Expresses empathy for the situation and the patient's bitter disappointment (gonorrhoea contracted from ex-husband may be the cause of current situation)
- Explains rationale for recommending laparoscopic assessment of pelvis and possible salpingectomy in preparation for IVF (self funded as not eligible for NHS funded IVF)
- Conveys suggested management plan (IVF) and offers hope
- Recommends laparoscopy and possible tubal surgery before self-funded IVF
- Recommends the RCOG's Patients Information Leaflet, e.g. laparoscopy leaflet
- Encourages and welcomes her partner to attend consultation in the future

Communication with colleagues

- Referral to specialist reproductive medicine team
- Involvement of counsellors

Patient safety

- Confirms patients details at the start of the task
- Understands that laparoscopy maybe associated with risks
- May need referral to specialist fertility clinic for further treatment/advice
- Ability to balance risks of tubal surgery and IVF treatment
- Presents the pros and cons of proposed management in a balanced way
- Recognises the limits of their clinical abilities and refers appropriately
- Highlights all governance issues and necessary actions to reduce risks and mishaps in future
- Identifies any allergies and demonstrates safe and accurate prescription techniques

Applied clinical knowledge

- Appreciates different causes of tubal blockage, e.g. gonorrhoea or *Chlamydia trachomatis* infections, pelvic sepsis from other causes, endometriosis and adhesions from CS
- Interprets and explains the clinical findings accurately
- Justifies investigations and management options and demonstrates a rationale for each
- Synthesises a comprehensive and well-organised management plan, based on the history and investigations and takes into consideration the various factors
- Demonstrates a sound and comprehensive evidence-based clinical knowledge, especially of NICE and ESHRE Guidelines

Examiner score sheet		
Information gathering		
Standard not met	Standard partly met	Standard met
0	1	2
Communication with patients and families		
Standard not met	Standard partly met	Standard met
0	1	2
Communication with colleagues		
Standard not met	Standard partly met	Standard met
0	1	2
Patient safety		
Standard not met	Standard partly met	Standard met
0	1	2
Applied clinical knowledge		
Standard not met	Standard partly met	Standard met
0	1	2

Examiner Expectations and Basis for Assessment

Information gathering

- Takes comprehensive and focused history
- Interprets results provided for both female and male partners and requests for appropriate additional tests if necessary
- Summarises discussions succinctly at an appropriate level at regular intervals and checks that the patient/couple understands at appropriate intervals

---

Communication with patients and families

- Introduces self and role
- Gives information about infertility, investigations and treatment options in incremental steps, using patient-friendly language and avoiding jargon
- Honest around benefits, side effects, complications and outcomes of fertility treatments
- Understands the psychological needs of the partner as well as the infertile woman
- Has an understanding of the psychological issues and sensitivities surrounding infertility and IVF treatment

---

Communication with colleagues

- Knows when and who to refer to for further management – in this case, referral to the reproductive medicine team for IVF
- Involves counselling support team for IVF

Patient safety

- Confirms patients details at the start of the task
- Knowledgeable of risk management and clinical governance and regulatory processes in relation to infertility, including issues of confidentiality
- Understands the need to consider the welfare of the child in providing fertility treatment
- Understands the risks of multiple pregnancies associated with fertility treatment

---

Applied clinical knowledge

- Knowledgeable of the treatment of infertility, including surgical management of tubal disease based on NICE guidelines
- Sound evidence-based clinical knowledge of ovulation induction and assisted conception and gamete donation, including the risks and limitations of these treatments
- Ability to critically appraise medical literature in relation to infertility treatment
- Has an understanding of the role of HEFA and the NHS funding restrictions and rationing of assisted conceptions (couple do not qualify for NHS funded IVF)
- Has an understanding of the role of counselling for the infertile couple
- Understands current literature on the management of infertility (NICE guidelines, ESHRE and HEF Guidance)

Reference: Fertility problems: assessment and treatment. NICE Clinical guideline [CG156] 20 February 2013. Last updated 06 September 2017

Task 12: Pelvic Organ Prolapse. Module 14 – Urogynaecological and Pelvic Floor Problems

Candidate's Instructions

This is a structured discussion assessing:

- Information gathering
- Communication with patients and families
- Communication with colleagues
- Patient safety
- Applied clinical knowledge

You are the ST5 in the gynaecology clinic, working alongside your consultant. You are about to see a patient whose referral letter is enclosed. Rather than obtaining history from the patient, you will have a discussion with the examiner using the information provided in the GP's letter.

The Surgery
Coxtail Road
Barton upon Trent
BX12 8FG

Dear Mr Ashijubi,
I would be grateful if you could see this 67-year-old with symptoms of genital prolapse. She has had the symptoms for the past 12 months but says these have gradually got worse.

Yours sincerely

Dr Jason Gusehr MBBS, MRCGP, DCH

You have 10 minutes in which you should study the referral letter from the GP and then have a structured discussion with the examiner who has four questions to use. The examiner should guide you on time management for each of the questions.

Examiner's Instructions

Familiarise yourself with the candidate's instructions. Use the following four questions to guide you to conduct a structured discussion with the candidate. Please use discretion to advice the candidate on timings so that they are able to cover all the questions.

1. What specific information would you like to ask from the patient?
2. What examination will you undertake to determine the degree of prolapse – explain in detail?
3. Justify the investigations you will recommend for her?
4. What complications may arise from the treatment of this patient?

A good candidate should cover the following:

Information gathering

- Parity with details of the pregnancies and birth, including birthweights
- Past medical and surgical history – e.g. diabetic on treatment
- Any systemic illness that could make prolapse worse, e.g. abdominal mass, occupation and chronic obstructive airway disease
- Weight and BMI
- Ascertains the extent of the symptoms and how these affect the quality of life
- Any associated urinary symptoms – dissect these into those of incontinence secondary to prolapse or genuine incontinence

Communication with patients and families

- Introduces self and role
- Explains findings to patient
- Discusses the treatment options, including surgery, drugs and physiotherapy
- Ideal – vaginal hysterectomy and sacrocolpopexy/sacrospinous fixation
  - Pros and cons of hysterectomy and sacrospinous fixation
  - Pros and cons of vaginal hysterectomy and abdominal sacrocolpopexy
- Complications of different treatment options – hysterectomy and anterior and posterior and vault repair; Vagina hysterectomy and repair
- Non-surgical options
  - Pessaries – ring and shelf pessaries – pros and cons

Communication with colleagues

- Involvement of continence adviser in treatment
- Referral to urogynaecology

Patient safety

- Confirms patients details at the start of the task
- Empowers the patient to choose a treatment option

- Explicit on the success rates and recurrence
- Use of drugs – safe prescription

Applied clinical knowledge

- Assessment of genital prolapse using POP-Q score
- Discusses anatomy of the prolapse and treatment
- Discusses the rationale for investigations and complications of various treatment options
- Evidence of familiarity with current literature on pelvic organ prolapse – RCOG Green-top Guideline and NICE guideline

Examiner score sheet		
Information gathering		
Standard not met	Standard partly met	Standard met
0	1	2
Communication with patients and families		
Standard not met	Standard partly met	Standard met
0	1	2
Communication with colleagues		
Standard not met	Standard partly met	Standard met
0	1	2
Patient safety		
Standard not met	Standard partly met	Standard met
0	1	2
Applied clinical knowledge		
Standard not met	Standard partly met	Standard met
0	1	2

Examiner Expectations and Basis for Assessment

Information gathering

- Takes comprehensive urogynaecology history, focusing on symptoms of incontinence relating these to the surgery, excluding co-morbidities (diabetes and hypertension)
- Requests notes for review
- Undertakes appropriate investigations and interprets results, e.g. urinalysis and fluid diary
- Interprets cystometry, imaging and fluid balance charts in order to reach a diagnosis and develop a management plan

---

Communication with patients and families

- Introduces self and role and then discusses the rationale for the plan of care – examination, investigations and treatment in a measured approach
- Demonstrates an ability to give information about urogynaecological examination, investigations and treatment in manageable amounts, using patient-friendly language and avoiding jargon
- Discusses honestly the pros and cons of treatment options, including clinical uncertainty about long-term outcomes of vault prolapse treatment options
- Demonstrates an understanding of the psychological issues and sensitivities surrounding vault prolapse surgery and incontinence

---

Communication with colleagues

- Describes the differential diagnoses of urinary symptoms and formulates management plans
- Clearly communicates requirements and situation with staff, assistants and anaesthetists
- Involves specialist in the management of the symptoms

Patient safety

- Confirms patients details at the start of the task
- Has an understanding of the principles of safe surgery, including WHO safe surgery checklist
- Has an understanding of safe prescription in relation to urogynaecological problems such as detrusor overactivity and urodynamic stress incontinence
- Has an understanding of the contraindications and interactions of urogynaecological drugs and common medical co-morbidities

---

Applied clinical knowledge

- Knowledgeable of the complications of the surgical management options of urogynaecological disorders, including pelvic organ prolapse (in this case, sacrocolpopexy), acute voiding disorders, overactive bladder and stress urinary incontinence
- Ability to critically appraise the literature/evidence in relation to vault prolapse treatment options
- Familiarity with NICE guideline on urinary incontinence and ROCG Green-top Guideline on vault prolapse

Reference: *Urinary incontinence and pelvic organ prolapse in women: management. NICE guideline [NG123] 02 April 2019. Last updated 24 June 2019*

Task 13: Laparoscopic Sterilisation. Module 11 – Sexual and Reproductive Health

Candidate's Instructions

This is simulated patient task assessing:

- Information gathering
- Communication with patients and families
- Communication with colleagues
- Patient safety
- Applied clinical knowledge

You are an ST5 who is seeing a 32-year-old in the clinic with a request for sterilisation. The referral letter from the GP is given below.

You have 10 minutes in which you should:

- Take focused history
- Establish her suitability for sterilisation
- Counsel her about the procedure
- Plan the procedure

The surgery
London Road
Lisburn
LB14 7 WE

Dear Miss Sandra FRCOG,
Re: Ms Catherine Stonley – Age 32 years
This 32-year-old wishes to be sterilised. She has two children aged 4 and 2 years. All were normal vaginal deliveries. She is otherwise well and her last cervical smear was 2 years ago and was normal.
Thank you.

Yours sincerely

Dr Orihme Fazeka BSc, MBBS, MRCGP

Simulated Patient's Information

You are Catherine Stonley, a 32-year-old mother of two who is currently unemployed. You stopped working when you had your daughter. Prior to that, you were a supervisor in Sainsbury. You are not going to work until both your kids have gone to school.

You are not married but have been in a steady relationship for 7 years. You moved because your partner Greg Sinclair (age 30 years), who is builder with George Wimpey, was moved to this area. He is the father of your two children.

Your first child was a normal vaginal delivery 4 years ago. The pregnancy was uncomplicated, and she weighed 3.6 kg. The second was a normal vaginal delivery of an uncomplicated pregnancy 2 years ago. Your son weighed 4.1 kg.

Your periods are regular and the last one was 3 weeks ago. You are currently on microgynon but do not want to take this anymore as you have put on weight with it. Before you went on the pill, you were 67 kg but you now weighed 75 kg! The pill also makes you depressed, and you feel that you have been snapping at the children a lot since you went on it 1 year ago. Prior to that, your partner was using the condom. You definitely do not want any more children although your partner is not certain.

You are up to date with your smears. The last one was 2 years ago and was normal.

You do not suffer from any medical problems and have not had any surgery in the past. You are allergic to egg yolk.

You smoke 5–10 cigarettes per day and also take alcohol occasionally. Your partner smokes 20 cigarettes per day and drinks regularly. You are currently living in a three bedroom rented house but once you have sold your house in your previous residence, you plan to buy in this area.

Clinical Examiner's Instructions

Familiarise yourself with the candidate's instructions as well as the stimulated patient's information. Discuss with the lay examiner and agree upon a common approach to the assessment.

Lay Examiner's Instructions

Familiarise yourself with the candidate's instructions as well as the simulated patient's information. Score the candidate's performance in the two domains of information gathering and communication with patients and families.

A good candidate should cover the following:

Information gathering

- Focused history – number of children and obstetrics history, relationship and social history, including employment; past medical and surgical history, previous contraception; smear history, drug allergy and LMP
- Offers to perform a physical examination, including measuring BP
- Establishes why opting for sterilisation – including an understanding of the associated risks
- Considers other options, including vasectomy

Communication with patients and families

- Introduces self and role
- Discusses other options including LARC
- Discusses pros and cons of sterilisation – procedure, complications, considered permanent, failure rate and regret rate
- Provides information in a step-wise manner at an appropriate pace, ensuring a thorough understanding, and encourages and answers all questions
- Consents for procedure and add onto waiting list – give date for procedure

- Emphasises the need to continue with contraceptive pill until the period after sterilisation
- Provide RCOG Patient Information Leaflet or other leaflet

Communication with colleagues

- Confirms decision with the consultant
- Links up with waiting list coordinator/clerk
- Ensures anaesthesia is informed, especially if any risks of general anaesthesia (in this case, allergic to egg yolk)

Patient safety

- Confirms patients identify at the start of the task
- Contraception until next period after procedure
- Identifies the best time to perform the procedure (during menstruation)
- Establishes drug allergy and allergy (to eggs that could affect anaesthesia)
- Follows WHO safe surgery checklist at the time of surgery (this is not particularly applicable at this stage but may be in cases of discussions around this task)

Applied clinical knowledge

- Uses the RCOG Green-top Guideline on female sterilisation to provide failure rates of procedure and knows what counselling to offer
- Discusses alternatives to sterilisation like copper intrauterine device and subdermal (Nexplanon) and intrauterine progestogens (Mirena)
- Discusses vasectomy as an alternative (failure rate 1:2,000 versus 1:200)
- Discusses complications of laparoscopy – 1:500 of major complication
- Demonstrates an understanding of the current literature on providing sterilisation to women – Faculty of Family Planning and RCOG Guideline
- Familiar with NICE Guidelines on LARC
- Demonstrates an understanding that decision is that of the patient though partner may want more children

Examiner score sheet		
Information gathering		
Standard not met	Standard partly met	Standard met
0	1	2
Communication with patients and families		
Standard not met	Standard partly met	Standard met
0	1	2
Communication with colleagues		
Standard not met	Standard partly met	Standard met
0	1	2

Patient safety		
Standard not met	Standard partly met	Standard met
0	1	2
Applied clinical knowledge		
Standard not met	Standard partly met	Standard met
0	1	2

Examiner Expectations and Basis for Assessment

Information gathering

- Takes comprehensive sexual and relevant history, with respect to the request for sterilisation
- Requests appropriate investigations (e.g. examination including abdominal, pelvic and BP measurement)
- Identifies the reasons for wanting to change contraception or be sterilised

Communication with patients and families

- Introduces self and role
- Able to communicate in a non-judgemental way on the choice of the patient
- Discusses the various options to sterilisation
- Able to communicate the pros and cons of sterilisation, including the fact that it should be considered permanent although could be reversed but not on the NHS (with associated increased risk of ectopic pregnancy and no guarantee of success)
- Describes clearly and logically the approach to sterilisation, including obtaining consent and the need for contraception until a period after sterilisation

Communication with colleagues

- Communicates with the consultant to ensure that decision is endorsed
- Liaises with other colleagues where appropriate (in this case, anaesthetist – in view of allergy to egg yolk – propofol may not be a suitable anaesthetic)
- Liaises with family planning if appropriate to provide more information about the availability of the alternatives, including vasectomy

---

Patient safety

- Confirms patients details at the start of the task
- Demonstrates an understanding of the risk of sterilisation (failure rate – 1:200) and increased risk of ectopic if failure
- Ascertains allergy and how this may affect the sterilisation

---

Applied clinical knowledge

- Knowledgeable of the current literature on the provision of sterilisation services in the UK
- Demonstrates an understanding of NICE guidelines on LARC and RCOG Green-top Guidelines on female sterilisation
- Knows to use the RCOG Patient Information Leaflet on sterilisation
- Understands the UKMEC
- Communicates that the decision is of the patient's and not the partner's but carefully discusses this

---

Reference: *Female sterilisation. The Royal College of Obstetricians and Gynaecologists. Consent Advice No. 3 February 2016*

Task 14: Referral Letters. Module 9 – Gynaecological Problems

Candidate's Instructions

This is a structured discussion task assessing:

- Information gathering
- Communication with patients and families
- Communication with colleagues
- Patient safety
- Applied clinical knowledge

You are the ST5 who has been asked by your consultant's secretary to come and undertake some tasks on her behalf. You have four referral letters to review and categorise them as one of the following:

(a) Routine – to be seen within 4–8 weeks
(b) Soon – to be seen within 2–4 weeks and
(c) Urgent – to be seen within 2 weeks

In addition, you should mention (1) any additional investigation(s) that should be performed on each of the patient (if appropriate) following their visit to the clinic and (2) the most likely diagnosis/pathology and treatment.

You have 10 minutes in which you should:

- Read each letter and categorise it into routine, soon or urgent
- Decide which additional investigation should be undertaken when the patient comes to the clinic
- Provide a possible working diagnosis based on the information on the letter

Examiner's Instructions

Familiarise yourself with the instructions to the candidates. You should guide the candidate on the use of their time. Each letter should take approximately 2 minutes. Candidates are at liberty to review the letters in any order.

Referral Letter Number 1

Date

Dear Doctor,

I would welcome a gynaecological assessment of this 18-year-old student (Susan Jones), who came to see me very concerned that she has not started menstruating. She is the second of her mother's two children. She has some vague lower abdominal pain which is intermittent but there was nothing abnormal found on examination. Her secondary sexual characteristics are well developed (breast, axillary and pubic hair).
Many thanks for seeing her.

Yours sincerely

Dr Josephine Plumb

Referral Letter Number 2

Date

Dear Doctor,

I would be grateful if you could see Mrs TK, who is 37 years old, for a gynaecological assessment. She previously presented 10 years ago with oligomenorrhoea and subsequently amenorrhoea. She has associated problems with morbid obesity and hirsutism but no biochemical confirmation of polycystic ovary syndrome. She was seen by a gynaecologist at that time and treated briefly with Dianette. The emphasis then was very much on weight reduction to improve her symptoms.

She has presented again today with a 3-month history of unpredictable and very heavy periods.

She continues to have problems with morbid obesity (her weight has increased to 150 kg). She is a moderate smoker and not normally on medication.

I have given her some norethisterone to take, but she and I are both keen that she has a gynaecological review and would welcome any advice you can give us on further investigation and management.
Many thanks for seeing her.

Yours sincerely

Dr P Frances

Referral Letter Number 3

Date

Dear Doctor,

I would be grateful if you could arrange to see Mrs Joan Tyler, a 42-year-old teacher whose recent cervical smears have shown to be persistently low-grade dyskaryotic changes. Her smear history is as follows:

November 2003	**Normal**
December 2006	**Low-grade dyskaryosis**
June 2006	**Normal**
November 2009	**Normal**
December 2012	**Normal**
December 2015	**Low-grade dyskaryosis (low-grade dysplasia) – Reflex HPV test – negative**

I examined her and found a large cervical erosion on the posterior lip of the cervix which bled easily on contact. She does not have any coital/post-coital or intermenstrual bleeding.

She has had four normal vaginal deliveries and a spontaneous miscarriage at 10 weeks gestation.

She has a history of recurrent urinary tract infections and is allergic to penicillin and plaster but is not on any regular medications.
Many thanks for your help.

Yours sincerely

Dr Jenny Timpson DRCOG, MBChB

Referral Letter Number 4

Date

Dear Doctor,

I would appreciate it if you could arrange to see this 38-year-old woman, who presented to us with secondary amenorrhoea of 18 months duration. She had a normal vaginal delivery

2 years ago and breastfed for 6 months. Since weaning her baby off breast milk, she has remained amenorrhoeic. In addition, she continues to produce milk although she has not breastfed for the past 18 months. She describes her libido as poor but does not have any other complaints.

On examination, I was able to demonstrate obvious galactorrhoea but nothing else was abnormal. I therefore took the liberty of performing a hormone profile the results of which are enclosed.

Yours sincerely

Dr Elaine David MRCG, DCH, MBBS

Results

	Result	Normal range
LH (U/L)	6.2	(2.5–9.0)
FSH (U/L)	5.8	(3.0–9.0)
Prolactin (miu/L)	2,679	(50–400)
(miu/L)	5.2	(0.3–5.0)
Free T4 (pmol/L)	9	(9–25)

Examiner score sheet		
Information gathering		
Standard not met	Standard partly met	Standard met
0	1	2
Communication with patients and families		
Standard not met	Standard partly met	Standard met
0	1	2
Communication with colleagues		
Standard not met	Standard partly met	Standard met
0	1	2
Patient safety		
Standard not met	Standard partly met	Standard met
0	1	2
Applied clinical knowledge		
Standard not met	Standard partly met	Standard met
0	1	2

Letter No	Category	Additional investigations	Possible working diagnosis
1	Routine	Ultrasound scan of the pelvis/MRI	Mullerian abnormality; imperforate hymen
2	Soon/ urgent	FSH/LH/Testosterone/SHBG/FAI/Ultrasound scan ± endometrial biopsy/FBC	PCOS with endometrial hyperplasia
3	Urgent	Colposcopy and biopsy	Cervical ectropion/cervical cancer
4	Soon	Prolactin/MRI or CT of the brain	Hyperprolactinaemia

Examiner Expectations and Basis for Assessment

Information gathering

- Identifies additional information/appropriate investigations
- Discusses appropriate investigations for each of the patients and the information to be obtained from the investigation
- Synthesise the information provided in each letter and then uses it correctly in planning the management

Communication with patients and families

- Ability to communicate to each patient the need for further investigations and when to come to the clinic
- An ability to explain the rationale for classifying case as routine, soon or urgent

Communication with colleagues

- Ability to prioritise the letters appropriately into urgent, soon (semi-urgent) and routine (non-urgent) cases
- Ability to form a logical differential diagnosis for each of the cases
- Provides appropriate amount of detail to ensure management plans are clear and easily understood by colleagues
- Ability to identify additional expertise required for each case as it's prioritised

Patient safety

- Aware of possible consequences of a delay in seeing patient on the waiting list
- Has an understanding of the need for additional investigations to ensure correct diagnosis and treatment

Applied clinical knowledge

- Knowledgeable of various common gynaecological problems
- Ability to critically appraise the information provided in the letters to arrive at a diagnosis
- An ability to initiate appropriate investigations to confirm diagnosis and make management plans
- Has a working knowledge of the roles of other members of the multidisciplinary team to ensure best care for the patient (in discussing the additional precautions to be taken)
- Knowledgeable to an appropriate level for various NICE/RCOG Guidelines on general gynaecology and the governments recommendation for waiting times for oncology cases

16

Paper V

Task 1: Cytomegalovirus Infection. Module 4 – Antepartum Care

Candidate's Instructions

This is a simulated patient task assessing:

- Information gathering
- Communication with patients and families
- Communication with colleagues
- Patient safety
- Applied clinical knowledge

You are an ST5 and are about to see Mrs Martha Poloski, who is 12 weeks pregnant. She was seen by the GP last week complaining of fever, muscle pain and generally feeling unwell. The GP took some blood for investigations, including a viral screen on the advice of your consultant. The results of these investigations have been shown to the consultant who has asked that you see the patient as she is away.

Results of investigations

CMV – IgM – positive high titre, CMV – positive – low titre
Parvovirus B19 – IgM – negative, IgG – negative
Toxoplasmosis – IgG – negative, IgM – negative

You have 10 minutes in which you should:

- Obtain focused history
- Explain the results and justify any investigations you will like to undertake
- Establish and answer any questions the patient may have
- Discuss the plan of care and agree it with the patient

Simulated Patient's Information

You are Mrs Poloski, a 34-year-old in your second pregnancy. You saw the GP when you were 8 weeks pregnant and were placed on folic acid 400 µg daily. Two week later you felt unwell with a fever, a dripping nose and muscle aches. You went to the GP who did a series of blood test, including a viral screen. You were off work for 1 week but now feel much better and ready to go back to work. You had a phone call from the GP's surgery yesterday, asking that you come to the hospital today.

Your periods have always been regular, and the last one was 10 weeks ago. You had an ultrasound scan at 8 weeks and were told your dates are correct. This is a planned pregnancy.

You are otherwise healthy having had a normal vaginal delivery of your son 2 years ago. You are not aware of any problems with your marriage, and there is no family history of hypertension or multiple pregnancies.

You delivered your son 2 years ago at the same hospital, following an uncomplicated pregnancy, managed most of the time by the midwife as you were low risk.

You do not smoke but drink alcohol occasionally. You are generally very well and do moderate exercises such as walking. You have no known allergies

Action for the simulated patient

You are very concerned about the phone call. The GP's surgery just said you needed to be seen urgently in the hospital.

If not covered, you could ask the following questions:

1. How do you get CMV infection?
2. What is the implication of this infection on my baby and my health?
3. How can you know that my baby is infected or not?
4. How will you monitor the baby and for what?
5. What if the baby is infected? What will happen to my baby?
6. When will you deliver me and what will happen to the baby after?

A good candidate will cover the following:

Information gathering

- History of symptoms of infection – chronology of symptoms (e.g. onset of body aches, fever, sore throat, dripping nose, any known contacts etc.)
- Reviews investigations (serology and imaging)
- Ascertains concerns about infection
- Past obstetric history

Communication with patients and families

- Introduces self and role
- Discusses and explains the results of the investigations
- Explains the need to do further test, such as the avidity test and what it means
- The need for follow-up with ultrasound scan – 5 weeks after primary infection in fetal medicine unit

Communication with colleagues

- Communication with virology department/virologist
- Liaises with fetal medicine and neonatologist if appropriate
- Liaises/referral to fetal medicine for ultrasound scan to exclude CMV specific abnormalities (usually about 5 weeks after the primary infection)

Patient safety

- Ensures patients identify is confirmed at the start of the task
- Empowers the patient to make the right decisions
- Weighs the pros and cons of any invasive testing to check fetal infection and timing (at least 5 weeks after primary infection), e.g. amniocentesis, including timing, to reduce false negatives (recognises that fetal blood sampling is unreliable)
- Monitors and knows what to do if severely affected (risk versus benefits of interventions)

Applied clinical knowledge

- Demonstrates familiarity with most up-to-date literature on CMV as evidenced from discussions on diagnosis of *in-utero* infection (amniocentesis and when) and fetal imaging – 5 weeks from acute infection
  Complications – fetal and maternal (small for gestational age, microcephaly, hydrocephalus, hepatosplenomegaly and neonatal thrombocytopenia)
  Monitoring of the fetus – serial growth scans
  Diagnosis in an infected infant – cord blood for immunology

Examiner score sheet		
Information gathering		
Standard not met	Standard partly met	Standard met
0	1	2
Communication with patients and families		
Standard not met	Standard partly met	Standard met
0	1	2
Communication with colleagues		
Standard not met	Standard partly met	Standard met
0	1	2
Patient safety		
Standard not met	Standard partly met	Standard met
0	1	2
Applied clinical knowledge		
Standard not met	Standard partly met	Standard met
0	1	2

Examiner Expectations and Basis for Assessment

Information gathering

- Able to take concise and relevant history on infections (symptoms)
- Skilled in signposting and guiding the consultation based on chronology of symptoms and investigations
- Able to ensure that the patient understands and encourages questions

Communication with patients and families

- Introduces self and role
- Able to describe/explain to the patient the diagnosis and implications of CMV
- Able to tackle difficult or sensitive issues on CMV infections and potential implications, including severe congenital malformations (microcephaly and hydrocephaly)
- Able to give information to the patient on the impact of CMV on the fetus
- Discusses termination options and when to consider this
- Discusses serial monitoring of fetus

Communication with colleagues

- Provides appropriate amount of detail to ensure that the management plans are clear and easily understood by colleagues
- Able to communicate with colleagues in primary care and within the multidisciplinary team, including nurse specialist, virologist, physicians and fetal medicine
- Support groups – linking patient and family with these

Patient safety

- Confirms patients identify at the start of the task
- Aware of the safety of investigations and no specific therapy to improve the outcome for CMV infections
- Understands both the impact of pregnancy on CMV and the impact of CMV on the pregnancy and the fetus

---

Applied clinical knowledge

Demonstrates:

- A clear and logical approach to differential diagnosis or management plan for CMV in pregnancy
- Knowledge of antenatal and postnatal care, including the risks of maternal morbidity and mortality related to CMV
- An awareness of contemporary literature on CMV

Task 2: Fetal Growth Restriction: Module 4 – Antenatal Care

Candidate's Instructions

This is a simulated patient task assessing:

- Information gathering
- Communication with patients and families
- Communication with colleagues
- Patient safety
- Applied clinical knowledge

You are an ST5 in the clinic with your team consisting of your consultant, another trainee and two midwives. The midwife calls you to see a patient she has just seen and feels that the baby is small. The growth charts from the ultrasound scans are shown in Figure 16.1a–d.

You have 10 minutes in which you should:

- Obtain a focused history
- Explain and justify any investigations you will like to undertake
- Establish and answer any questions the patient may have
- Discuss the plan of care and confirm it with the patient

Simulated Patient's Information

You are Mrs Julie Bent, a 30-year-old customer relation officer (CRO) in your first pregnancy at 34 weeks. Your husband is Tony, a 41-year-old police officer. You have been married for 2 years, and this was a planned pregnancy.

You now smoke 5–10 cigarettes per day, having cut down from 20–25 per day because of the pregnancy. You drink alcohol occasionally. Your weight has always been on the high side (your last BMI was 32 kg/M²) but you are in general very fit and walk on an average of 1 mile per day even in pregnancy. You are taking vitamin D and iron tablets (which cause constipation) because of low iron levels.

You booked for antenatal care at 12 weeks when you had a dating and NT ultrasound scan as well as all the usual tests, including HIV, and all these were normal. You had the test for Down syndrome and your risk was low. At 20 weeks, you had a scan which was also normal. You were asked whether you were on aspirin after the scan but you said no. You did not know why this was asked

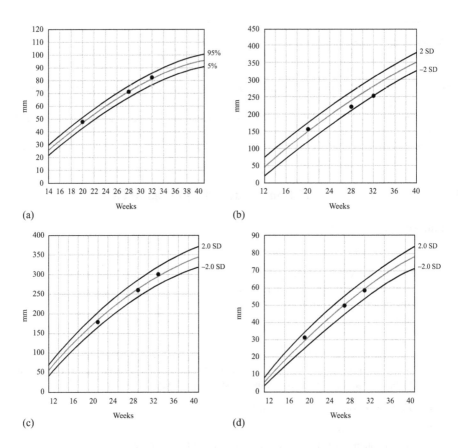

Figure 16.1   (a) Biparietal diameter (see further Lai FM et al., Reference charts of foetal biometry in Asians. Singapore Med J. 1995 Dec; 36(6):628–36). (b) Abdominal circumference (see further Hadlock F P et al., Estimating fetal age: computer-assisted analysis of multiple fetal growth parameters. Radiology. 1984 Aug; 152(2):497–501). (c) Head circumference (see further Westerway S C et al., AustNZJO&G. 2000; 40(3):297–302). (d) Femoral length (see further Westerway SC et al., AustNZJO&G. 2000; 40(3):297–302).

but the midwife did not follow it up so you really did not give it any further thoughts. The baby has been moving very well, and you have had no problems so far. You had an ultrasound scan at 28 weeks and were told that the baby was on the small side but that there was nothing to worry about. You saw your midwife regularly and yesterday were told to go to the hospital to see the consultant because the baby measured small. You had another ultrasound at 32 weeks and again the baby was said to be small but healthy.

If not covered, you should ask the following questions:

- What is wrong with my baby?
- What tests will you do on the baby now?

- How will you monitor my baby?
- When will I deliver?
- How will I deliver?
- Will my baby have any problems after it's born?

A good candidate should cover the following:

Information gathering

- Obtains good history that identifies the risk factors of small for the gestational age – smoking, comment about aspirin at 20 weeks scan and symptoms of hypertension/pre-eclampsia
- Ascertains when early ultrasound scan was done
- Reviews notes or asks to review notes for the results of the ultrasound at 20 weeks
- Ascertains concerns and questions the patient has
- Examination – checks BP and reviews urinalysis

Communication with patients and families

- Introduces self and role
- Discusses the plans of care – ultrasound scan to check growth, liquor volume and Dopplers of fetal vessels and monitoring and timing of the delivery
- Explains how the diagnosis of small for the gestational age is made (based on crossing of centile lines)
- Discusses the implications of the baby being small

Communication with colleagues

- Involvement of MDT – neonatologist and fetal medicine

Patient safety

- Confirms patients details at the start of the task
- Empowers the patient to participate in her care – education on perceived fetal movements and other symptoms suggesting deterioration (e.g. those of pre-eclampsia or abruption)
- Explores and addresses issues that the patient is anxious about
- Balances risks of preterm delivery (consider steroids if delivery is before 34 weeks) and associated neonatal complications with those if intrauterine complications form growth restriction

Applied clinical knowledge

- Explains the possible factors associated with small for the gestational age in this woman
- Explains the rationale for further scans and monitoring
- Explains the decision on timing of delivery and how to deliver
- Discusses the risks to the fetus *in-utero* and *ex-utero*
- Demonstrates an understanding of RCOG SGA Guidelines in discussion

Overall process should include:

History

- Smoker
- Ultrasound scan and findings
- No other risk factors
- Weight a risk factor but not major

Investigations and monitoring

- Ultrasound scan for biometry and liquor volume
- Doppler of the umbilical artery, middle cerebral artery and ductus venosus when indicated
- Frequency of ultrasound scan will depend on the measurements but likely to fortnightly
- Frequency of Dopplers will depend on whether normal, or not
- Timing of delivery and how to deliver

When to deliver

- Static growth
- Abnormal Dopplers
- Gestation reaches 37 weeks
- How to deliver will depend on the presentation and the severity of growth abnormality
- If abnormal Dopplers, better by ELLSCS, but if normal, aim for induced vagina delivery

Potential risks to the baby in-utero

- Intrauterine fetal death – need to monitor movements and present if reduced rather when they have stopped
- Neonatal feeding problems
- Neonatal breathing problems
- Bowel problems – necrotising enterocolitis

Examiner score sheet		
Information gathering		
Standard not met	Standard partly met	Standard met
0	1	2
Communication with patients and families		
Standard not met	Standard partly met	Standard met
0	1	2
Communication with colleagues		

Standard not met	Standard partly met	Standard met
0	1	2
Patient safety		
Standard not met	Standard partly met	Standard met
0	1	2
Applied clinical knowledge		
Standard not met	Standard partly met	Standard met
0	1	2

Examiner Expectations and Basis for Assessment

Information gathering

- Able to take concise and relevant antenatal history – relevant to fetal growth restriction
- Skilled in signposting and guiding the antenatal consultation
- Able to ensure that the patient understands and encourages questions
- Initiates appropriate and timely investigations (e.g. fetal Dopplers and CTG), whose results will inform the decision on time of delivery

Communication with patients and families

- Introduces self and role
- Able to discuss investigations, follow-up and plan for antenatal care
- Able to succinctly summarise discussions with antenatal patients
- Discusses with honesty the uncertainty about the timing of delivery and sensitively about smoking cessation

Communication with colleagues

- Has a clear and logical approach to differential diagnosis and management plan for patients with fetal growth restriction
- Communicates appropriate amount of detail to colleagues to ensure that the management plans are clear and easily understood by the colleagues
- Able to communicate with other specialties, e.g. obstetric anaesthetics and midwifery colleagues, including specialist midwives and neonatologists
- Documents an agreed management plan in the notes for colleagues

---

Patient safety

- Confirms patients details at the start of the task
- Aware of the safety of investigations and therapeutics during pregnancy, including safe prescription, for example, corticosteroids
- Able to clearly plan for complications of prolonged admission for fetal monitoring, for example, venous thromboembolism

---

Applied clinical knowledge

- Knowledgeable of antenatal care, including fetal growth restriction
- Able to interpret clinical examination findings and results of investigations in the context of fetal growth restriction
- Aware of the risks and benefits of various different management options, balancing the needs of the mother and fetus (delivery versus continuation of pregnancy)
- Familiar with current literature on fetal growth restriction, including RCOG Green-top Guideline on management of small for gestational age

---

Reference: The investigation and management of small-for-gestational age fetus. The Royal College of Obstetricians and Gynaecologists Green-top Guideline No. 31 February 2013. Minor revisions January 2014

Task 3: Vascular Lower Segment at Emergency Caesarean Section for Fetal Distress. Module 3 – Core Surgical Skills

Candidate's Instructions

This is a structured discussion task assessing:

- Communication with colleagues
- Patient safety
- Applied clinical knowledge
- Communication with patients and families

You are the ST5 covering the labour ward of your unit. You and your consultant were doing a ward round and you were called to see a 30-year-old G2P1 in labour at 39 weeks of gestation who was at 5 cm dilatation with intact membranes and a pathological CTG. The consultant asked that you proceed to deliver the baby by caesarean section.

This woman whose BMI is 33 kg/M2 had a normal vaginal delivery 3 years ago at term. This was an uncomplicated pregnancy and the placenta was described as being anterior and high on ultrasound scan.

The patient had an epidural which has been topped up for the caesarean section. You open the abdomen and find a very vascular lower segment. There are huge vessels all over the lower segment.

You have 10 minutes in which to discuss with the examiner four questions about the management of the patient, both during the CS and after.

Examiner's Instructions

Familiarise yourself with the candidate's instructions.

Use the following four questions to guide the discussion you will have with the candidate. Provide some guidance on how much time the candidate spends on each question.

A good candidate should cover the following:

What will be your immediate action?

- Inform anaesthetist, scrub team and the rest of the theatre team
- Inform consultant
- Request for cross-match of six units of blood and inform blood bank
- Request for a second IV line with large bore cannula (16FG)
- Explain to the patient as under epidural
- Ask for uncross-matched blood to be in theatre (group O negative)

How will you approach the rest of the surgery?

- This is an emergency so proceed to deliver the baby (most likely incision in the lower segment as the placenta is anterior and incision in the upper segment) – a vertical upper segment incision may also suffice
- Incision over large vessels – may clamp vessels prior to making incision
- Deliver the baby and apply Green-Armytage and other artery forceps to stem bleeding
- Deliver placenta, and with the consultant, secure bleeding vessels
- If unsuccessful, proceed to hysterectomy
- Leave drain in the peritoneal cavity
- Replace blood loss quickly and effectively (may need to do a point-of-care Hb and check coagulation)
- Leave an indwelling catheter for input output
- Transfer patient to ITU as she would have lost more than 1.5 litres of blood

What will your post-operative management be?

- Monitor using Modified Obstetric Early Warning Score (MEOWS)
- Antibiotics – for 5 days
- Thromboprophylaxis
- Input and output monitoring chart
- Complete incident form
- Debrief patient
  - If hysterectomy – offer counselling and support
  - If not hysterectomy – counsel about implications for subsequent pregnancies – high risk of recurrence

What clinical governance issues will you deal with post-operatively?

- Inform risk management team to undertake a root cause analysis
- Debrief patient and family
- Identify areas that require addressing from the risk management report and institute steps to address – may include multidisciplinary meetings and training
- Communicate with the patient and the family the outcome of the risk management report (duty of candour)
- Offer to further debrief with consultant

Examiner score sheet		
Information gathering		
Standard not met	Standard partly met	Standard met
0	1	2
Communication with patients and families		
Standard not met	Standard partly met	Standard met
0	1	2
Communication with colleagues		
Standard not met	Standard partly met	Standard met
0	1	2
Patient safety		
Standard not met	Standard partly met	Standard met
0	1	2
Applied clinical knowledge		
Standard not met	Standard partly met	Standard met
0	1	2

Examiner Expectations and Basis for Assessment

Communication with colleagues

- Informs theatre team (anaesthetist, nurses and midwives) of findings and implications
- Informs and calls consultant
- Informs blood bank and asks for activation of the massive haemorrhage protocol
- Informs oncologist – may require more than hysterectomy
- Completes incident form – informs risk management team
- Communicates with GP and community midwife
- Asks for more support– anaesthetist, obstetrician and others (radiologist, vascular surgeon etc.)

Patient safety

- Activates massive haemorrhage protocol
- Ensures uncross-matched blood is available
- Asks for a second large bore cannula to be inserted (secures IV line)
- Requests for four to six units of cross-matched blood
- Hysterectomy not delayed
- Post-operative fluid management and transfer to ITU
- Takes steps to minimise DVT

Communication with patients and families

- Informs the patient and the partner at the time of surgery (as under regional)
- Debriefs the patient
- Communicates findings from the risk management team to the patient honestly

Applied clinical knowledge

- Demonstrates knowledge of management of vascular lower uterine segment
- Knowledgeable of RCOG Green-top Guidelines on placenta praevia and management of PPH

Reference: Placenta praevia and accreta: diagnosis and management. *The Royal College of Obstetricians and Gynaecologists Green-top Guideline No. 27a September 2018*

Task 4: Request for Elective CS for Non-Medical Reasons. Module 7 – Managing Delivery

Candidate's Instructions

This is a simulated patient task assessing:

- Information gathering
- Communication with patient and families
- Communication with colleagues
- Patient safety
- Applied clinical knowledge

You are an ST5 in the antenatal clinic and have been asked by the midwife to see a 21-year-old nursery assistant in her first pregnancy at 36 weeks of gestation, who is requesting for an elective caesarean section.

You have 10 minutes in which you should:

- Take an appropriate history
- Counsel the patient on her request
- Answer any questions she may have

Clinical Examiner's Instructions

Familiarise yourself with the candidate's instructions and use the standard marking sheet to score them on the five domains. Discuss with the lay examiner and agree on a common approach to assessment.

Lay Examiner's Instructions

Familiarise yourself with the candidate's instructions as well as the simulated patient's information. Score the candidate's performance on the two domains of information gathering and communication with patients and families. Discuss with the clinical examiner and agree on how to approach the assessment.

Simulated Patient's Information

You are Ms Stacy Scrimbs, a 21-year-old nursery assistant, who is having your first pregnancy. The pregnancy has so far been uncomplicated. You have been reading lots of stuff about pregnancy and delivery, and you do not want to have a vaginal delivery. You are so frightened of complications like a tear, having to be rushed for a caesarean and more importantly you have had a dream to the effect that you lost your son in a normal vaginal delivery. Your friend, who was a few months ahead of you in her pregnancy, was induced and ended up with a very difficult delivery. Her baby was admitted to the neonatal unit with brain haemorrhage.

You booked for antenatal care at 12 weeks and had all the tests during pregnancy, and these were normal. You had an ultrasound scan last week, and the baby was said to be growing normally. Its estimated weight was 2.6 kg.

Your due date is in 4 weeks but you do not want to go into labour. You have been discussing this with the midwife in the community for the past 4 weeks, and she has been trying to convince you to have a vaginal deliver as there are no contraindications and the baby is not big.

You do not have any medical problems, and your blood pressure has been normal throughout pregnancy. You iron levels have also been normal.

You have not had any surgery in the past and are not allergic to anything that you know of.

You smoke, although you have cut down quite a lot in this pregnancy. You currently smoke about two to three cigarettes per day.

Your partner Chris Smith is 26 years old and a teacher. He is very supportive. This was an unplanned pregnancy as you had been going out for 6 months when you got pregnant. He did not want the pregnancy but you refused to have an abortion. You live together in a one bedroom terrace house, close to both your parents who are supportive of the pregnancy. You plan to go back to work soon after delivery as you have not been working for long to be able to get a prolonged maternity leave.

If not covered, you should ask the following:

- I plan to have two more children. Should it be a problem if I have a caesarean section?
- I have read that the risk of a caesarean section is similar to those of a vaginal delivery. Is this true?
- Why should I not have a CS? It is my body and I do not want to have a tear in my vagina.
- Can you guarantee that if I went for a vaginal delivery, it will be successful and I will not have a tear?

A good candidate should cover the following:

Information gathering

- Reviews the notes and investigations, including the ultrasound scan report
- Obtains history of pregnancy and the rationale for the decision to have a CS
- Attempts to understand the logic behind the decision
- Able to bring out the psychological impact of the friend's complicated pregnancy on her decision, showing empathy/displaying understanding
- Asks about other relevant information – social history, support after delivery and plans for future deliveries

Communication with patients and families

- Introduces self and role
- Discusses the pros and cons of vaginal delivery versus CS
- Complications of CS – haemorrhage, risk of hysterectomy and implications for baby (emerging information suggests increased long-term health problems)
  - Risk of placenta praevia in subsequent pregnancy and hysterectomy
  - Reduced fertility
  - Risk of adhesions and chronic pelvic pain
  - Prolonged recovery and need for additional support at home
  - May not be able to go back to work quickly
- Vaginal delivery
  - Early recovery
  - No guarantee that may not end up with an emergency CS
  - No guarantee that will not have a perineal tear
  - Increased risk of bladder complications and long-term genital prolapse

Communication with colleagues

- Refers to consultant for second opinion
- May ask for psychiatric input to deal with the fear of poor outcome
- Anaesthetic review

Patient safety

- Confirms patients details at the start of the task
- Excludes known allergies
- Screens for MRSA

Applied clinical knowledge
- NICE guideline – no difference between elective CS and vaginal delivery in terms of benefits versus risks
- Familiar with the complications of CS
- Able to use information leaflet from RCOG and other sources
- Knowledgeable on the timing of elective CS

Examiner score sheet		
Information gathering		
Standard not met	Standard partly met	Standard met
0	1	2
Communication with patients and families		
Standard not met	Standard partly met	Standard met
0	1	2
Communication with colleagues		
Standard not met	Standard partly met	Standard met
0	1	2
Patient safety		
Standard not met	Standard partly met	Standard met
0	1	2
Applied clinical knowledge		
Standard not met	Standard partly met	Standard met
0	1	2

Examiner Expectations and Basis for Assessment

Information gathering

- Able to obtain history of pregnancy
- Reviews notes and investigations
- Obtains the history of request and why
- Obtains social, past medical, surgical and allergic history
- Able to obtain information on support after delivery, planned family size and return to work

Communication with patients and families

- Introduces self and role
- Discusses the pros and cons of vaginal versus CS
- Discusses the timing of CS
- Anaesthesia
- Recovery post delivery
- Gives time to consider decision

Communication with colleagues

- Refers to consultant for review of decision (second opinion)
- Considers referral to psychiatrist for review of mental state and to address anxieties from the friend's experience
- Refers to anaesthetic clinic
- Feedback to nurse and GP

Patient safety

- Confirms patients details at the start of the task
- Blood group and antibodies checked
- Blood transfusion acceptable, and if not (say Jehovah Witness), make alternate care plans
- Safe prescription after excluding allergy

Applied clinical knowledge

- Demonstrates knowledge of NICE guideline on CS
- Familiar with current literature on the timing of CS and the emerging evidence that CS is associated with increased morbidity on the babies
- Increased fertility rate post CS

Reference: *Caesarean section. NICE Clinical guideline [CG132] 23 November 2011. Last updated 04 September 2019*

Task 5: HIV in Pregnancy. Module 5 – Maternal Medicine

Candidate's Instructions

This is a simulated patient task assessing:

- Information gathering
- Communication with patients and families
- Communication with colleagues
- Patient safety
- Applied clinical knowledge

You are the ST5 in the antenatal clinic, and the midwife has brought a set of notes to you for the next patient. She will like you to see the patient as the consultant is away today. She was seen here last week, and the results from that visit are given below.

Results of investigations for Ms Jenny Mngwana

1. Full blood count
   a. Hb = 125 g/L
   b. WCC = 10 × 10⁹/L
   c. Lymphocytes = 2 × 10⁹/L
   d. Platelets = 345 × 10³/L
2. Rubella immunity – immune
3. Syphilis serology – negative
4. Blood group – O Rhesus positive, no atypical antibodies found
5. HIV – positive IgG antibodies (from fourth generation test)

You have 10 minutes in which you should:

1. Obtain focused history
2. Discuss the patient's results with her
3. Plan her antenatal care
4. Answer any questions that she may have

Simulated Patient's Instructions

You are Ms Jenny Mngwana, a 32-year-old care assistant, who attended to book for antenatal care 1 week ago at 10 weeks. You had your routine blood tests done as well as an ultrasound scan. The scan showed a single baby that agreed with your dates. You are due to have an ultrasound scan and blood test here in 2 weeks' time. You are 11 weeks today. You then had a phone call 4 days ago to come to the clinic to see the consultant as soon as possible to discuss some of the results of your test. You were not able to come until today.

This is your first pregnancy. You are originally from Zimbabwe but have been living in the UK for the past 12 years. Your partner Tsubeli, who is 36 years old, is also from Zimbabwe and joined you 2 years ago. He is a supply maths teacher to a local secondary school.

You used the combined pill for 6 years but stopped 2 years ago after you broke up with your previous partner. Your partner was using the condom until 6 months ago when he stopped, and you started depending on the fertile period method of contraception as your periods were relatively regular.

You have not had any medical problems in the past. You are currently taking folic acid – you started taking it once you had a missed period. This is not a planned pregnancy but it's welcomed. You and your partner are very happy and looking forward to the arrival of the baby.

Neither of you smokes but you both drink alcohol. Since you found out about the pregnancy, you have not had alcohol. You have never used drugs either in the form of tablets, smoke or injections. You are not sure whether your partner has done drugs before.

You have not had any sexually transmitted infections in the past and know of no such infections in your partner's past. Before your present partner, you were in a relationship for 6 years but broke off 2 years ago after finding out that your then partner had a string of girlfriends and a wife in London.

You are up to date with your smears and have no known allergies.

You have an older sister back in Zimbabwe, who had a son last year. He was diagnosed with Down syndrome 6 months after birth when they found that he was not growing well and had a heart problem. You are very worried whether Down syndrome is inherited.

If not covered, you should ask the following questions:

1. Why am I HIV positive?
2. How will I be managed?
3. I will like to be tested for Down syndrome as my sister has a child with Down syndrome and I will not want to have one.
4. Will I be able to have a normal vaginal delivery?
5. What are the chances of my baby being infected with HIV?

Examiner's Instructions

Familiarise yourself with the candidate's instruction and simulated patient's information. You have 10 minutes in which to assess the candidate in the domains on the marking sheet.

Lay Examiner's Instructions

Familiarise yourself with the candidate's instructions and simulated patient's information. Discuss how to assess the candidate with the clinical examiner.

A good candidate should cover the following:

Information gathering

- Able to obtain information about the pregnancy – unplanned but welcomed
- Offers to review notes to see results of investigations and ultrasound scan report
- Confirms social history
- Confirms family history – partner from high risk area for HIV (his HIV status unknown), sister has child with Down syndrome and broke up because partner had multiple relationships and a wife in London
- Establishes history of no previous recreational drugs (smoking, intravenous or tablets)

- Obtains information about drug history and allergy
- Sexual history – no previous history of sexually transmitted infections, number of sexual partners and contraception
- Initiates appropriate investigations (viral load, CD4 count, liver function test and screening for sexually transmitted infections) and ART resistance status of virus
- Initiates investigations for aneuploidy test (biochemistry and NT around this time); may consider NIPT (in view of anxiety over having a baby with Down syndrome)
- Screens for gestational diabetes at 16 and 24 weeks by OGTT
- Screens for opportunistic infections

Communication with patients and families

- Introduces self and role
- Informs patient about the positive HIV test in a very sensitive way, demonstrating empathy
- Gives time for the patient to react
- Does not ask for someone to be with the patient during breaking of news as this will demonstrate insensitivity
- Discusses implications of test – need for further investigations (screening for sexually transmitted infections, liver function test and viral resistance to ART)
- Asks to inform the partner – either by herself or invite the partner to come to hospital to be informed by HIV team and screening
- Counsels about the need for and timing of commencement of cART (antiretroviral therapy) based on viral load and CD4 count. Best to start before 16 weeks and aim for viral load of less than 50 and normal CD4 count by 36 weeks
- Informs patient that the greatest risk for vertical transmission is from 36 weeks' gestation and intrapartum
- Discusses the management of baby – requires neonatal ART duration of which will depend on whether the patient is very low, low, moderate or high risk
- Breastfeeding contraindicated
- Briefly mentions neonatal screening for vertical transmission

Communication with colleagues

- Discusses with/informs consultant
- Refers to GUM/HIV multidisciplinary team (GUM/HIV physician, consultant with special interest in HIV/infectious diseases in pregnancy, specialist midwife and clinical psychologist)
- Neonatal referral and flagging in notes – positive blood borne infection (to indirectly inform all staff involved in care)
- Communicates with the GP and the community midwife
- Involves contact tracing team if possible that HIV may have come from previous partner
- Provides positive reinforcement that cART is now almost associated with normal life (so many people with HIV now have a near normal life)

Patient safety

- Confirm patients details at the start of the task
- Establishes that there is no drug/other allergy
- Institutes cART appropriately having discussed the benefits
- Institutes appropriate vaccination

- Demonstrates an understanding of when to inform the partner and screens him
- Counsels about sexual intercourse – use of condom until partner has been screened and found to be positive

Applied clinical knowledge

- Discusses the implications of HIV in pregnancy – the impact of pregnancy on HIV and vice versa
- Discusses the management and the need for MDT
- Able to introduce prenatal screening for aneuploidy and the difficulties if an invasive test is required and the viral load is high

Examiner score sheet		
Information gathering		
Standard not met	Standard partly met	Standard met
0	1	2
Communication with patients and families		
Standard not met	Standard partly met	Standard met
0	1	2
Communication with colleagues		
Standard not met	Standard partly met	Standard met
0	1	2
Patient safety		
Standard not met	Standard partly met	Standard met
0	1	2
Applied clinical knowledge		
Standard not met	Standard partly met	Standard met
0	1	2

Examiner Expectations and Basis for Assessment

Information gathering

- Offers to review record and results
- Obtains information on pregnancy – unplanned
- Able to obtain information on sexual history
- Obtains information on social and drug history, including allergies
- Enquires after contraception and sexual transmitted infection
- Obtains information on family history and identifies history of Down syndrome and anxieties

- Initiates appropriate investigations, including aneuploidy screen and invasive testing, if required, or NIPT
- Familiar with the recent BASHH and RCOG Guidelines on HIV in pregnancy

Communication with patients and families

- Introduces self and role
- Discusses the results – in a sensitive way and showing empathy
- Discusses implications and risks of vertical transmission, co-existing infections and medical disorders of pregnancy, e.g. diabetes mellitus and risk of preterm birth
- Offers plan of management, including investigations
- Structured approach to informing the partner and the screening, including previous partner if current partner is negative
- Provides information at a steady pace and ensures understanding and encourages and answers all questions – also recognising and reacting all verbal clues

Communication with colleagues

- Refers to consultant for additional counselling
- Refers to GUM/HIV team (MDT Team) and signposting to appropriate consultant team (consultant with special interest in HIV/infectious diseases and specialist midwife)
- Consultation with the neonatologist
- Informs the GP and the community midwife
- Documents in the notes that blood borne infection (flagging up with other staff)
- Identifies neonate for neonatal screen and ART after delivery

Patient safety

- Confirms patients details at the start of the task
- Ascertains drug allergy
- Offers counselling on safe sex until the partner is screened
- Discusses the implications for the patient and the baby of HIV
- Screens for opportunistic infections and gestational diabetes
- Discusses on the mode of delivery
- Avoidance of breastfeeding after delivery

Applied clinical knowledge

- Demonstrates knowledge of the current literature on management of HIV in pregnancy
- Familiar with the recent BHIVA and RCOG Guidelines on HIV in pregnancy
- Demonstrates familiarity with screening for aneuploidy and its application in women with blood borne disorders (that are vertically transmitted)
- Counsels about the mode of delivery and avoidance of breastfeeding after delivery

Reference: British HIV Association guideline for the management of HIV in pregnancy and postpartum 2018 (2019 second edition)

Task 6: Prioritisation in Gynaecology. Module 9 – Gynaecological Problems

Candidate's Instructions

This is a structured discussion task assessing:

- Information gathering
- Communication with colleagues
- Communication with patients and families
- Patient safety
- Applied clinical knowledge

You are the ST5 in your unit and have been asked to look at the waiting list of your consultant. For each case on the list, you need to determine:

a. The appropriateness of the procedure
b. The category of the case (routine, soon or urgent)
c. The suitable venue for the case – day or inpatient
d. Any additional precautions necessary

Waiting List

a. A 29-year-old who presented with vulval itching and a whitish vaginal discharge and in whom nothing was found on examination for an examination under anaesthesia and biopsy of the vulva

b. A 79-year-old on the list for biopsy of vulva for an indolent ulcer on the vulva which bleeds occasionally

c. Mrs TT is on the list for a diagnostic hysteroscopy. She is 45 years old, diabetic and presented with heavy and irregular periods. An endometrial biopsy was not possible

d. Mrs BS is a 56-year-old on the waiting list for a diagnostic laparoscopy for an adnexal mass, which was described on ultrasound as containing papillae and partly solid and cystic areas. Her CA125 was 140 iu

e. A 36-year-old mother of three on the list for laparoscopic sterilisation as she is not able to tolerate any other form of contraception

f. A 60-year-old with uterovaginal prolapse was seen in the clinic and placed on the list for a vaginal hysterectomy and pelvic floor repair. She has a mild cystocele and also complains of urinary incontinence

You have 10 minutes in which you should:

Read through each case and then determine

- The appropriateness of the procedure
- The category of the case (routine – to be done within 4-6 weeks, soon to be done within 2-4 weeks or urgent to be done within 2 weeks)
- The suitable venue for the case – day or inpatient
- Any additional investigations/precautions necessary

Case No	Appropriate (Yes/No)	Category and venue (in-patient/ Day case)	Additional information/alternative management if appropriate	Additional investigation/ precautions
a	No	Not applicable	History to exclude dermatological disorders and Screen for STI. May require referral to Genito-urinary Medicine	High vaginal swab for culture
b	Yes	Urgent Day-case and	Exclude any co-morbidities/ systemic disease – how fit is she?	MRI of the pelvis, urea and electrolyte, full blood count
c	Yes	Urgent and day care	How well controlled is her diabetes? Any contraindications to being a day-case? Parity and history of PCOS? What is her weight	Urea and electrolytes (U&E), full blood count (FBC), First on the list and inform anaesthetist to review
d	No	Urgent In-patient	Referral to oncologist and for an MDT Requires a staging laparotomy as RMI is high	CT/MRI of the abdomen, pelvis and CXR FBC, U&E, liver function test
e	Yes	Routine Day-case	Any period problems (cyclicity and quantity) Current contraceptive Offer LARC (Long active reversible contraception such as Nexplanon/ Mirena or Copper intrauterine device). Discuss male sterilisation	Pregnancy test
f	Yes	Routine In-patient	Sexually active? Any bowel problems Review by urogynaecologist	Urine for urinalysis Urodynamics U&E and FBC

Examiner score sheet

Information gathering		
Standard not met	Standard partly met	Standard met
0	1	2
Communication with patients and families		
Standard not met	Standard partly met	Standard met
0	1	2
Communication with colleagues		
Standard not met	Standard partly met	Standard met
0	1	2
Patient safety		
Standard not met	Standard partly met	Standard met
0	1	2
Applied clinical knowledge		
Standard not met	Standard partly met	Standard met
0	1	2

Examiner Expectations and Basis for Assessment

Information gathering

- Discusses the various cases focusing on the additional information required to plan management
- Synthesises the information provided in each case logically to justify decisions on investigations and venue of treatment
- Requests appropriate investigations for each of the cases to facilitate decision on care

Communication with patients and families

- Able to communicate to each patient or about each patient clearly on the management pathway and rationalise it
- Able to explain the rationale for decision on management including timing of procedure, venue and additional investigations
- Able to explain clearly the rationale behind changing decision on care pathway

---

Communication with colleagues

- Demonstrates an ability to prioritise cases appropriately
- Describes the differential diagnoses and formulates an appropriate management plan
- Demonstrates an ability to prioritise cases appropriately into routine, soon and urgent, based on the NHS definition of cases and the rationale for such a classification

---

Patient safety

- Demonstrates clearly an understanding of the limits of their clinical abilities, and demonstrates an understanding of when to refer to other specialties (gynaecology oncology urogynaecology genito-urinary medicine) and involve senior colleagues and other disciplines
- Demonstrates clearly an understanding of safe prescription if applicable and special circumstances,
- Demonstrates an understanding of the principles of safe surgery – right surgery at the right place and right time

---

Applied clinical knowledge
Demonstrates:

- Knowledge of the treatment of gynaecological disorders
- Knowledgeable on the common gynaecological disorders and their management
- An understanding of referral pathways in complex gynaecological disorders
- An understanding of the NHS recommended timelines for management especially suspected oncology cases

---

Task 7: Combined Hormonal Contraception. Module 11 – Sexual and Reproductive Health

Candidate's Instructions

This is a structured discussion task assessing:

- Information gathering
- Communication with patients and families
- Communication with colleagues
- Patient safety
- Applied clinical knowledge

You are the ST5 in the clinic with your consultant. You have been informed that a 27-year-old is attending for contraception advice. She is a mother of three and is very keen to go on the combined hormonal contraception. Her last menstrual period was 1 week ago. Below is the referral letter from the GP.

Brookes Side Surgery
St Peters
Leicester, LE20 17 UP

Dear Mr Al-Magdi,
Thanks for seeing this 27-year-old mother of three, who wishes to go on hormonal contraception. She has had three normal vaginal deliveries; the last one was 9 months ago. She works as a secretary for one of the consultants in surgery in the hospital.

Yours sincerely

Dr Ahmed Mustafa MBChB, DRCOG, DCH, MRCGP

The examiner will have a conversation with you based on a series of questions. There are four questions, which you should cover in the 10 minutes. The examiner will ask you to move on after about 2 minutes to ensure that you cover all the four questions.

Examiner's Instructions

Familiarise yourself with the candidate's instructions.
   Use the following four questions to form the basis of a discussion with the candidate. You should time each question and move the candidates on after approximately 2 minutes to make sure that the task is completed.

1. What information will you ask from the patient that will determine whether she is suitable for combined hormonal contraception?
2. What options will you offer her and what are the advantages and disadvantages of these options?
3. She opts for the contraceptive patch. What will you be telling her about how to take it and the precautions when it slips off or there is a delay in replacing it?
4. What if she forgets to take the patch off to start a new cycle?

A good candidate should cover the following:

1. *What information will you ask from the patient that will determine whether she is suitable for the combined hormonal contraception?*
   - Menstrual cycle – regular or not?
   - Previous hormonal use and why combined hormonal contraception?
   - Sexual history and history of the pelvic inflammatory disease
   - How long she wishes to use contraception for?
   - Medical history – headaches especially migraines with aura, high blood pressure, overweight, heart disease in family, hypercholesterolaemia, thrombophilia or previous VTE
   - Motivation to remember to take daily, weekly or monthly

- Cervical cytology – last cervical smear
- Physical examination – blood pressure and weight

2. *What options will you offer her and what are the advantages and disadvantages of these options?*
   - Combined oral contraceptive
     — Taken daily – main disadvantage – remembering to take it daily. Once becomes habit, less likely to forget
   - Combined transdermal hormonal contraception (the patch)
     — Taken once weekly – advantage of only changing it once a week, however, easy to forget to change or may not know when it slips off
   - Combined hormonal ring
     — Taken once monthly – compliance better, may forget to change ring

3. *She opts for the contraceptive patch. What will you be telling her about how to take it and the precautions when it slips of or there is a delay in removing it?*
   - How to use the patch:
     — Start during first 5 days of period – the first Sunday after period starts. Advisable to use a backup method of contraception, e.g. condoms for the first 7 days of using the patch as it can take time to become effective
     — Apply the patch to a clean and dry area of skin where it won't be rubbed by tight clothing. It can be worn on the stomach, buttock, upper back or upper outer arm. Do not place it on the breast
     — Make sure the patch sticks; no make-up, cream, lotion, etc. should be applied to the skin where the patch is placed. Press down firmly on the patch for 10 seconds when applying, and make sure the edges stick well
     — The patch stays in place for 1 week if applied properly, even if during exercise, shower or swim
     — A new patch is put on once a week for 3 weeks. No patch is worn on the fourth week, and this is when periods occur
     — The patch should be changed on the same day each week
   - The patch should not be off for more than 7 days in a row. After the seventh day, a new patch is applied to restart the 4-week cycle, even if you still have your period
   - Missed patch/slipped off
     — Important questions:
       — When in the cycle did this slip off? When was it noticed? Has it slipped off completely? Any retrieved patch?
       — Protect until next period
   Patch off less than 24 hours
     — Reapply the patch or put a new patch on as soon as possible
     — Patch change day will remain the same
     — Make a cycle of three patches
       During week 1
   Patch has been off for 24 hours or less:
     — Apply a new patch as soon as possible
     — Keep it on until the next scheduled patch change day
     — Make a cycle of three patches

— Use backup birth control (i.e. condoms) for the next 7 days and consider using emergency contraception

During week 2 or 3

Patch has been off for less than 72 hours (3 days):
— Apply a new patch as soon as possible
— Keep same patch change day
— Finish the cycle of patches and start a new cycle of three patches with no patch-free week

Patch has been off for more than 72 hours (3 days):
— Apply a new patch as soon as possible
— Keep your same patch change day
— Finish the cycle of patches and start a new cycle of three patches with no patch-free week
— Use backup birth control (i.e. condoms) for 7 days and consider using emergency contraception

4. *What if she forgets to take the patch off to start a new cycle?*

If patch 3 is on for more than 9 days:
- This is the patch-free week and will not decrease the effectiveness of the patch unless worn past the next patch cycle.

If patch 1 or 2 is on for 9 to 12 days:
- Apply a new patch
- Keep the same patch change day
- Finish the cycle of patches and start a new cycle of patches without a patch-free week

If patch 1 or 2 is on for 12 or more days:
- Apply a new patch
- Keep the same patch change day
- Finish the cycle of patches and start a new cycle of patches without a patch-free week
- Use backup birth control (i.e. condoms) for 7 days and consider using emergency contraception

Examiner score sheet		
Information gathering		
Standard not met	Standard partly met	Standard met
0	1	2
Communication with patients and families		
Standard not met	Standard partly met	Standard met
0	1	2
Communication with colleagues		
Standard not met	Standard partly met	Standard met
0	1	2

Patient safety		
Standard not met	Standard partly met	Standard met
0	1	2
Applied clinical knowledge		
Standard not met	Standard partly met	Standard met
0	1	2

Examiner Expectations and Basis for Assessment

Information gathering

- Obtains detailed menstrual and sexual history
- Takes detailed medical and surgical history
- Confirms reproductive history
- Enquires after previous contraceptive use and why the chosen method
- Reviews any results in previous records or initiates appropriate investigations including BP and weight

Communication with patients and families *(not relevant in this particular task but useful in same scenarios but with a simulated patient)*

- Introduces self to patient and the role they are to play
- Discusses the various options – pros, cons and the way these are used
- Provides information at a reasonable pace and in enough detail to ensure understanding and at the same time encourages questions and provides answers
- Summarises discussion and agreed upon option (making decisions with the patient)

Communication with colleagues

- Recognises when to refer, i.e. recognises limits of own abilities
- Communicates with the GP after the agreed method of contraception has been agreed and provides with details of follow-up with by the GP or the hospital

Patient safety

- Ensures that the allergy is confirmed or excluded
- Safe prescription – contraception
- Informs what to do with missed contraception

- No contraindications to chosen method of contraception
- Monitors for side effects of the chosen method

Applied clinical knowledge

- Knows the different forms of combined hormonal contraception (oral, transdermal and transvaginal)
- Knowledgeable about the current literature on contraception, including NICE and Faculty of Sexual and Reproductive Health Guidelines

Task 8: Ectopic Pregnancy. Module 12 – Early Pregnancy Care

Candidate's Instructions

This is a patient simulated task assessing:

1. Information gathering
2. Communication with patients and families
3. Communication with colleagues
4. Patient safety
5. Applied clinical knowledge

You are an ST5 on call and have been asked to see a patient who has been referred by the GP to the early pregnancy assessment unit (EPAU) of your hospital.

London Road Surgery
Brent Town
Lowfield
LO2 9PG

Dear Dr,
Re: Ms June Snowforth Age: 25 years
Please kindly see as an emergency this patient who came to the surgery this morning with sudden onset of lower abdominal pain. Her periods are 1 week late. She is very tender in the lower abdomen and a pregnancy test is positive. Her vital signs are stable. I suspect that she may have an ectopic pregnancy.
Thank you

Yours sincerely

Dr Angela Burke MBBS, MRCGP, DCH

You have 10 minutes in which you will:

- Take focused history
- Initiate appropriate investigations
- Discuss management with the patient
- Plan a follow-up

Simulated Patient's Information

You are a 25-year-old sales person with a travel agency. You saw your GP earlier today with lower abdominal pain and some vaginal bleeding which started 2 hours ago. The GP examined you and also did a urine pregnancy test and then referred you to the hospital.

You are single but have a steady boyfriend. You developed lower abdominal pain which was initially on the left side but is now all over your lower abdomen. The pain is sharp, and the only time you have some relief is if you remain still. You have not felt dizzy and do not have any shoulder tip pain. Shortly after the pain started, you noticed a brownish red discharge coming from your vagina. This is now red but is not heavy.

Your periods are irregular, and the last one was about 5 weeks ago. They last for 4–5 days with heavy bleeding but no clots on days 1 and 2. You go from 5–6 weeks in between periods. They have always been like this since your first period at the age of 13 years. You do not have any pain with your periods and do not bleed in between periods.

You have never used any contraceptives in the past but your boyfriend uses the condom on a regular basis. You were invited to have your first smear test a year ago, and this was normal.

You were treated for a pelvic infection 3 years ago. You seem to recall that it was thought to be chlamydia infection and after that you were advised not to use any intrauterine contraception. You believe that this infection was given to you by your then boyfriend. You broke up with him after that and have been very careful with anyone you have a relationship with. You have been going out with Tom for the past 9 months. He works in the same company with you as a manager. He is 35 years old. You both smoke and drink alcohol. You are allergic to penicillin.

If not covered, you should ask the following questions:

- What is the cause of the ectopic pregnancy?
- Can the pregnancy be removed and the tube preserved?
- What if I do not want surgery? Are there any non-surgical options?
- What type of surgery will I have?
- What are the chances of it happening again and how can I prevent it?

A good candidate should cover the following:

Information gathering

- Takes comprehensive focused history – onset of pain, symptoms of rupture (dizziness, shoulder tip pain and fainting), history of *Chlamydia trachomatis* treatment, LMP and cycles and social factors – smoking and alcohol
- Offers to examine – general, abdominal and pelvis
- Initiates appropriate investigations – urine pregnancy test, FBC, group and save, quantified HCG and transvaginal ultrasound scan

Communication with patients and families

- Introduces self and role to patient and explains the suspected diagnosis and the rationale for investigations
- Discusses treatment options – medical versus surgical and the various types of surgical management – pros and cons
- Provides information at a reasonable pace and in such a manner that the patient comprehends and encourages and answers all questions
- Obtains consent for surgery if surgical treatment is the chosen option

Communication with colleagues

- Links with imaging, laboratory, anaesthesia and theatre staff (book patient on the emergency list)
- Informs senior on call and junior as would require assistant in theatre
- Feedback to GP

Patient safety

- Confirms patients details at the start of the task
- Explains the risk of rupture and haemorrhage and need for IV line and IV fluids
- Discusses the risks of medical management, including complications of methotrexate
- Safe prescription having ascertained allergy and contraindications to methotrexate

Applied clinical knowledge

- Demonstrates knowledge of current literature on the management of ectopic pregnancy
  - Medical treatment – criteria – clinically stable, hCG 1,500–5,000, USS gestational sac <35 mm and no active fetal heart beat
  - Methotrexate – IM and then monitor hCG on days 4 and 7 – decrease >15% continue monitoring, decrease by <15% TVS and repeat in 32–75% of cases. Success rate 65–95% May need repeating
  - hCG monitoring until <15 iu
- Surgery – laparoscopic – salpingectomy or salpingotomy
  - Salpingotomy, if unruptured, and tube will be preserved
  - Need to follow-up with hCG
  - Contralateral tube damaged
  - Salpingectomy
    - Contralateral tube normal
    - Tube ruptured
- Contraception – avoid IUDs
- Recurrence – 1:10
- From above shows familiarity with NICE and RCOG Green-top Guidelines

Examiner score sheet		
Information gathering		
Standard not met	Standard partly met	Standard met
0	1	2

Communication with patients and families		
Standard not met	Standard partly met	Standard met
0	1	2
Communication with colleagues		
Standard not met	Standard partly met	Standard met
0	1	2
Patient safety		
Standard not met	Standard partly met	Standard met
0	1	2
Applied clinical knowledge		
Standard not met	Standard partly met	Standard met
0	1	2

Examiner Expectations and Basis for Assessment

Information gathering

- Takes comprehensive focused history identifying symptoms of ectopic
- Offers to perform an examination to define cardiovascular status (stable or not)
- Initiates appropriate investigations that would help make diagnosis and plan management (urine pregnancy test, hCG quantification, FBC, group and safe and transvaginal ultrasound scan)
- Summarises and ensures that the patient understands

Communication with patients and families

- Introduces self and role
- Able to communicate clearly with the patient the possible diagnosis and the management plan
- Sensible approach to breaking bad news, including implications for future pregnancies (showing empathy)
- Able to discuss management options clearly – pros and cons

Communication with colleagues

- Able to work with colleagues in laboratory, anaesthesia, imaging (ultrasound scan) and operating theatre

- Able to clearly describe an agreed management plan to colleagues, including the use of SBAR
- Recognises the need to liaise with consultant/senior on call
- Feedback to the GP with diagnosis and management, including a follow-up plan

---

Patient safety

- Confirms patients details at the start of the task
- Takes the necessary steps to prevent deterioration and complications – IV line and start on fluids
- Appropriate management, recognising limitations of one's own abilities and calling consultant/senior when appropriate
- Safe prescription excluding allergies especially to methotrexate
- Understands the principles of WHO safe surgery checklist (note that this does not apply when communicating with patient)

Applied clinical knowledge

- Knowledge of early pregnancy complications, particularly ectopic pregnancy
- Demonstrates an understanding of the medical and surgical management of ectopic pregnancy
- Able to present management options – including the advantages and disadvantages of each of the options
- Demonstrates an understanding of the recurrence rate and impact of ectopic pregnancy on contraception and future pregnancies
- Knowledgeable of current literature, especially RCOG and NICE guidelines on ectopic pregnancy

---

Reference: *Ectopic pregnancy and miscarriage: diagnosis and initial management. NICE guideline [NG126] 17 April 2019*

Reference: *Diagnosis and management of ectopic pregnancy. The Royal College of Obstetricians and Gynaecologists Green-top Guideline No. 21 November 2016*

Task 9: Diagnostic Laparoscopy. Module 2 – Core Surgical Skills

Candidate's Instructions

This is a structured discussion task assessing (this could also be a teaching station or a patient simulated station):

- Information gathering
- Communication with colleagues

- Communication with patients and families
- Patient safety
- Applied clinical knowledge

You are an ST5, working with Mr Garfield. Today is his operating list, and one of the patients on the list is a 30-year-old nurse for a diagnostic laparoscopy for chronic lower abdominal pain. She is a mother of one, who has been trying for a baby for the past 2 years. The consultant is conducting a pre-operative ward round and has asked you to see this patient as you will be performing the laparoscopy.

You have 10 minutes in which you will have a structured conversation with the examiner who has five questions that will be used to discuss the management of the patient.

Examiner's Instructions

Familiarise yourself with the candidate's instructions.

Use the following five questions as a guide to conduct a structured discussion with the candidate. You should give guidance on time management so that all the questions can be attempted.

1. How will you conduct a pre-operative ward round on this patient?
2. She is in theatre for surgery and is now asleep. What would be the approach to her diagnostic laparoscopy?
3. What in her history will make you take additional steps to minimise visceral injury?
4. If the risk of bowel injury is significant, how may you overcome this?
5. What will be your management of the patient until she is discharged from the hospital?

A good candidate will cover the following:

1. *How will you conduct a pre-operative ward round on this patient?*
   - Introduce yourself
   - Review the notes to familiarise yourself with the history and indication for the procedure, checks any investigations that were done and confirm results are available, and if not, ask for them
   - Ascertain that the symptoms at the initial presentation when booked for laparoscopy have not changed and the patient is still happy to go ahead
   - Confirm an understanding of the procedure and risks by patient
   - Ask for LMP and ensure that a pregnancy test has been done (check for result)
   - Confirm that a consent has been given and dated, and if not, obtain consent
   - Briefly discuss post-operative course and assure that these will be affirmed after the procedure
   - Encourage questions and answer accordingly
2. *She is in theatre for surgery and is now asleep. What would be the approach to her diagnostic laparoscopy?*
   - WHO safe surgery checklist (introductions of members of the theatre team, confirm procedure being performed, check patients details, equipment, surgical precautions etc.)
   - Position patient in the lithotomy (Lloyd-Davis) position
   - Clean the vagina and empty bladder
   - Perform a pelvic examination and then insert a uterine manipulator
   - Clean the abdomen and apply drapes

- Connect the CO_2 tubing to the inflator and the light source to the stack system
- Check that the gas flow and pressure are normal and also check that the Veress needle is patent
- Make an incision in the infra-umbilical region
- Insert the Veress needle and check that it's in place (this can be done with a syringe with saline or pressure of flowing the gas)
- Once assured that it is in peritoneal cavity, increase flow rate and pressure to 30 cm of H_2O and aim to achieve at least 3 L pneumoperitoneum
- Remove the needle and extend the incision to introduce either a 5 or 10 mm trocar. Remove the cannula and introduce the laparoscope
- Once in the peritoneal cavity, ensure that the bowel has not been injured by directly inspecting underneath the umbilicus
- Under direct vision, insert a 5 mm trocar just above the umbilicus and introduce a probe through it
- Perform a thorough inspection (take appropriate records by means of photographs) of the abdomen in the nine quadrants, lifting the ovaries to inspect the ovarian fossa and the pouch of Douglas
- Deflate the abdomen as much as possible and remove the suprapubic trocar under direct vision to ensure there is no bleeding. Remove the infra-umbilical trocar and close up the incisions (if you've used a 10 mm scope, you should use a J-needle to close the deeper part of the infra-umbilical incision and then close the skin subcutaneously)

3. *What in her history will make you take additional steps to minimise visceral injury?*
   - Previous pelvic infections
   - Previous surgery, especially laparotomy and CS
   - Inflammatory bowel disease, e.g. Crohn's disease
   - Low BMI

4. *If the risk of bowel injury is significant, how may you overcome this?*
   - Entry through Palmer's point
   - Open laparoscopy
   - Make sure senior colleague is available or assists in the procedure

5. *What will be your management of the patient until she is discharged from the hospital?*
   - Complete the operation notes and suggest options for management to be discussed
   - Write to her GP
   - Prescribe adequate pain relief
   - See patient after she has recovered from anaesthesia and explain the procedure and findings
   - Discuss management option
   - Discharge home with an appointment to see in the outpatient. May start treatment if she is happy to do so

Examiner score sheet		
Information gathering		
Standard not met	Standard partly met	Standard met
0	1	2

Communication with patients and families		
Standard not met	Standard partly met	Standard met
0	1	2
Communication with colleagues		
Standard not met	Standard partly met	Standard met
0	1	2
Patient safety		
Standard not met	Standard partly met	Standard met
0	1	2
Applied clinical knowledge		
Standard not met	Standard partly met	Standard met
0	1	2

Examiner Expectations and Basis for Assessment

Information gathering

- Able to confirm the symptoms that led to the planned laparoscopy
- Identifies the risk factors for bowel injury from history
- Reviews investigations results and initiates appropriate investigations that will help with surgery
- Asks after LMP
- Confirms that a pregnancy test has been done and consent has been obtained

Communication with patients and families

- Confirms patients identify at the start of the task
- Informs the patient in detail of the procedure, its complications and course of post-surgical recovery
- Gives enough information in a staged approach with enough details and ensures understanding and encourages questions and answers them at each stage
- Explains post-operative findings and treatment options
- Discusses and agrees on a follow-up plan

Communication with colleagues

- Identifies when and what to communicate to various members of the team – anaesthetist, theatre nurses and stack operator

- Knows when to call for help from senior colleagues (knows the limitations of own skills)
- Feedback to the GP after procedure with findings and a clear plan for follow-up and management

Patient safety

- Ensures patient is not pregnant
- Safety checks of equipment
- Demonstrates safety steps throughout laparoscopy
- Ensures WHO safe surgery checklist
- Safe prescription after establishing drug allergy
- Ensures the positioning of patient, including checking at every stage for the safety of equipment and procedure
- Meticulous assessment of bowel during entry as well as the nine quadrants of the peritoneal cavity and bleeding ports during removal of equipment

Applied clinical knowledge

- Knowledgeable of the causes of chronic pelvic pain
- Familiar with surgical process of diagnostic laparoscopy
- Knowledgeable of the current literature on laparoscopy
- Familiar with RCOG Green-top guidelines on safe entry in laparoscopy and visceral injuries at laparoscopy and BSGE guidelines

Reference: Preventing entry-related gynaecological laparoscopic injuries. The Royal College of Obstetricians and Gynaecologists Green-top Guideline No. 49 May 2008

Task 10: Waiting List in Gynaecology. Module 9 – Gynaecological Problems

Candidate's Instructions

This is a structured discussion task assessing:

- Information gathering
- Communication with patients and families
- Communication with colleagues
- Patient safety
- Applied clinical knowledge

You are the ST5 in your unit and have been asked to look at the waiting list of your consultant. For each case on the list, you need to determine:

a. The appropriateness of the procedure
b. The category of the case – routine (to be done within 4–6 weeks, soon to be done within 2–4 weeks and urgent to be done within 2 weeks)
c. The suitable venue – day case or inpatient
d. Any additional investigations or information required or precautions necessary

You have 10 minutes in which you should:

- Read the details of each of the case
- Decide appropriateness of the procedure
- Categorise it as suitable to be done as day or inpatient
- Discuss any additional investigations or information required or precautions to be taken

Waiting List

1. A 10-year-old with a blood-stained vaginal discharge of 3 months duration on the list for an EUA
2. A 80-year-old with a simple ovarian cyst measuring 10 × 15 cm for laparotomy. The cyst was identified incidentally at ultrasound scan for suspected carcinoma of the colon which has not been confirmed. She is living on her own but frail
3. A 66-year-old on the list for an abdominal hysterectomy and bilateral salpingoophorectomy for hyperplasia of the endometrium with focal areas of atypia
4. A 33-year-old with primary infertility and associated deep dyspareunia on the list for a diagnostic laparoscopy and dye test
5. A 26-year-old on the list for a diagnostic laparoscopy for deep dyspareunia and menorrhagia. She is severely asthmatic and uses Ventolin and Becotide to control her asthma
6. A 40-year-old with invasive carcinoma of the cervix on the waiting list for examination under anaesthesia. She is hypertensive and suffers from severe arthritis affecting the T-mandibular joint

A good candidate will cover the tasks as detailed in the table below.

Case No	Appropriate (yes/no)	Category an inpatient/day care	Additional information/alternate management if inappropriate	Additional investigations
1	Yes	Urgent Day case	Drug history, cyclicity of bleeding? Pubertal milestones and trauma; sensitivity about abuse Admit onto paediatrics ward (ideally on a paediatrics list)	FBC
2	No	Not applicable	Interventional radiology and percutaneous drainage (frail 80-year-old living on her own)	CA125 and calculate RMI

3	Yes	Urgent/ inpatient	Review notes for risk factors for endometrial cancer (obesity, nulliparity, history of PCOS, diabetes, hypertensive and fibroids)	FBC, U&E and ECG
4	Yes	Routine/day case	Semen analysis for partner; investigations for ovulatory dysfunction; when was the last screen for *Chlamydia trachomatis,* and if not, within last 3 months screen (if not and cannot be done, administer IV antibiotics at time of procedure) Check LMP prior to day of procedure	Complete investigations on the left column if not done
5	Yes	Routine/day case	Review medical treatment tried, and if not, consider hormonal suppression until asthma is well controlled. How well controlled is the asthma – anaesthetist to review	Assessment by pulmonologist and anaesthetist
6	Yes	Urgent/day case	Review by anaesthetist to determine the type of anaesthesia – maybe given a regional (e.g. spinal), involve ENT	FBC, U&E, LFT, CXR, MRI of pelvic and CT of abdomen/USS of kidneys

Examiner score sheet		
Information gathering		
Standard not met	Standard partly met	Standard met
0	1	2
Communication with patients and families		
Standard not met	Standard partly met	Standard met
0	1	2
Communication with colleagues		
Standard not met	Standard partly met	Standard met
0	1	2
Patient safety		
Standard not met	Standard partly met	Standard met
0	1	2
Applied clinical knowledge		
Standard not met	Standard partly met	Standard met
0	1	2

Examiner Expectations and Basis for Assessment

Information gathering

- Discusses appropriate investigations for each of the patients and the information to be obtained from the investigation
- Synthesises the information provided in each letter and then uses it correctly in planning and management

---

Communication with patients and families

- Able to communicate to each patient the need to obtain additional information, including further investigations
- Able to explain the rationale for classifying case as routine, soon or urgent

---

Communication with colleagues

- Ability to prioritise each case appropriately into urgent, soon (semi-urgent) and routine (non-urgent) cases
- Able to synthesise the information in enough detail to ensure management plans are clear and easily understood by the colleagues involved in the care of the patient, e.g. those requiring additional input (ENT and respiratory physician/pulmonologist)
- Ability to identify additional expertise required for each case as it's prioritised

---

Patient safety

- Aware of the possible consequences of a delay in seeing a patient on the waiting list
- Appropriate precautions to take for each case to minimise complication

---

Applied clinical knowledge

- Knowledgeable of various common gynaecological problems
- Ability to form a logical differential diagnosis for each of the cases

- Ability to critically appraise the information provided in the letters to arrive at a diagnosis
- An ability to initiate appropriate investigations to confirm diagnosis and make management plans
- Has a working knowledge of the roles of other members of the multidisciplinary team to ensure best care for patient (in discussing the additional precautions to be taken)
- Knowledgeable to an appropriate level of various NICE/RCOG Guidelines on general gynaecology and the governments recommendation for waiting times for oncology cases

Task 11: Gynaecology Prioritisation Board. Module 9 – Gynaecological Problems

Candidate's Instructions

This is a structured discussion task assessing:

- Information gathering
- Communication with colleagues
- Patient safety
- Applied clinical knowledge

You are the gynaecology Specialist Trainee 5 on call. You have been handed the following problems at 8.00 am on Monday. There is only one theatre in the unit, which deals with elective and emergency cases. You have a list with your consultant, which starts at 9.00 am. You have the following staff available – a career ST1 (3 months into his first post) and three nurses, one of who can take blood.

You have 10 minutes in which you should:

- Study each of the cases on the list below
- Identify what is the task for each patient
- Delegate staff to each task
- Prioritise the order in which the task should be undertaken

List of Cases on the Unit

1. A 22-year-old with 6 weeks amenorrhoea, abdominal pain and vaginal bleeding. She presented at 6.30 am. Her Hb is 126 mg/L. Pregnancy test on the ward is positive. She is suspected to have an ectopic pregnancy. She is clinically stable

2. Mrs Green presented 45 minutes ago at 10 weeks amenorrhoea with vaginal bleeding. She was initially stable but has been in severe pain for the past 20 minutes and is now in shock. She is continuing to bleed very heavily. When she was examined on admission, the cervical os was opened

3. Mrs MJY, 78 years old, had surgery for ovarian cancer yesterday. She is still unable to drink. Her drip has tissued, and it is time for her intravenous antibiotics

4. Mrs TTO is 14 weeks pregnant and has presented with urinary retention for the past 24 hours. She is yet to be seen by a doctor

5. Mrs Bailey has attended for surgery and is yet to be consented. She is the first on the list which starts at 8.30 am

6. A 50-year-old woman, who had a vaginal hysterectomy yesterday for prolapse, has not passed urine. Her blood pressure is 90/60 mmHg and her pulse is 120 bpm. She has a vaginal pack and has not been reviewed

7. A 22-year-old admitted with an acute onset abdominal pain, which initially was intermittent but is now constant. Abdominal examination was difficult because of tenderness and guarding. Her FBC shows significant leucocytosis. Her temperature is 37.6°C

Case No	Tasks	Delegated to	Order
1	IV access, group and safe, ultrasound scan (TVS), serum HCG and book theatre	ST1 insert IV cannula, take bloods and book USS as well as theatre	6
2	Speculum examination to check if products are in the cervix and remove, IV access and group and safe; book theatre if necessary Check if Jehovah Witness	ST5 (myself)	1
3	Resite IV and administer antibiotics	ST1	7
4	Empty bladder Ultrasound scan	Nurse to empty bladder	3
5	Obtain consent Inform patient, theatre staff and consultant that surgery will be delayed	ST5 (myself) – to obtain consent Nurse – to ring theatre and inform of the delay	4
6	Review vital signs quickly Abdominal examination Check pack if soaked through FBC and cross-match blood Book theatre for exploration, inform consultant and obtain consent Check input/output for fluid balance	ST5 to obtain consent and book theatre	2
7	Ultrasound scan Consent for surgery and book theatre for laparoscopic ovarian detorsion/cystectomy	ST1 – book for USS ST5 to obtain consent for surgery and book theatre	5

Examiner score sheet		
Information gathering		
Standard not met	Standard partly met	Standard met
0	1	2
Communication with colleagues		
Standard not met	Standard partly met	Standard met
0	1	2
Patient safety		
Standard not met	Standard partly met	Standard met
0	1	2
Applied clinical knowledge		
Standard not met	Standard partly met	Standard met
0	1	2

Examiner Expectations and Basis for Assessment

Information gathering

- Able to digest patient information and use it to define tasks to be undertaken
- Able to sought additional information to complement the given information to signpost management

Communication with colleagues

- Has an understanding of the limits of one's own competence and when to call for senior help or involve other specialties
- Team work – identifies easily the multidisciplinary teams involved in the care of various gynaecological problems
- Prioritises appropriately
- Works within a multidisciplinary team and knows the skills mix within the team and is able to delegate appropriately

---

Patient safety

- Understands the risks from complications of the abnormal result if untreated and treatment options
- Has an understanding of the risk management and clinical governance processes in relation to gynaecological investigations and interpretation
- Ability to critically appraise results within the context of the information given
- Able to work in a stressful environment and prioritise appropriately

---

Applied clinical knowledge

- Knowledge of the current literature on common gynaecological problems, routine investigations, interpretation and treatment
- Able to critically appraise the literature, including guidelines (NICE and RCOG Green-top) and scientific papers
- Has a working knowledge of the roles of other members of the multidisciplinary team

---

Task 12: Perforation of the Uterus at Evacuation of Products of Conception. Module 3 – Post-Operative Care

Candidate's Instructions

This is a structured discussion task assessing:

- Communication with colleagues
- Communication with patients and families
- Patient safety
- Applied clinical knowledge

You are the ST5 on call covering emergency gynaecology. On call with you is a consultant who is at home (20 minutes from the hospital).

You admitted a 25-year-old teacher in her first pregnancy at 10 weeks with bleeding and abdominal pains. The bleeding is severe, and when you examined her, you found a closed cervical os with active bleeding. An ultrasound scan showed a gestational sac in the lower uterine segment with a fetal pole and absent fetal heart beat. This is confirmed by an emergency ultrasound performed by the sonographer. She continued to bleed heavily, and on this basis, you decided to take the patient to theatre for evacuation of retained products of conception.

You dilated the cervix to size 8 mm Hegar and start the process of evacuation. You insert the cannula, start suction but discover that the cannula goes much further than you would expect. You suspect perforation of the uterus.

You have 10 minutes to have a structured discussion with the examiner, who has four questions for a discussion with you on the management of this patient now and after surgery.

Examiner's Instructions

Familiarise yourself with the candidate's instructions.

Use the following four questions to guide the discussion you will have with the candidate. Provide some guidance on how much time the candidate spends on each question.

1. What immediate action will you take?
2. How will you approach the rest of the surgery?
3. What will your post-operative management be?
4. What clinical governance issues will you deal with post-operatively?

A good candidate would cover the following:

What immediate action will you take?

- Stop the procedure
- Disconnect the suction pump (switch it off) but leave the tube in-situ with no further suction
- Inform anaesthetist, scrub nurse and the rest of the theatre team
- Inform and call the consultant/senior gynaecologist on call

How will you approach the rest of the surgery?

- Perform a laparoscopy
- Check for visceral injury – if present – can this be repaired laparoscopically (involved appropriate specialty)
- Complete suction under direct vision with scope inside to ensure that no bowel is involved
- Prescribe antibiotics

What will your post-operative management be?

- Monitor overnight
- Complete incident form
- Debrief patient about incident
- Counsel about implications of perforation for future pregnancies (consider as a classical incision and therefore should be a CS with all subsequent deliveries)
- Communicate with GP – the complications and a clear logical plan for a follow-up and management of any complications

What clinical governance issues will you deal with post-operatively?

- Complete incident form (Datix) to notify the risk manager
- Debrief patient after surgery prior to discharge from hospital and arrange a follow-up to complete the process and answer questions
- Undertake root cause analysis
- Communicate the risk management review findings with the patient honestly (duty of candour)
- Communicate with GP

Examiner score sheet		
Information gathering		
Standard not met	Standard partly met	Standard met
0	1	2
Communication with patients and families		
Standard not met	Standard partly met	Standard met
0	1	2
Communication with colleagues		
Standard not met	Standard partly met	Standard met
0	1	2
Patient safety		
Standard not met	Standard partly met	Standard met
0	1	2
Applied clinical knowledge		
Standard not met	Standard partly met	Standard met
0	1	2

Examiner Expectations and Basis for Assessment

Communication with colleagues

- Informs anaesthetist and theatre team of suspicion of perforation
- Informs consultant/senior colleague on call
- Completes incident form and thus informs the risk manager and team
- Informs the GP upon discharge from the hospital

Patient safety

- Knows when to stop suction but leave the tube in-situ
- Laparoscopy – understands why this is necessary
- Takes appropriate steps to complete the evacuation and offers antibiotics
- Aware of the risk of bleeding from the perforation, and hence need to monitor for some time before discharge from hospital
- Includes the risk of subsequent pregnancy in counselling

Communication with patients and families

- Informs the patient after the procedure
- Provides the risk management review report to the patient and family
- Discusses the implications for subsequent pregnancies – treat as a classical CS
- Counsels on the symptoms to watch out for on discharge – abdominal pain and fever

Applied clinical knowledge

- Knows the current literature on the management of early pregnancy complications
- Familiar with RCOG Green-top and NICE Guidelines on early pregnancy complications

Index

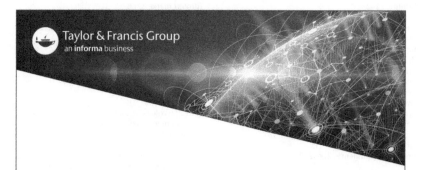